DATE DUE

NOV 2 9 1994	
DEC 3 1 1995	
JAN 0 5 1997	

GAYLORD

PRINTED IN U.S.A.

Issues in Reproductive Management

Lawrence S. Neinstein, M.D.
Associate Professor of Pediatrics and Medicine
University of Southern California School of Medicine

Associate Director
Division of Adolescent Medicine
Childrens Hospital of Los Angeles

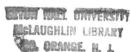
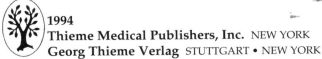
1994
Thieme Medical Publishers, Inc. NEW YORK
Georg Thieme Verlag STUTTGART • NEW YORK

Thieme Medical Publishers, Inc.
381 Park Avenue South
New York, New York 10016

ISSUES IN REPRODUCTIVE MANAGEMENT
Lawrence S. Neinstein, M.D.

Library of Congress Cataloging-in-Publication Data

Neinstein, Lawrence S.,
    Issues in reproductive management / Lawrence S. Neinstein.
        p.   cm.
    Includes bibliographical references and index.
    ISBN 0-86577-505-2 (Thieme Medical Publishers).—ISBN
3-13-119001-9 (Georg Thieme Verlag)
        1. Pregnancy—Complications.   2. Chronic diseases in pregnancy.   3. Infertility,
Female—Etiology.   4. Contraception—Complications.   I. Title.
        [DNLM: 1. Contraception.   2. Pregnancy.   3. Chronic Disease.   WP 630
N4141 1994]
    RG572.N43   1994
    618.3—dc20
    DNLM/DLC
    for Library of Congress   93-33909
                                                                       CIP

Important note: Medicine is an ever-changing science. Research and clinical experience are continually broadening our knowledge, in particular our knowledge of proper treatment and drug therapy. Insofar as this book mentions any dosage or applications, readers may rest assured that the authors, editors, and publishers have made every effort to ensure that such references are strictly in accordance with the state of knowledge at the time of production of the book. Nevertheless, every user is requested to carefully examine the manufacturers' leaflets accompanying each drug to check on his own responsibility whether the dosage schedules recommended therein or the contraindications stated by the manufacturers differ from the statements made in the present book. Such examination is particularly important with drugs that are either rarely used or have been newly released on the market.

Some of the product names, patents, and registered designs referred to in this book are in fact registered trademarks or proprietary names even though specific reference to this fact is not always made in the text. Therefore, the appearance of a name without designation as proprietary is not to be construed as a representation by the publisher that it is in the public domain.

Printed in the United States of America.

5 4 3 2 1

TMP ISBN 0-86577-505-2
GTV ISBN 3-13-119001-9

Contents

Preface

In discussions that I have had with family practitioners, gynecologists, pediatricians, internists, nurses, and nurse practitioners, it has become clear to me that there is considerable confusion about the interaction of chronic illnesses and reproductive needs. There has been an explosion of knowledge in the past 20 to 30 years in the medical management of many medical conditions. This has led to a larger population of women in the reproductive age group that have a chronic medical condition. However, the special concerns of fertility, pregnancy, and contraception in these women has too often been ignored.

With the ever-increasing complexity of the medical management of various chronic diseases, it becomes critical to examine the relationship between these conditions and reproductive function. Too often the answers to some of these relationships are hidden deep in the medical literature. It is usually difficult to find a practical discussion of these relationships in one source. Over the years, I have had significant involvement with teens and young adults with chronic illnesses and have dealt with their reproductive needs. This involvement has made me increasingly aware of these women's needs and how often these needs are neglected. It was these concerns that led me to write this book.

The objective of this book is to provide insight into the interrelationships between many special conditions (including chronic illnesses, disabilities, adolescence, and women over 35) and fertility, pregnancy, and contraception. I will explore in my discussions the effects of these conditions on pregnancy and vice versa. I will also examine the relationship between these conditions and contraceptive devices.

Unfortunately, in many of these areas there is little hard research to guide decision-making. I have tried to review what is known and what advice experts give to practitioners. There is still considerable controversy in many issues related to chronic illnesses, pregnancy, and contraception. I have tried to point out the controversy when it exists and give to the practitioner the best directions and options available.

Much of this book is directed toward chronic medical conditions such as diabetes mellitus, epilepsy, cystic fibrosis, congenital heart disease and inflammatory bowel disease. I have focused the chapters into specialty areas. Some conditions included are not chronic medical conditions, but I have incorporated them because of the important reproductive concerns related to these states. This includes women at both ends of the reproductive age group, adolescents and women over 35.

The text is written to give practical solutions to difficult questions for the busy practitioner. In addition, each section has a summary so that recommendations are reviewed for easy reference. Also included are detailed references to the medical studies that recommendations are based on. This will allow the interested practitioner ready access to the original research papers.

I believe this book is a practical, valuable resource for clinicians who deal with reproductive issues in women. I also think the text will be useful to both primary care practitioners and specialists.

I would like to thank several people for their help in the preparation surrounding this book. I would like to thank Anita Nelson, M.D., for her tremendous support in the undertaking of this manuscript. She has reviewed the manuscript in detail and given many helpful suggestions. In addition she has contributed an enlightening foreword. I am thankful to Richard MacKenzie, M.D., for his encouragement in the pursuit of this undertaking over the past several years. I would like to thank Cathy Perez for secretarial help in the preparation of this manuscript. I would further like to thank my many colleagues, including attending staff, fellows, and house officers who have read and commented on various sections of this manuscript. I am grateful to Doreen Keough for her extensive efforts in tracking references for this manuscript.

Gratitude is also extended to my publisher, Mr. Philip van Tongeren, and Thieme Medical Publishers, Inc., for making this edition possible. They recognized the special need for a book in this area of reproductive health care. I would especially like to thank Elyse Dubin, my production manager, for her support and assistance.

Last, I lovingly thank my wife Debra and my children, Yael, Aaron, and David, for their support and understanding during the compilation of this book. Numerous times, they lost their computer time to my needs in compiling this book. I thank them all for their patience.

Foreword

The twentieth century has seen a revolution in women's health care. Maternal mortality rates have plunged, due in great part to reduction in the three big obstetrical risks of hemorrhage, infection, and hypertension. Tremendous strides have been made in prenatal care, enabling women with medical problems to have successful pregnancies. Diabetes management in pregnancy is a case in point. Prior to the introduction of insulin, overt diabetics could not successfully carry pregnancies. Fetal death rates approached 100%. Maternal mortality rates were also staggering. Today, not only can women with diabetes conceive and carry to viability, but with tight glucose control, the risk of fetal malformation in those infants can be no different from infants of nondiabetic mothers. In family planning, the pace of change has been impressive. One hundred years ago couples had very limited access to effective birth control. Abstinence, withdrawal, lactation, and some version of periodic abstinence were the only officially approved methods. Condoms were intended for prevention of STD transmission (although some couples stretched the meaning of STD to include unintended pregnancies). Today we have a wide variety of contraceptive choices — both reversible and irreversible. Some of the newer reversible methods are at least as effective as sterilization. The impacts of these safe and effective contraceptive devices have been felt worldwide. Birth rate is down; volitional delays in childbearing are obvious as many women establish their careers before starting their families. Family size has markedly decreased.

Although healthy women in this country today have potential access to a veritable cornucopia of birth control methods, by historical standards there remains a very important minority of women with limited information about their contraceptive choices: women with chronic medical diseases.

All medical research is conducted, perforce, on healthy women. The clinical trials exclude women with any possible medical problems. So postmarketing monitoring studies focus again on healthy women. The entire FDA approval process is constructed around the premise that contracepting women are healthy. The standards of safety, the balance of risks and benefits, do not even compare the risks associated with contraceptive use against the risks associated with pregnancy but de facto assume sexual abstinence. Nowhere in the equations are there considerations of the risks and benefits of pregnancy protection in women with medical problems.

Much of the information we have available about fertility-associated risks (both pregnancy and contraceptive risks) is contained in small case series published in specialty journals. For example, an expert in lupus may come to grips with the sexuality of his patients and collect some clinical experience with pregnancy or contraceptive complications and summarize them in the rheumatology journals. Similarly, a cardiologist may have a small series of women with tetralogy of Fallot who have reached reproductive age and face the risks of childbearing and/or contracepting and may share that information with his colleagues in circulation.

What has been needed for quite some time is a compendium of these small reports summarizing the known data about the risks and benefits of reproductive choices for women with chronic medical conditions. A careful discussion of the consequences of any reproductive choice made by women with special conditions would be extremely helpful. Dr. Neinstein has provided us such a tool. In this volume he thoughtfully presents all the information about the impact of the disease upon a woman's fertility and pregnancy and counters that with information about the impact of pregnancy upon her disease. Having set the stage, he completes the picture by providing available data about the impact of her condition on the major methods of contraception and the reverse impact of the contraceptive's impact on the woman's disease.

Dr. Neinstein also provides valuable interpretation into the applicability of the available data in modern settings. For example, older studies about the impact that high-dose oral contraceptives have on heart disease may have limited predictive value for the woman who is taking today's lower-dose birth control pill. However, more modern studies may not be available.

As more women with serious medical problems and genetic disorders are surviving past reproductive ages, this balanced, thorough approach to the whole arena of fertility and fertility control challenges facing women with medical conditions is valuable to primary care providers with limited experience with some of these rarer diseases as well as to the specialist who sometimes is less familiar with reproductive issues. The work also focuses the spotlight on areas needing more research. It serves as a recording of our current knowledge as well as a chronicle of our ignorance. Hopefully, it will motivate practitioners and scientists together to extend further the reach of our understanding in these areas.

Anita Nelson, M.D.
Assistant Professor of Obstetrics and Gynecology
UCLA School of Medicine
Medical Director of Women's Health Care
Harbor-UCLA Medical Center

*To my wife Debra
and my children,
Yael, Aaron, and David*

1

Introduction

By the age of 18, approximately 10% of all individuals will have experienced a serious chronic physical disorder.[1,2] The mean age at first intercourse in the United States is approximately 16 years for boys and 17 years for girls.[3] Thus, a great many young adults with a chronic illness will be exposed to the risks of pregnancy and will need counseling regarding pregnancy and contraception.

Individuals with a chronic illness must deal with many issues throughout their life. Many of these issues, including medical treatment and psychological adjustment, are reviewed in depth in the scientific literature. Despite the fact that individuals with a chronic illness often have active sex lives, reproductive issues, particularly the area of sexuality and family planning, are neglected areas for individuals with chronic diseases such as diabetes mellitus, cardiac disease, and inflammatory bowel disease. As Glass and Padrone summarize: "Illness and disability remove the patient from accustomed personal, social and sexual interactions, changing the entire life pattern. Feelings of self-worth and attractiveness are threatened at a time when need for intimacy and belonging is greatest, causing a sense of loneliness and isolation."[4]

This book focuses primarily on the following issues:

- What are the effects of the disease or disease treatment on fertility?
- What are the risks and effects of pregnancy on a particular disease?
- What are the effects of the disease or its treatment on a pregnancy and the offspring?
- What are the risks of the various contraceptive devices with individuals with different chronic illnesses?
- What are the interactions between devices and drugs used for family planning and the medications used for treating various chronic disease states?

1

It would be easier if the answers to all of these questions were simple and based on large, well-controlled studies. However, data for many of these questions are not available and so answers must be based on the best information in the medical literature.

Recommending contraception for healthy individuals is a continual challenge for physicians and other health care practitioners. However, the challenge becomes even more formidable when the task is complicated by the individual's chronic illness. Physicians are in a frequent quandary as to whether hormonal contraception, an intrauterine device, or another method is appropriate for an individual with a chronic illness and who may be on multiple medications. Even though there may not always be a "best answer," practitioners should be prepared to address these issues.

Much of the information provided regarding contraception focuses on hormonal contraceptives and the intrauterine device. These are the contraceptive methods that most likely would affect these individuals or interact with medications utilized. However, while oral contraceptives have been around for over two decades, most of the research has been conducted in healthy women. In addition, the amount of estrogen and progesterone in oral contraceptives has been reduced dramatically over the past 20 years. The effect of this reduction may be either positive or negative. On one hand, the reduction in the hormones reduces the metabolic effects and makes them less likely to interact and complicate a chronic illness. However, if there is a factor that reduces bioavailability of the oral contraceptive, either due to the illness or due to a medication, the efficacy of the hormone may fall. The following terms are utilized in this book in referring to hormonal contraceptives:

- **Hormonal contraceptives:** This group includes combined oral contraceptive pills, progestin-only pills, the Norplant device, and depomedroxyprogesterone acetate (DMPA).
- **Oral contraceptives:** This group includes both combined estrogen/progestin oral contraceptives and progestin-only oral contraceptive pills.
- **Combined oral contraceptives:** This group includes the combination estrogen/progestin oral contraceptive pills.
- **Progestin-only contraceptive pill:** This group includes the progestin-only oral contraceptive pill.
- **Progestin-only contraceptives:** This group includes the progestin-only pill, DMPA, and the Norplant device.

In general, barrier methods including condoms, spermicides, diaphragms, and contraceptive sponges do not have significant adverse effects on chronic illnesses. However, the actual effectiveness of these devices is less than that of oral contraceptives, intrauterine devices, and long-acting progesterones. Table 1–1 summarizes the typical and lowest reported failure rates during the first year of use of different contraceptive methods and first-year continuation rates. The lower effectiveness rates for

Table 1–1   Typical and Lowest Reported Failure Rates During First Year
of a Contraceptive Method and First Year Continuation Rates, United States

| | PERCENTAGE OF WOMEN EXPERIENCING ACCIDENTAL PREGNANCY IN FIRST YEAR OF USE | | PERCENTAGE OF WOMEN CONTINUING USE AT 1 YEAR[a] | |
Method	*Typical*[b]	*Lowest Reported*[c]	*Excluding Pregnancy*	*Including Pregnancy*
Chance	85	85		
Spermicides[d]	21	3	55	43
Periodic abstinence	20		84	67
Calendar	9	14[e]		
Ovulation method	3	11[e]		
Symptothermal	2	12[e]		
Postovulation	1	2[e]		
Withdrawal	18	7[e]		
Cap[f]	18	8	77	63
Sponge				
Parous women	18	14	73	60
Nulliparous women	28	28	73	53
Diaphragm[f]	18	2	69	57
Condom[g]	12	4[e]	73	64
IUD			75	73
Progestasert	1.9	2		
Copper T380A	0.5	0.8		
Pill	3		75	73
Combined		0		
Progestogen only		1.1		
Injectable progestogen			70	70
DMPA	0.3	0		
Implants			90	90
Norplant (6 capsules)	0.04	0		
Norplant-2 (2 rods)	0.03	0		
Female sterilization	0.4	0		
Male sterilization	0.15	0		

[a]Among couples attempting to avoid pregnancy, the percentage who continue to use a method, under the alternative assumptions that no one becomes pregnant ("Excluding Pregnancy" column) and that the proportion becoming pregnant is given by second column ("Including Pregnancy" column).
[b]Among typical couples who initiate use of a method (not necessarily for the first time), the percentage who experience accidental pregnancy during the first year if they do not stop use for any other reason.
[c]In the literature on contraceptive failure, the lowest reported percentage who experience accidental pregnancy during the first year following initiation of use (not necessarily for the first time) if they did not stop use for any other reason.
[d]Foams, creams, jellies, and vaginal suppositories.
[e]Rate is probably too low, since many studies report a Pearl index. The Pearl index utilizes data over a long period of time. When this occurs, the failure rate drops with time as users become more familiar with the method and as less-effective users drop out.
[f]With spermicidal cream or jelly.
[g]Without spermicides.
Adapted from Hatcher HA, et al. Contraceptive Technology, 1990-1992, 15th ed. New York, Irvington Publishers, 1990.

barrier methods can be a significant consideration for women who may be at high risk if she were to become pregnant. Of all the barrier methods, condoms have the best observed effectiveness rate. Latex condoms have the additional benefit of providing some protection against the transmission of many sexually transmitted diseases including *Neisseria gonorrhoea, Chlamydia trachomatis,* cytomegalovirus, herpes simplex virus, hepatitis B virus (HBV), and human immunodeficiency virus (HIV). Natural membrane condoms do not stop HBV and HIV. In fact, because of the concern of acquired immunodeficiency syndrome (AIDS), condom use has risen from 38 to 60% from 1984 to 1987.[5]

There are some general principles for the practitioner to keep in mind when considering contraceptive and pregnancy care in individuals with a chronic illness.

1. Ability to conceive: What are the individual's chances of getting pregnant or of being fertile?
2. Appropriate timing for a pregnancy: At what age or at what stage in the disease process should the individual become pregnant? Family and psychosocial factors may also affect this decision.
3. Preconception care: Visits by women with a chronic illness should be viewed as an opportune time to provide overall preconception care. This includes optimizing the woman's health prior to any planned pregnancy.
4. Diagnostic tests: Does the pregnancy or the contraceptive method planned have significant interactions with laboratory tests needed to follow the individual's course? Plan for performing any needed tests that might be altered before the pregnancy or contraception is started.
5. Contraception: How much of a risk is the contraceptive method to the mother? Are there any drug interactions between the contraceptive planned and the medications that the individual is using? How acceptable is the contraceptive method to both partners?
6. Medical treatment: Are there any changes in the diet or medications that need to be made before a pregnancy is started?
7. Pregnancy risks: What are the risks to the mother of pregnancy and the risks to the offspring of the disease or its treatment? Have these risks been explained to the woman and her partner?
8. Prenatal care: If a pregnancy is planned, can appropriate prenatal care be arranged?

New Contraceptives

Contraceptive technology is changing with various new contraceptive devices recently developed or approved. Several new condoms are in various stages of development or production. One new condom available, called Pleasure Plus (International Prophylactics, Inc.), has a bulbous tip that does not constrict the upper shaft and head of the penis. This condom seems to overcome some of the concerns with regard to sexual comfort and pleasure. Another condom in development is a nonlatex condom, Tactylon from Tactyl Technologies. It provides protection against viral particles but is not associated with allergic reactions in those individuals sensitive to latex. There is also a polyurethane, roll-on condom in clinical trials that is thinner and stronger than latex condoms and has better heat transmission. There has also been significant progress in the development of the female condom. There are several vaginal sheaths condoms in development or recently approved by the Food and Drug Administration (FDA). One is the Reality female condom, a polyurethane sheath manufactured by Wisconsin Pharmacal and another a latex sheath called the Women's Choice Condomme manufactured by M.D. Personal Products. These products contain a sheath with two flexible rings, one inserted into the vagina and the open ring lays outside the labia. The other female condom in development is the Bikini condom manufactured by Reddy Health Care. This product is worn like underwear but contains a latex pouch attached to it.

Available hormonal contraceptives have also recently changed with the availability of the Norplant device, injectable DMPA, and the addition of combined oral contraceptives with new progestins. One of the newest contraceptive devices available in the United States is the Norplant implant. The Norplant implant was introduced in the United States in January of 1991.[6] The device consists of a flexible implant with six capsules containing 36 mg of levonorgestrel in each capsule. The capsules are 34 mm by 2.4 mm in diameter and made of polydimethylsiloxane tubing. They are placed subdermally on the inside portion of the upper arm through a small incision under local anesthetic. The device is inserted in a nonpregnant woman within the first 5 days of a menstrual cycle or within 5 days of an abortion, miscarriage, or delivery of a baby, except in breast-feeding mothers when the insertion can be done at 6 weeks postpartum. A newer system, Norplant-2, consists of only two capsules, each measuring 44 mm in length and containing 35 mg of levonorgestrel with an effective period of about 3 years. Experience to date suggests that the efficacy of the Norplant-2 is equivalent or better than that of the original Norplant implant.[7] It is expected to be on the market in the next several years.

The Norplant implant works through a combination of preventing ovulation in about 50% of cycles, thickening the cervical mucus, and decreasing the thickness of the endometrium.[6] The effectiveness rate is about 0.2 per 100 users at 1 year. This compares with a failure rate in typical women of about 0.3 per 100 users with 150 mg of medroxyprogesterone acetate (Depo-Provera), 2.3 to 3.5 per 100 users with the combination oral contraceptive pill, 9.5 per 100 users with the progestin-only oral contraceptives, and 0.7 per 100 users with the new-generation intrauterine device. After removal, fertility returns quickly, with an 18% pregnancy rate by 1 month, 49% by the fourth month, 73% by the sixth month, and 86% by the end of 1 year.[6] No congenital abnormalities have been associated with its use. The continuation rate is 80 to 98% at end of year 1 and about 30% after 5 years.

The most frequent complaint in about 60 to 70% of women with the Norplant implant is the associated menstrual problems including a change in the frequency and amount of menstrual bleeding and amenorrhea. In most women the number of days of bleeding increases but the amount of blood loss per day decreases.[8-11] About 25% of women have amenorrhea for up to 90 days. The menstrual problems decrease in severity after the first 6 to 12 months. Another 10% of women have been found to develop an ovarian cyst that usually requires no treatment and resolves spontaneously.[8-11] Other complaints and problems have included weight gain or loss, nausea, dizziness, headache, nervousness, acne, hirsutism, pain or itching at the implant site, depression, hypertension, and anemia.[6] Headache, in one evaluation, was the most frequent single problem, leading to 21% of medically removed implants.[7] The potential advantages of the Norplant implant in women with chronic illnesses include that it has no estrogen side effects, the contraceptive dose is low with a constant release, and there is less reliance on user compliance.

DMPA was developed in the 1960s and is sold in more than 90 countries worldwide. It has been used by an estimated 30 million women worldwide but was only recently approved in the United States for contraceptive purposes. It is a highly effective form of contraception given at 3-month intervals, providing protection for at least 3 months. It also continues to provide contraceptive protection even if the woman is several weeks late in receiving her next injection.

The most common and troublesome side effect of DMPA has been menstrual irregularities. Over two-thirds of women taking DMPA have no regular cycles in the first year of use.[12,13] With continued use, women may either become amenorrheic, have irregular bleeding, or have changes in the duration and amount of their menstrual flow.[14] The most common of these menstrual changes is amenorrhea, which occurs in over half of the women using DMPA. Very heavy or prolonged bleeding can occur but is very uncommon.

Other occasionally reported side effects include weight gain, dizziness, headaches, depression, and decreased libido. Although the contraceptive effect is reversible, women may not ovulate or conceive until several months after the injections are stopped. The median time to conception after the last DMPA injection is 10 months.[14]

DMPA appears to have less effect on the cardiovascular system than combination oral contraceptives.[14] There appears to be little, if any, increased risk of hypertension and blood clotting. DMPA has been reported to have some adverse effect on glucose tolerance.[14-18] The medication appears to have no significant effects on total cholesterol although high-density-lipoprotein (HDL) levels may decrease.[14-18] DMPA has been shown to increase the risk of mammary gland tumors in beagle dogs, but the risk of breast, cervical, ovarian, endometrial, and liver cancer has not been demonstrated to be increased in humans.[18] While not documented, there is still some concern about the risk of breast cancer for young women who use DMPA for extended periods of time.[14,18]

Before the year 2000, at least five new methods using only progestins are also likely to be marketed in the United States. These include a biodegradable implant placed under the skin that will remain active for about 1 year, injectable microspheres of hormones that dissolve slowly over 1 to 6 months, and a vaginal ring of levonorgestrel that releases hormones for 3 months. Other methods that are being investigated include luteinizing hormone–releasing hormone agonists, RU 486 (a progesterone antagonist), and an antifertility vaccine.

New combination oral contraceptives pills containing the progestins norgestimate and desogestrel have been approved in the United States. These progestins are from a group of three new progestins developed and in use in Europe during the 1980s, including desogestrel, gestodene, and norgestimate. All three are gonanes and are related to levonorgestrel. Oral contraceptive pills with these compounds appear to have an efficacy and side effects similar to those of other low-dose combination pills. There has been some discussion that these new progestins may have less androgenic effects, including a more favorable low-density-lipoprotein (LDL) to HDL ratio, than other progestins including norgestrel and norethindrone.[18] However, the clinical significance between these new pills and other low-dose pills is not yet certain.

References

1. Pless IB, Doubleas JWB. Chronic illness in childhood: Part I: Epidemiological and clinical characteristics. Pediatrics 1971;47:405–14.
2. Pless IB, Roghmann K. Chronic illness and its consequences: Results from three epidemiological surveys. J Pediatr 1971;79:351–9.
3. Teenage Pregnancy: The Problem Hasn't Gone Away. New York, The Alan Guttmacher Institute, 1981.
4. Glass DD, Padrone FJ. Sexual adjustment in the handicapped. J Rehabil 1978;44:43–7.
5. Kulig JW. Adolescent contraception: Nonhormonal methods. Pediatr Clin North Am 1989;36:717–30.
6. Flattum-Riemers J. Norplant: A new contraceptive. Am Fam Physician 1991;44:103–10.
7. Sivin I. International experience with Norplant and Norplant-2 contraceptives. Stud Fam Plann 1988;19:81–94.
8. Bardin CW. Long acting steroidal contraception: An update. Int J Fertil 1989;34:88–95.
9. Liskin L, Blackburn R. Hormonal contraception: New long-acting methods. Popul Rep [K] 1987;3:K57–87.
10. Shoupe D, Mischell DR. Norplant: Subdermal implant system for long-term contraception. Am J Obstet Gynecol 1989;160:1286–92.
11. Fakeye O, Balogh S. Effect of Norplant contraceptive use on hemoglobin, packed cell volume and menstrual bleeding patterns. Contraception 1989;39:265–74.
12. Castle WM, Sapire KE, Howard KA. Efficacy and acceptability of injectable medroxyprogesterone: A comparison of 3 monthly and 6 monthly regimens. S Afr Med J 1978;53:842–5.
13. Swenson I, Khan AR, Jahan FA. A randomized, single blind comparative trial of norethindrone enanthate and depo-medroxyprogesterone acetate in Bangladesh. Contraception 1980;21:207–15.
14. Population information program: Hormonal contraception: New long acting methods. Popul Rep [K] 1987;3:58–87.
15. Liew DF, Ng CS, Yong YM, Ratnam SS. Long-term effects of Depo-Provera on carbohydrate and lipid metabolism. Contraception 1985;31:51–64.
16. Fajumi JO. Alterations in blood lipids and side effects induced by Depo-Provera in Nigerian women. Contraception 1983;27:161–75.

17. Liew DF, Ng CS, Heng SH, Ratnam SS. A comparative study of the metabolic effects of injectable and oral contraceptives. Contraception 1986;33:385–94.
18. Hatcher RA, Stewart F, Trussell J, Kowal D, Guest F, Stewart GK, Cates W. Contraceptive Technology: 1990–1992. 15th rev ed. New York, Irvington Publishers, 1990.

2

Pulmonary Diseases

Asthma

Asthma is a common chronic illness affecting almost 3% of women in the childbearing age, and is probably the most common respiratory disorder among pregnant women. Asthma complicates about 1% of pregnancies during either gestation, labor, or early puerperium.[1]

Effect of Pregnancy on Asthma

There are numerous hormonal and mechanical factors that occur during pregnancy that could potentially affect a woman's asthmatic condition. Hormonal factors during pregnancy that might benefit a woman with asthma include the rise in cortisol levels to two to three times normal[2,3] and the smooth muscle-relaxing effect of increased progesterone levels.[4] Hormonal factors that might worsen asthma during pregnancy include an increase in prostaglandin F2α during late pregnancy and labor, which can act as a bronchoconstrictor, and an increase in progesterone, which can compete for glucocorticosteroid receptor sites on smooth muscle.[5] Detrimental mechanical factors secondary to an enlarging uterus include changes in respiratory function, particularly a decrease in functional residual capacity, residual volume, diffusion capacity, and carbon dioxide tension (pCO_2).[4,6] In addition, there is the possible increase in gastroesophageal reflux secondary to more pressure on the stomach, which could stimulate asthma attacks.[5]

Overall, pregnancy does not seem to have a consistent effect on asthma with the exception being those women with severe disease.[7] There have been numerous studies that have examined this question. Reviewing studies involving 1037 women with asthma, Turner et al. found that 49% had no change in their condition, 29% improved, and 22% worsened.[8] Gluck and Gluck, in reviewing nine studies involving 1087 pregnancies, found similar results, with 41% of the women having no change in their asthma, 23% becoming worse, and 36% improving.[7] It was noted in this review that the condition of the women with more severe asthma prior to pregnancy was more likely to deteriorate. The levels of IgE were also helpful in predicting prognosis in that those with decreasing levels were likely to improve and those with unchanged or increasing IgE levels had a worse asthma course. In a prospective study of women with asthma, Schatz et al. also found similar responses in that 33% had no change, 28% improved, and 35% became worse.[9] Any changes in these women for the better or worse reverted back to prepregnancy levels by 3 months postpartum, which did suggest that pregnancy had an effect on asthma in some of these women. It was also noted in this study that the women's asthma condition seemed to behave similarly from pregnancy to pregnancy.

Data vary on the timing during pregnancy in which asthma symptoms change. Overall, worsening seems to occur mainly between 28 and 36 weeks of gestation while improvement tends to occur in the last 4 weeks of gestation. Asthma attacks usually do not occur in the last 4 weeks of pregnancy and in most controlled individuals, do not occur during labor. In a prospective study, symptom scores, peak flow, and bronchodilator use were correlated to time periods of pregnancy.[10] In women with mild and moderate asthma in this study, an improvement was found to be more likely during pregnancy, particularly in the last trimester, but 33% had postpartum deterioration. Severe asthmatics were at the greatest risk of deterioration, particularly late in pregnancy. In summation, except in women with severe asthma, pregnancy does not appear to be a significant risk factor and there does not appear to be an increase in maternal mortality if the asthma is well controlled.[1]

Effect of Asthma on Pregnancy

There have been several studies that have examined the effect of asthma on the course and outcome of pregnancy. In an evaluation of 277 asthmatic patients, there was no difference in birthweight or Apgar scores, but there was an increase in perinatal death as compared to controls.[11] However, some studies have demonstrated a higher rate of low-birthweight infants in women with asthma.[12–14] In general, mild asthma does not seem to be associated with maternal or fetal problems. On the other hand, pregnancy in women with severe asthma is more likely to result in either maternal death, neonatal death, intrauterine growth retardation, preterm birth, and low birthweight.[15–17] The control of asthma in these women seems the best predictor of pregnancy outcome, regardless of the use of medication including steroids. Studies have indicated that women with uncontrolled asthma have children with low birthweight and that there is a direct relationship between the mean birthweight and the mean percent predicted forced expiratory volume in 1 second (FEV$_1$).[15–18] In fact, in 16 women with severe asthma who Gordon et al. evaluated, there were four perinatal deaths, five low-birthweight newborns, and two neurologically abnormal infants.[11] Greenberger and Patterson also demonstrated that there was a decrease in birthweight only if an episode of status asthmaticus occurred during gestation.[16] Stenius-Aarniala et al. noted that when asthma was managed closely, perinatal mortality and morbidity were not increased. However, they did note that preeclampsia occurred more frequently.[17] Apter et al. examined the pregnancy outcome in 21 adolescents with severe asthma who were aggressively managed during 28 pregnancies. With this management there were no maternal or fetal deaths or evidence for intrauterine growth retardation.[19] Overall, there is no increase in perinatal mortality if asthma is well controlled; however, with severe hypoxia in the mother (pO$_2$ < 60 mm Hg), fetal mortality is increased.

Asthma Medications and Pregnancy

None of the studies noted above found an increased incidence of congenital malformations despite the use of multiple medications.[15–17] The methylxanthines are considered a safe medication and are not associated with fetal malformation.[5] Doses should be maintained on the low side in order to prevent nervousness in the newborn. Beta-agonists have not been reported to have any adverse fetal effects. The inhaled route is recommended, when feasible, to expose the fetus to lower serum levels, compared to levels obtained with the oral route. If needed, steroids and cromolyn also appear safe during pregnancy. Fitzsimons et al. studied 56 pregnancies in 51 women treated for severe asthma with long-term prednisone or beclomethasone dipropionate.[15] There were no malformations found. There was a slight increase in the prevalence of low-birthweight infants compared to the general population. However, there was a significant decrease in birthweights when women with status asthmaticus were compared to those without a history of status asthmaticus during pregnancy. The safety of inhaled beclomethasone to treat severe asthma was examined in a study by Greenberger and Patterson.[16] There was no increase in the incidence of fetal and neonatal mortality, abortion, or congenital malformations. When controlled, asthma does not appear to have a significant negative outcome on pregnancy or the newborn. The risk to the mother and infant is in uncontrolled asthma. Thus, while no drug is absolutely safe, sufficient medication should be used to avoid asthma exacerbations and in particular, status asthmaticus. Methylxanthines, beta-agonists, steroids, and cromolyn are all indicated to control asthma. However, iodides are contraindicated in pregnancy as they concentrate in the fetal thyroid and are teratogenic. Preconception care should involve optimizing a woman's asthmatic condition utilizing the lowest doses of medications to accomplish this task.

Asthma and Contraception

While pregnancy does not appear to place women at significant risk, are there interactions between asthma, antiasthma medications, and contraceptives that could adversely affect a woman's asthma? Unfortunately, the literature is sparse on reporting the effects of hormonal contraceptives on asthma. Progesterone could potentially be of benefit as it can relax smooth muscle.[20] Benyon et al., in fact, reported on three women with premenstrual exacerbations of asthma who did not respond to conventional therapy but responded to intramuscular progesterone.[21] Progesterone receptors are located on nasopharyngeal passages and the lungs and thus may be responsible for premenstrual exacerbations of rhinitis, sinusitis, and asthma.[22] However, the receptors may need pharmacological doses rather than physiological doses of progesterone to stimulate them. Since oral contraceptives contain small doses of progesterone and lower circulating endogenous progesterone levels, they may not have much effect on asthma. Pauli et al., in a study of 11 asthmatic and 29 controls, could not find a relationship between premenstrual symptom worsening and levels of circulating estradiol and progesterone.[23] Juniper et al. also evaluated airway responsiveness and spirometry data in 16 pregnant women with asthma and found no correlation between changes in airway responsiveness and estrogen and progesterone levels.[24]

Actual clinical trials examining effects of oral contraceptives on symptoms are minimal and involve primarily case reports of allergic rhinitis. Horan and Lederman commented on one patient with respiratory symptoms including nasal congestion, sneezing, coughing, and dyspnea which cleared only after discontinuing the pill.[25] Oral contraceptives were also reported to be related to 50 cases of vasomotor rhinitis in another report.[26] Symptoms in these patients resolved after stopping oral contraceptives. Clearance of bronchodilating agents including theophylline and aminophylline may be reduced by between 30 and 40% in oral contraceptive users.[27,28] Thus, in asthmatic women on oral contraceptive pills, initial doses of theophylline and aminophylline should be reduced by one-third.[28]

There is one other consideration in the use of oral contraceptives in women with asthma. Many of the most common clinical manifestations of an asthma attack, including shortness of breath, tachypnea, and tachycardia, are the same manifestations of a pulmonary embolus. While this potential confusion may complicate the use of oral contraceptives in these women, it is not a contraindication to their use. The patient and the practitioner need to be aware of the possible confusion.

No reports have been made on interactions between DMPA or the Norplant device and asthma. It would appear that these forms of contraception would also appear to be safe in women with asthma. While the intrauterine device would appear to be as safe in women with asthma as in those without asthma, there is one potential problem. There have been reports of an occasional pregnancy in women with an intrauterine device who are also on steroids.[28–30] This potential interaction needs further study as it has potential impact on all intrauterine device users taking steroids regardless of their underlying illness. In addition, the immunosuppressive actions of steroids might increase the potential risk of uterine infections in women with an intrauterine device.

Summary

1. Asthma itself does not appear to affect pregnancy unless the asthma is poorly controlled.
2. Treatment during pregnancy should be aggressive enough to control asthma, as asthma exacerbations can affect both the mother and the newborn.
3. Medications used to control asthma do not appear to cause additional morbidity or mortality during pregnancy.
4. There does not appear to be any contraindications to the use of hormonal contraceptions in women with asthma. However, the practitioner needs to be aware of the decreased clearance of theophylline and amino-phylline in women on oral contraceptives, requiring a reduction of between 30 and 40% in theophylline and aminophylline doses. The practitioner should also keep in mind the possible confusion between the signs and symptoms of pulmonary embolus and exacerbation of asthma.
5. The possibility exists of a worsening of allergic rhinitis with the use of hormonal contraceptives.
6. While the intrauterine device is not contraindicated during asthma, the practitioner should be aware of the possible lessening of contraceptive efficacy in women on steroids and the theoretical increased risk of infectious complications.

Cystic Fibrosis

More and more individuals with cystic fibrosis are now living into the childbearing age, with a median survival age of 20 to 22 years.[31,32] Cystic fibrosis occurs in 1 in 1000 to 2000 live births in the United States and is the most frequent lethal hereditary disorder in white populations, with 1 in 20 being carriers.[31,33] Contraceptive and sexuality counseling is often over-looked in these teens and young adults, particularly those who may be maturationally delayed. In a study by Cromer et al. of teens with cystic fibrosis, 43% were sexually active and 100% felt that they would have a sexual relationship at some point.[34] Despite this, only 21% had ever talked with a physician about sexuality issues or concerns. In addition, while 57%

planned to have children and 84% felt that their children might be at increased risk of having cystic fibrosis, only 16% had talked with a physician about the chances of transmitting cystic fibrosis to their offspring.

Fertility

Cystic fibrosis has an effect on the fertility in both men and women with this condition. Approximately 95% of males with cystic fibrosis are sterile.[35] Some women have fertility problems but not to the same degree as males.[36,37] The cause of infertility in women is thought to be related to the change in cervical mucus. Normally a 93 to 96% hydration of cervical mucus is necessary for sperm migration while cervical mucus in individuals with cystic fibrosis contains less than 80% water at midcycle.[37] Other alterations in cervical mucus include a low sodium concentration and changes in the electrolytes.[31] Kredentser et al. reported a case of a 23-year-old woman with cystic fibrosis and infertility in which the infertility was overcome with intrauterine insemination.[37]

Pregnancy and Cystic Fibrosis

Pregnancy can be of significant risk to the patient with cystic fibrosis, with older studies reporting a perinatal mortality rate of 11% and a maternal mortality rate of 12% within 6 months of delivery.[38] However, this maternal mortality rate was no higher than the rate in those women with cystic fibrosis who were not pregnant. Cohen et al. reviewed the results of a survey of 100 pregnant women with cystic fibrosis from multiple centers in the United States and Canada.[39] The results suggest that the outcomes for the mother and the infant are related to the severity of the mother's disease as determined by the presence or absence of pancreatic involvement, pulmonary hypertension, and the level of vital capacity. In another study, four factors were associated with a favorable outcome of pregnancy for both mother and infant: good nutritional status as measured by weight for height, good Schwachman-Kulczycki clinical score, good pulmonary function with normal lung volumes and only mild to moderate airway obstruction, and chest roentgenograms that appeared nearly normal.[40] Women without these findings tended to have worse postpartum courses and to deliver their infants prematurely. The maternal course was little affected by pregnancy in women with good lung function and good nutritional status. Women with mild cystic fibrosis seem to have normal morbidity and mortality for both themselves and their children.[37] There are no reports of a higher-than-normal incidence of fetal malformations.

Women with cystic fibrosis should be involved in genetic, pregnancy, and contraceptive counseling. They need to be aware that any pregnancy carries a risk to their respiratory status. The effect of the pregnancy depends a lot on the severity of their underlying disease. These individuals require extensive prenatal and postpartum care including managing any associated diabetes closely.

Contraception and Cystic Fibrosis

Research on the effects of hormonal contraceptives in relationship to cystic fibrosis has been minimal. Two possible side effects have been written about in relationship to hormonal contraceptive use in these women. Progesterone can cause a decrease and thickening of cervical mucus.[36] If progesterone has the same effect on bronchial mucus, it could cause a deterioration in the woman's pulmonary status. Dooley et al. described two women who had rapid deterioration of their respiratory status after starting oral contraceptives.[41] They also noted an endocervical polyp that appeared with the initiation of oral contraception and regressed with discontinuance of the pill. On the other hand, the only study of oral contraceptive use in women with cystic fibrosis did not find an exacerbation of pulmonary disease.[42] This study examined the effects of Ovral 28 (ethinyl estradiol and norgestrel) for a 6-month period on 10 women with cystic fibrosis aged 15 to 24 years. There were no significant changes in subjective pulmonary symptoms or in pulmonary function tests at 2-, 4-, and 6-month intervals. None of these individuals developed a cervical polyp. While 4 of the women had exacerbations of their pulmonary problems during the study period, this was at a similar rate as before their use of oral contraceptives. This study utilized a potent progestin so one might expect even less effects with lower-dose pills. However, this was only one short-term study involving a small number of individuals. This area deserves further research as does the use of newer hormonal devices such as the Norplant device. As in individuals with asthma, respiratory problems associated with cystic fibrosis could be confused with a pulmonary embolism. Most individuals with cystic fibrosis are on long courses of antibiotics. Potential interactions between antibiotics and oral contraceptives are discussed elsewhere (see Chapt. 16).

Because of the potential severe complications of oral contraceptives in individuals with cystic fibrosis if pulmonary problems were to occur, oral contraceptives should be used with extreme caution. Further studies would be helpful in giving better guidance in the care of these individuals. There are no data available on the interaction of intrauterine devices and individuals with cystic fibrosis.

Summary

1. Cystic fibrosis lowers the fertility rates in me and women, but predominantly in men.
2. Pregnancy can have a detrimental effect on the course of women with cystic fibrosis and the effect correlates with the severity of disease.

3. Hormonal contraceptives could potentially worsen cystic fibrosis by altering bronchial mucus; however, in the one small, short-term study that was conducted, this was not found to occur.
4. Oral contraceptives could be used but with caution in women with cystic fibrosis. Progestin-only pills containing lower hormonal doses may be preferable to combination oral contraceptives.
5. Pregnancy and family planning counseling should not be forgotten in men and women with cystic fibrosis.

Sarcoidosis

The most common interstitial lung disease to complicate pregnancy is sarcoidosis.[38] This disease involves noncaseating granulomas that can affect virtually every organ, but most commonly the lung. There is no evidence that fertility is altered by sarcoidosis.[38] Usually sarcoidosis does not worsen with pregnancy and may improve.[43,44] However, women with active disease during pregnancy are at risk for an exacerbation within 3 to 6 months postpartum. There is no evidence that sarcoidosis has a negative impact on the course of a pregnancy.[43,44] No interactions between sarcoidosis and any contraceptive devices have been reported. Naturally, if significant liver involvement is present, hormonal contraceptives would be contraindicated.

A final consideration for women with a pulmonary disease of any nature who are on antibiotics, such as women treated with rifampin for tuberculosis, is the possible interaction between antibiotics and oral contraceptives. This is discussed in Chapter 16.

References

1. Huff RW. Asthma in pregnancy. Med Clin North Am 1989;73:653–60.
2. O'Connell M, Welsh G. Unbound plasma cortisol in pregnant and Enovid-E treated women as determined by ultrafiltration. J Clin Endocrinol 1969;29:563.
3. Demey-Ponsart E, Foidart JM, Sulon J, Sodoyez JC. Serum CBG, free and total cortisol and circadian patterns of adrenal function in normal pregnancy. J Steroid Biochem 1982;16:165–9.
4. DiMarco AF. Asthma in the pregnant patient: A review. Ann Allergy 1989;62:527–33.
5. Salinger L, Low MB. Asthma in pregnancy. NAACOGS Clin Issu Perinat Womens Health Nurs 1990;1:165–76.
6. Lewis PJ, Boylan P, Friedman LA, Hensby CN, Downing I. Prostacyclin in pregnancy. Br Med J 1980;280:1581–2.
7. Gluck JC, Gluck PA. The effects of pregnancy on asthma: A prospective study. Ann Allergy 1976;37:164.
8. Turner ES, Greenberger PA, Patterson R. Management of the pregnant asthmatic patient. Ann Intern Med 1980;6:905–18.
9. Schatz M, Harden K, Forsythe A, Chillingar L, Hoffman C, Sperling W, Zeiger RS. The course of asthma during pregnancy, post partum, and with successive pregnancies: A prospective analysis. J Allergy Clin Immunol 1988;81:509–17.

10. White RJ, Coutts II, Gibbs CJ, MacIntyre C. A prospective study of asthma during pregnancy and the puerperium. Respir Med 1989;83:103–6.
11. Gordon M, Niswander KR, Berendes H, Kantor AG. Fetal morbidity following potentially anoxigenic obstetric conditions. VII. Bronchial asthma. Am J Obstet Gynecol 1970;106:421–9.
12. Bahna SL, Bjerkedal T. The course and outcome of pregnancy in women with bronchial asthma. Acta Allergol 1972;27:397–406.
13. Greenberger PA. Pregnancy and asthma. Chest 1985;87(suppl):85S–7S.
14. Schatz M, Patterson R, Zeitz S, O'Rourke J, Melam H. Corticosteroid therapy for the pregnant asthmatic patient. JAMA 1975;233:804–7.
15. Fitzsimons M, Greenberger P, Patterson R. Outcome of pregnancy in women requiring corticosteroids for severe asthma. J Allergy Clin Immunol 1986;8:349–53.
16. Greenberger PA, Patterson R. Beclomethasone dipropionate for severe asthma during pregnancy. Ann Intern Med 1983;98:478–80.
17. Stenius-Aarniala B, Piirila P, Teramo K. Asthma and pregnancy: A prospective study of 198 pregnancies. Thorax 1988;43:12–8.
18. Schatz M, Zeiger RS, Hoffman CP. Intrauterine growth is related to gestational pulmonary function in pregnant asthmatic women. Kaiser Permanente Asthma and Pregnancy Study Group. Chest 1990;98:389–92.
19. Apter AJ, Greenberger PA, Patterson R. Outcomes of pregnancy in adolescents with severe asthma. Arch Intern Med 1989;149:2571–5.
20. Asthma, progesterone, and pregnancy (editorial). Lancet 1990;335:204.
21. Beynon HL, Garbett ND, Barnes PJ. Severe premenstrual exacerbations of asthma: Effect of intramuscular progesterone. Lancet 1988;2:370–2.
22. Dalton K. Progesterone for premenstrual exacerbations of asthma (letter). Lancet 1988;2:684.
23. Pauli BD, Reid RL, Munt PW, Wigle RD, Forkert L. Influence of the menstrual cycle on airway function in asthmatic and normal subjects. Am Rev Respir Dis 1989;140:358–62.
24. Juniper EF, Daniel EE, Roberts RS, Kline PA, Hargreave FE, Newhouse MT. Improvement in airway responsiveness and asthma severity during pregnancy. A prospective study. Am Rev Respir Dis 1989;140:924–31.
25. Horan JD, Lederman JJ. Possible asthmogenic effect of oral contraceptives. Can Med Assoc J 1968;99:130–1.
26. Morrison IC. Oral contraceptives: A new syndrome. Med J Aust 1964;2:691.
27. Back DJ, Orme JL'E. Pharmacokinetic drug interactions with oral contraceptives. Clin Pharmacokinet 1990;18:472–84.
28. Goldzieher JW. Hormonal Contraception: Pills, Injections and Implants. 2nd ed. London, Ontario, EMIS-Canada, 1989, pp 44–9.
29. Zerner J, Miller BA, Festino MJ. Failure of an intrauterine device concurrent with administration of corticosteroids. Fertil Steril 1976;27:1467–8.
30. Mennuti MT, Shepard TM, Mellman WJ. Fetal renal malformation following treatment of Hodgkin's disease during pregnancy. Obstet Gynecol 1975;46:194–6.
31. MacMullen NJ, Brucker MC. Pregnancy made possible for women with cystic fibrosis. MCN Am J Matern Child Nurs 1989;14:196–8.
32. Huang NH, Schidlow DV, Szatrowski TH, Palmer J, Laraya-Cuasay LR, Yeung W, Hardy K, Quitell L, Fiel S. Clinical features, survival rate and prognostic factors in young adults with cystic fibrosis. Am J Med 1987;82:871–9.
33. Plotz EJ, Patterson PR, Streit JH. Pregnancy in a patient with cystic fibrosis (mucoviscidosis) and diabetes mellitus. Am J Obstet Gynecol 1967;98:1105–10.
34. Cromer BA, Enrile B, McCoy K, Gerhardstein MJ, Fitzpatrick M, Judis J. Knowledge, attitudes and behavior related to sexuality in adolescents with chronic disability. Dev Med Child Neurol 1990;32:602–10.
35. Seale TW, Flux M, Rennert OM. Reproductive defects in patients of both sexes with cystic fibrosis: A review. Ann Clin Lab Sci 1985;5:152–8.
36. Burki NK. Pulmonary Diseases. New York, Medical Examination Publishing, 1982.
37. Kredentser JV, Pokrant C, McCoshen JA. Intrauterine insemination for infertility due to cystic fibrosis. Fertil. Steril 1986;45:425–6.
38. Noble PW, Lavee AE, Jacobs MM. Respiratory diseases in pregnancy. Obstet Gynecol Clin North Am 1988;15:391–428.

39. Cohen LF, Di Sant'Agnese PA, Friedlander J. Cystic fibrosis and pregnancy. A national survey. Lancet 1980;2:842–4.
40. Palmer J, Dillon-Baker C, Tecklin JS, Wolfson B, Rosenberb B, Burroughs B, Holsclaw DS Jr, Scanlin TF, Huang NN, Sewell EM. Pregnancy in patients with cystic fibrosis. Ann Intern Med 1983;99:596–600.
41. Dooley RR, Braustein H, Osher AB. Polypoid cervicitis in cystic fibrosis patients receiving oral contraceptives. Am J Obstet Gynecol 1979;118:971–4.
42. Fitzpatrick SB, Stokes DC, Rosenstein BJ, Terry P, Hubbard VS. Use of oral contraceptives in women with cystic fibrosis. Chest 1984;86:863.
43. Haynes de Regt R. Sarcoidosis and pregnancy. Obstet Gynecol 1987;70:369–72.
44. O'Leary JA. Ten year study of sarcoidosis and pregnancy. Am J Obstet Gynecol 1962;84:462–6.

3

Neurological Diseases

The most common neurological problems in young adults and the best-studied areas in relation to pregnancy and contraception include epilepsy, multiple sclerosis, and migraine headaches.

Seizure Disorders

Seizure disorders are a relatively common occurrence in individuals of reproductive age. Approximately 1 in every 200 pregnancies occur in women with epilepsy, resulting in about 20,000 children born each year to epileptic women in the United States.[1] Besides the seizures themselves, these individuals are often on one or more medications that can have a significant impact on pregnancy and on hormonal contraceptive agents.

Infertility

Fertility may be affected in individuals with epilepsy through effects on the hypothalamic-pituitary-gonadal axis either through the seizures themselves or through antiepileptic medications.[2-4] However, once conception occurs, the live birthrates of these individuals are normal.[2] Oligospermia has been reported in two men on valproic acid.[4] However, after the doses were reduced to 150 mg daily from over 1000 mg, the sperm parameters returned to normal, with one of the two men succeeding in a pregnancy after 5 years of a childless marriage.

Effects of Pregnancy on Seizure Disorders

Numerous studies have examined the risk of pregnancy in women with a seizure disorder. Bardy conducted a large prospective study of 154 pregnancies in 140 women with epilepsy.[5] In this study, electroencephalography (EEG) was done both during pregnancy and in the nonpregnant state. Most individuals had no change in their background EEG activity or paroxysmal activity during pregnancy. Of 34 women with a change, 50% had an increase in paroxysmal EEG activity and 50%, a decrease. Bardy also reviewed the literature prior to 1982 involving 2684 pregnancies from 35 different studies.[5] The results showed that in 46% of women there was no change in seizure activity with pregnancy, in 34% there was an increase, and in 20% there was a decrease.[5,6] The percentages of women that had increased seizures in these studies varied widely from 4 to 75%. Bardy et al. also studied EEGs of epileptic women in late pregnancy and in the nonpregnant state and found no differences in the number of epileptic interictal discharges.[7] In another study of 136 pregnancies in 122 women with epilepsy, 50% had no change in their seizures while 37% had an increase and 13% a decrease.[8] In 34 of the 50 pregnancies associated with an increase in seizures, the increase was associated with sleep deprivation or noncompliance with medications. In a more recent review of the literature, Donaldson found a reported increase in seizure activity in 50% of women with epilepsy during pregnancy, no change in 42%, and a decrease in 8%.[9] A bias arising in most of these studies involves the method used to evaluate the seizures. Seizures prior to pregnancy are recalled retrospectively, while those after pregnancy are recorded prospectively. Thus, there may be a problem with the recall of seizures prior to pregnancy. Another confounding bias is the treatment changes for seizures that often occur after a pregnancy is diagnosed.

Many factors that may affect the frequency of seizure activity during pregnancy have been implicated. Estrogen and progesterone changes with pregnancy may alter convulsive thresholds in some women.[10–12] In one study of pregnant women with epilepsy, those women with increased seizures did in fact have significantly higher estrogen levels and lower progesterone levels.[13] A decrease in antiepileptic serum levels during pregnancy has been demonstrated from either an increase in hepatic or renal clearance,[14–17] malabsorption of the drug,[16,18] weight gain,[16,19] increased volume of distribution from the added volume of fetal tissue,[16,20] alterations in plasma protein binding,[21] or noncompliance.[8] The fear of taking drugs by the mother and of giving drugs by the physician may very well be the main cause of an increase in seizure activity during many pregnancies.

While the effect of pregnancy on seizures is highly variable, the greater the severity of epilepsy prior to pregnancy, the more likely that seizures will become worse.[22] This was also supported in a study that showed that 70% of women with severe epilepsy deteriorated during pregnancy.[23]

Effect of Epilepsy on Pregnancy

While overall there may be small increases in certain complications of pregnancy in women with epilepsy, the differences between women with and those without epilepsy appear to be small and not consistent from study to study. The most comprehensive study examining the interactions of epilepsy's effect on pregnancy and the fetus is the Collaborative Perinatal Project of the National Institute of Neurological and Communicative Disorder and Stroke.[24] In this study, 54,000 pregnant women were followed through pregnancy and until their children were 7 years old. The rate of complications of pregnancy and labor and postpartum hemorrhage was doubled in those women with seizures. In addition, the prevalence of low birthweight, infant mortality, and neonatal seizures was increased in the children of women with epilepsy. However, this study did not examine anticonvulsant drug levels and hormone levels in relation to complications. Andermann et al., in a study of women at Montreal Neurologic Institute, found no increase in pregnancy complications including spontaneous abortion, toxemia, and prematurity.[25] While the weights of infants of mothers with epilepsy were similar to those of controls, the weights were less if adjusted for age of gestation. While Andermann and coworkers did not find an increase in infant mortality, perinatal mortality was increased threefold. Yerby found a higher rate of preeclampsia, cesarean sections, low birthweight, and low Apgar scores in pregnancies of women with epilepsy.[26] Except for some of the women in Andermann's study, the data from these preceding studies were obtained retrospectively. Two small prospective studies have been performed. Battino et al. examined prospectively a small group of 59 pregnant women with epilepsy.[27] They found no increase in pregnancy complications compared to the general Italian population. Bag et al. also conducted a small prospective study and attempted to correlate complications with serum anticonvulsant drug and hormone levels.[13] Two of the women in the study had spontaneous abortions and both had high levels of estrogen. Neither women had experienced seizures during the first trimester. One infant in the study had a ventricular septal defect and this woman's anticonvulsant drug levels were high. Thus, while there is some evidence of a small increase in certain complications, a more complete answer to this question requires a large, well-controlled, prospective study. There is also growing evidence that epilepsy by itself carries a genetic risk for congenital malformations.[21,28]

Anticonvulsant Medications and Pregnancy

Another major concern for women with epilepsy is the effect of anticonvulsant medications on their offspring. Since not all "seizures" are related to epilepsy, it is important during preconception and prenatal evaluation to reconfirm the diagnosis and the need for maintenance with antiepileptic drugs. Anticonvulsant medications could possibly cause birth defects through direct drug effects, drug interactions, drug metabolites, or folate deficiency secondary to the medication. Major concerns have included spina bifida, cleft lip and palate, and congenital heart defects. Past reports have also indicated that children born to mothers on anticonvulsants have pharyngeal hypoplasia as well as craniofacial and digital dysmorphic features (fetal hydantoin syndrome).[29,30] Bossi found that women on anticonvulsants had a twofold increase in the rate of congenital malformations in their offspring, as compared to untreated and control women.[31] Cleft lip and palate was the most common malformation.[31] Table 3–1 lists the frequency of various congenital malformations in children of women treated with anticonvulsants during pregnancy. Kelly reviewed 16 studies examining this question and found a 17.9% rate of malformations in treated mothers compared with 5% in untreated mothers and 2.1% in control women.[32] However, most of these studies were not well controlled. Gailey et al. conducted a prospective, controlled study of 121 children of mothers with epilepsy compared to 105 control children.[28] They evaluated these children at age 5½ years for 80 minor physical anomalies including 9 features previously described as typical of fetal hydantoin syndrome. They also evaluated the mothers and fathers for these physical anomalies. There was an excess of minor anomalies, previously attributed to hydantoin, in both the mothers with epilepsy and their offspring. No other anomalies were more frequent in the study group. In addition, except for hypertelorism and digital hypoplasia, which were associated with phenytoin exposure, the other anomalies were found to be genetically linked to epilepsy and not related to drug exposure. The authors concluded that the risk of a developmental disturbance associated with phenytoin exposure seems much lower than that reported in prior studies.

Most anticonvulsants have been classified as either category C or D drugs. Category C drugs are those in which there are no controlled studies in women or animals, or studies in animals have shown adverse effects on the fetus. Such drugs should be used only if the benefit outweighs the risks. Category D drugs are those drugs in which there is positive evidence of fetal risk, but the drug may be indicated in some situations. Valproic acid (category D) does appear to cause a higher prevalence of neural tube defects, especially spina bifida, in infants exposed during the first trimester.[12,33,34] A prevalence of about 1 to 2% has been reported. It may also be associated with face, heart, and limb malformations. Trimethadione (category D) also has been linked to multiple teratogenic effects[35] with a rate as high as 50%, and is thus contraindicated for use in pregnancy.[36] Possible teratogenic effects include growth failure, mental retardation, and craniofacial, limb, and cardiac malformations. Carbamazepine (category C) has not generally been considered to be teratogenic. However, recently there have been reports of certain malformations in the offspring of mothers treated with carbamazepine alone during pregnancy.[37,38] These malformations have included facial dysmorphism (flat nasal bridge, arched palate, broad forehead, low-set ears), hypoplasia of fingers or toenails, spina bifida, congenital heart disease, and intrauterine growth retardation. It is not

Table 3–1   Frequency of Various Congenital Malformations
in Children of Women with Epilepsy Treated with
Anticonvulsants during Pregnancy

MALFORMATION	INCIDENCE (%)[a]
Orofacial clefts	1.8
Congenital heart disease	1.5
Skeletal abnormalities	1.0
Hypospadias	0.5
Anencephaly	0.3
Microcephaly	0.3
Neural tube defects	0.3
Intestinal atresia	0.3
Hydrocephalus	0.1

[a]Pooled data from several published series; includes 1726 pregnancies.
From Krumholz A. Epilepsy and pregnancy. In Goldstein PJ, ed. Neurological Disorders of Pregnancy. Mount Kisco, New York, Futura Publishing, 1986, pp 65–88.

entirely clear which, if any, of these are definitely associated with carbamazepine use.

In summary, while congenital anomalies do occur in infants born to women on anticonvulsant therapy, they appear less frequently than previously reported. Many of the minor anomalies appear linked to epilepsy itself and not related to medication use.[12,28] However, valproic acid used in the first trimester does appear to increase the risk of neural defects and phenytoin, with a small increased risk of hypertelorism and digital hypoplasia. As seizures and status epilepticus are associated with severe complications during pregnancy, medications should be utilized to control seizures in women who still have an active seizure disorder. Valproic acid should be avoided unless specific indications are present. The Commission on Genetics, Pregnancy, and the Child has recommended trying to control seizures with a single agent at the lowest effective dose.[39] Ideally, preconception health care would include evaluating a woman for the need of continued anticonvulsants and if needed, altering medications to the fewest number and lowest doses possible to control seizures. Multivitamins and folic acid should be used as some of the defects may be caused by folate deficiency. If valproic acid, carbamazepine, or both are used during pregnancy, then alpha-fetoprotein levels in the amniotic fluid should be measured followed by abdominal ultrasonography if abnormal alpha-fetoprotein levels are found. In addition, vitamin K_1 therapy, 20 mg/day, should be used in the last 4 weeks of gestation to avoid neonatal hemorrhage.

Seizures and Contraception

Since women with epilepsy are usually on at least one anticonvulsant, it is important for them to use a contraceptive that does not interact with their medication or alter the frequency of their seizures. The most studied areas in this regard have been the effect of estrogens and progesterones on epilepsy and the interaction between anticonvulsants and these hormones.

The relationship between hormones and seizures has been of interest for many years. In fact, Hippocrates wrote about a possible relationship between seizures and menstrual flow.[40] Evidence for a relationship has focused on either the effects of menses on seizures or the specific alterations of estrogens, progesterones, or oral contraceptives on EEG activity or seizures.

In 1881, Gowers noted that seizures increased during menstrual periods.[41] Lin et al. found that in women with either tonic clonic or absence seizures, spike and wave discharges were more common during menses.[42] Laidlaw, in a study of 50 institutionalized women with generalized tonic clonic seizures, noted that 72% had an exacerbation of their seizures either just before, during, or just after menses.[43] Thus, in these and in other studies, the seizure frequency increased either during the estradiol spike just before ovulation or at the time of a progesterone fall just before and during menses.[42–44] Shavit et al., however, suggested that some of the changes noted with menses could be related to changes in anticonvulsant medication clearance that might occur secondary to alterations in estrogen and progesterone levels.[45] They found that phenytoin levels fell during menses.[45]

Numerous studies have implicated estrogen in lowering seizure threshold in animals and humans.[46–57] Wooley and Timeras found that estrogen reduces the seizure threshold in rats.[46] Logothetis and Harner noted that intravenous estrogens given to women with epilepsy increased epileptiform activity.[47] Julien et al. reported that absence seizures could be induced in cats by applying estrogens to the sensory motor cortex.[48] Gevorkyan et al. hypothesized that estrogen may exert a proconvulsant effect either through a change in electrogenesis of neuron membranes or through an effect on the intracellular metabolism of neurons.[49] Their study in rats demonstrated that estrogen induced epileptic activity several minutes after being given and 3½ hours later, indicating two separate mechanisms.

Other studies have implicated progesterone to have anticonvulsant activity.[51–56] Progesterone increases the threshold of electrically induced convulsions in female rats and mice.[45,51,52] Intravenous progesterone suppressed epilepsy activity in four of seven women in one study[53] and 7 of 14 in another study.[54] In a study by Backstrom et al., intravenous progesterone decreased interictal EEG activity within a few seconds, suggesting a direct effect on neural membranes.[53] Recently, it was suggested that progesterone or one of its metabolites may interfere with gamma-aminobutyric acid (GABA) receptor activity similar to barbiturates[55] or increase the GABA inhibitory responses similar to benzodiazepines.[56]

The implication of these prior studies is that hormonal contraceptives including oral contraceptives, depomedroxyprogesterone acetate (DMPA), and Norplant implants could affect seizure activity. Several studies have explored the relationship between oral contraceptives and seizures in humans.[57–63] Espir et al. conducted a controlled crossover study of 20 epileptic women on regular anticonvulsant therapy who were taking Norinyl-1/50 (mestranol and norethindrone).[57] There were no significant changes in the frequency of seizures compared to when the women were taking a placebo. In another study, Toivakka studied 10 women without epilepsy and 11 women with epilepsy while on oral contraceptives.[58] EEGs were done before starting the pills and on the fourth day of three menstrual cycles. While the EEGs in the nonepileptic women were unchanged, the EEGs in 36% of the women with epilepsy worsened while on the pill. However, only 1 of the 11 women with epilepsy had an increased seizure frequency on oral contraceptives and that individual had decreased her medication just before the study began. Poser also found no increase in frequency of epileptic attacks when women with epilepsy were on oral contraceptives.[59] Diamond et al. found one adolescent with worsening seizure frequency among 10 studied who were on both anticonvulsants and oral contraceptives.[60] Dana-Haeri and Richens conducted a double-blind study of norethindrone and a placebo.[61] There was no difference in seizure frequency between patients receiving placebo compared to those on oral contraceptives. Mattson et al. evaluated the use of progestin-only contraceptives either orally or via injectable DMPA and demonstrated a modest improvement in seizure control.[62] Thus, in the small number of studies done, there does not seem to be evidence that hormonal contraceptives adversely affect seizure control. The effect of oral contraceptives may vary considerably from individual to individual and must be evaluated in each woman with epilepsy. The studies available suggest that a progesterone-only contraceptive might have more advantageous effects on seizures than a combination pill. However, as discussed in the next section, this potential advantage is countered by the lowered efficacy of the oral and Norplant device progesterone-only contraceptives when used in combination with anticonvulsants.

The other significant consideration with oral contraceptives in women with epilepsy is whether anticonvulsants have any interactions with oral contraceptives, or vice versa, that could affect medication efficacy. Kenyon first reported this problem in a case of a woman with epilepsy on phenytoin who became pregnant without a history of missing a pill.[63] The hypothesis being that anticonvulsants induced enzymes in the liver, leading to a more rapid metabolism of estrogen and progesterone with resultant contraceptive failure. Hempel et al. reported on six other contraceptive failures[64]; Janz and Schmidt, on three failures[65]; Belaisch et al., on three failures[66]; and Gagnaire et al., on three failures in women with epilepsy on both oral contraceptives and anticonvulsants.[67] Coulam and Annegers reviewed these studies and added four patients of their own.[68] They concluded that there was a 29-fold increase in the method failure from 0.07 to

2.00 in 884 women-months among women on both oral contraceptives and anticonvulsants. However, this still left the effectiveness rate at a very acceptable level. Sonnen reviewed the literature in 1983 regarding this problem and found 52 cases of contraceptive failure related to anticonvulsants.[69] However, he felt that the incidence was probably higher as 12 women in his own small clinic population had unplanned pregnancies while using the combination of oral contraceptives and anticonvulsants.[69] Back et al. examined all recorded cases in Great Britain between 1968 and 1984 and found 43 such pregnancies, of which 20 involved the use of phenobarbital, 25 phenytoin, 7 primidone, 6 carbamazepine, 4 ethosuximide, and 1 valproic acid.[70] Ethinyl estradiol levels were followed in two women taking phenobarbital and oral contraceptives and were found to drop 64 and 73%.[71] The interaction between anticonvulsants and oral contraceptives has usually been reported with either phenobarbital or phenytoin, although there have been reports of the problem in women receiving primidone or carbamazepine.[69,72]

The fall in hormonal levels has also been reported in women using Norplant implants and anticonvulsants.[73,74] In Haukkamaa's study, two of nine women using implants and anticonvulsants became pregnant within 1 year. The recommendation of Haukkamaa was not to use progestin-only pills or Norplant implants in women using anticonvulsants that affect steroid metabolism, and instead choose an oral contraceptive with 50 µg of ethinyl estradiol. Odlind and Olsson also reported on a woman who became pregnant while using the Norplant implant and phenytoin.[74] While using the Norplant, her plasma levonorgestrel levels were markedly below the levels found in healthy women with the Norplant device. In addition, while on phenytoin, the woman had regular ovulatory menstrual cycles, which stopped when phenytoin was discontinued. DMPA appears to be effective in women on anticonvulsants because the level of progesterone is much higher than with the progestin-only pill or the Norplant device.

The question has arisen as to whether there is a way of predicting which women might be more prone to a failure with this combination. Breakthrough bleeding has been suggested as a sign of insufficient contraceptive hormones.[69] However, no studies have validated this suggestion. Sonnen found that in women on both oral contraceptives and anticonvulsants, the frequency of breakthrough bleeding in 133 women ranged from 60 to 90% while on oral contraceptives with 30 to 50 µg of ethinyl estradiol.[69] In 10 of 12 women who had the estrogen content increased to 75 mg, breakthrough bleeding was eliminated. However, this study did not prove that these women were at less risk of contraceptive failure. Also, as the enzyme-inducing effect varies widely from individual to individual, it is difficult to predict an appropriate estrogen dose for any particular woman. Contraceptive Technology advises that women who are on phenytoin use an oral contraceptive with at least 50 µg of estrogen. This problem has not been reported with valproic acid or benzodiazepines, both of which have minimal enzyme-inducing effect. In one study, these medications had only a 6 and 0% prevalence of breakthrough bleeding, respectively.[69] However, while valproic acid has less enzyme induction potential, the practitioner needs to consider the higher teratogenic potential of valproic acid if a woman fails to use a contraceptive device appropriately.

One alternative for women using oral contraceptives and anticonvulsants is the addition of vitamin C. Back and associates showed a 47% increase in circulating ethinyl estradiol by adding 1 g of vitamin C daily orally, as ascorbic acid competes with ethinyl estradiol in the gastrointestinal tract wall for sulfate conjugation.[75] This allows for higher bioavailability of estrogen.

INTRAUTERINE DEVICE

There have been at least two reports of women with no prior seizure history who had grand mal seizures during intrauterine device insertion or removal.[76,77] Since intrauterine device insertion or removal can precipitate a neurovascular crisis including seizures and vasovagal syncope, the practitioner should be prepared for these complications.

Summary

1. Pregnancy has no effect on seizures in at least 50% of those with a seizure disorder. In other women it may make seizures worse or better. This may be related to changes in medication with pregnancy or changes in the metabolism of the medications with pregnancy. Those with severe seizure disorders are more likely to have a worsening of their condition with pregnancy.
2. A small increase in pregnancy complications has been reported in those women with epilepsy. However, the complication rates and types vary from study to study and the small prospective studies done to date do not seem to indicate a significant increase in pregnancy complications.
3. The risk of anticonvulsants to the fetus seems lower than previously reported. Many of the minor anomalies are probably more related to epilepsy itself than the anticonvulsants. However, phenytoin is associated with hypertelorism and digital hypoplasia, and valproic acid is associated with a higher prevalence of neural tube defects. Prior to a planned pregnancy, an attempt should be made to discontinue anticonvulsants in those women who have been seizure free for several years. In those women who need medication, the risk of seizures outweighs the risk of anticonvulsants. However, attempts should be made to put the women on monotherapy versus polytherapy. Phenytoin and carbamazepine are probably the drugs of choice for grand mal seizures while ethosuximide is the drug of choice for petit mal during pregnancy. Trimethadione and valproic acid should be avoided. Folic acid should be

used as a supplement in these women before conception and with pregnancy to lower the risk of spina bifida in the offspring.

4. While estrogens may have a proconvulsant effect and progesterones an anticonvulsant effect, hormonal contraceptives do not seem to have a significant impact on seizure disorders. However, anticonvulsants may interact with oral contraceptives and decrease their efficacy. Women on this combination of drugs should be advised of the small increased risk of pregnancy. They should be advised that breakthrough bleeding may be a sign of a higher risk of pregnancy. If this should occur, options include adding a barrier method, adding ascorbic acid, and increasing the dose of estrogen in the pill. Women should be advised not to stop oral contraceptives when spotting occurs. While most women can be started on a pill with 30 to 40 µg of ethinyl estradiol, if an unplanned pregnancy would cause significant hardship on the family, a higher dose of estrogen should be used to start. Because of this interaction, progestin-only contraceptives, including the progestin-only pill and Norplant implants, should probably be avoided in women on anticonvulsants that induce metabolizing enzymes of the liver, including phenytoin and phenobarbital. DMPA does not appear to be contraindicated in women on anticonvulsants because of the higher doses of progestins.

5. Women with epilepsy should be provided information on the interactions between epilepsy, pregnancy, and contraceptives.

Multiple Sclerosis

Multiple sclerosis as a chronic disease is of particular interest since young women are more affected than any other age group.

Fertility

Fertility rates have been reported to be unimpaired but pregnancy rates may remain lower in affected women compared to healthy women because some of those affected may choose not to have children secondary to their disability.[78,79] In men, sperm production has not been reported to be affected but problems could occur as a result of problems with erection or ejaculation.[79] One of the significant effects of this disease, its effect on sexuality, has until recently been unreported. Sexual dysfunction may be one of the most important early distressing manifestations of the disease.[79-84] Vas reported that 43% of men with multiple sclerosis stated that they were impotent and 46% complained of erectile dysfunction.[81] In another study, Lilius et al. found that 91% of 115 men and 72% of 134 women with multiple sclerosis reported a change in their sexual functioning, with half finding that their sexual activity either was unsatisfactory or had stopped.[84] The problem seems to be related to damage to the lower spinal cord and is correlated to damage in this area and not to either pyramidal or cerebellar damage or duration of the disease.[79] Both men and women with multiple sclerosis should be counseled to adapt to what gives them the most sexual pleasure.

Effect of Pregnancy on Multiple Sclerosis

Several studies have examined the effect of pregnancy on multiple sclerosis. Initial retrospective studies reported an increase in frequency of attacks in the postpartum period.[85–89] Birk et al. reviewed these studies and several others involving 935 pregnancies.[78] They found that about 10% of women experienced some worsening of symptoms during pregnancy but that 30% experienced a relapse in the postpartum period within 6 months of delivery. Four of the eight studies demonstrated an improvement prepartum, with six showing a worsening postpartum. Most concluded that there was no overall adverse effect on the course of multiple sclerosis. The relapse rate was about three times expected and was still twice expected at 6 months postpartum. The studies also indicated that an abortion might be associated with a risk of relapse. More recent studies demonstrated somewhat similar results. Nelson et al., in an interview study of 435 women, found that exacerbation rates were three times higher during the postpartum period, highest in the first 3 months postpartum.[90] Birk et al. conducted a small prospective study over a 2-year period in eight women.[91] During pregnancy, three improved, one had a possible increase in symptoms, and four had no change. Postpartum, six became worse and two had no change. Among the women who had worsening of their symptoms, about half had mild and transient problems while the other half had more severe and prolonged relapses. A similar response to pregnancy has been discussed in other immunological disorders including systemic lupus and myasthenia gravis. One explanation is the immunosuppressive effects of hormones or proteins that circulate at high levels during pregnancy such as estrogen, progesterone, corticosteroids, prolactin, alpha-fetoprotein and alpha-globulin.[90,91] As these disappear postpartum, an exacerbation may occur. No reports were encountered that studied whether treatment with immunosuppressants, such as steroids, in the postpartum period would decrease the risk of postpartum complications.

Weinshenker et al. examined the question of pregnancy on long-term disability in a retrospective population-based survey in Ontario, Canada.[92] This study failed to show a relationship between the degree of long-term disability and either the number of term pregnancies or the timing of pregnancy relative to the onset of multiple sclerosis. Thus, there may be a lack of association between short-term relapse and long-term outcome or disability. Stenager et al. found slightly different results in a study of 64 female patients on the Island of Funen.[93] In these women with multiple sclerosis, long-term disability was worse in women whose disease started before or in connection with a pregnancy. Overall, there seems to be a small reduction in disease activity, with pregnancy, with a high risk of at least short-term relapse in the postpartum period.

Effect of Multiple Sclerosis on Pregnancy

Multiple sclerosis does not appear to alter the course of pregnancy, labor, delivery, or the outcome of the pregnancy. There is no evidence of an increased rate of abortion, delivery complications, or congenital malformations.[78] The other consideration is the effect of medications used for the treatment of multiple sclerosis on the fetus. The most common drugs used for multiple sclerosis are corticosteroids. While corticosteroids are best avoided during pregnancy, they can be used if needed, without significant problems. There is a small risk of cleft palate, particularly if the drug is used in the first trimester, and fetal adrenal suppression, if it is used in high doses late in pregnancy.[78] Azathioprine and cyclophosphamide, other immunosuppressants, are discussed more fully in Chapters 11 and 13. Anticonvulsants may be used in some of these women and their effects on pregnancy were discussed earlier.

Multiple Sclerosis and Contraception

Sexuality and contraception are important topics to discuss with all men and women with multiple sclerosis. No methods are absolutely contraindicated. Barrier methods such as the condom or diaphragm may be difficult if there are problems with motor weakness or tremors in the upper extremities. However, the partner could help in these situations. The condom, by blunting sensation, may also be a problem in a man with multiple sclerosis, causing difficulties in maintaining an erection.

Oral contraceptives do not appear to have an effect on the long-term prognosis of women with multiple sclerosis in the two studies examining this question.[94,95] Poser and coworkers studied 179 women with multiple sclerosis of which 21% were on oral contraceptives.[95] Overall, there was no increase in attack rate of those on oral contraceptives. Of their patients who used the pill, 3 became worse, 9 improved, and 6 noted the beginning of symptoms during pill use. It is of significance that in this study, 54% of patients with multiple sclerosis did not use any contraception. Thus, the fear of contraceptive side effects may keep women away from contraceptive use. Some of these women may also need to be on long-term antibiotics for problems such as chronic urinary tract infection. The interaction of antibiotics with oral contraceptives is discussed in Chapter 16.

The intrauterine device might be a problem if adductor spasms of the thighs are present or other disabilities cause problems with menstrual hygiene. The intrauterine device might also be contraindicated if a woman had reduced abdominal sensation, thus not allowing her to notice early signs of inflammatory bowel disease.[79] The other problem with the intrauterine device would be the woman on concomitant steroids or immunosuppressants, leading to a possible decrease in efficacy, as discussed in Chapter 2, and immunocompromise increasing the risk of more serious uterine infections.

Summary

1. Fertility rates are not affected although pregnancy rates may be lower from fear of raising children with a disability.
2. A high percent of men and women with multiple sclerosis complain of sexual dysfunction, which appears related to the disease affecting the lower spinal column.
3. Pregnancy may cause a slight decrease in symptoms during the partum period, with a high risk of at least short-term exacerbation postpartum.
4. Pregnancies and the offspring in women with multiple sclerosis appear normal.
5. There are no contraindications to any contraceptive in individuals with multiple sclerosis. However, in certain situations, various contraceptives may cause problems. Those individuals with a physical handicap may have difficulty with barrier methods. Women on anticonvulsants need to be aware of the potential for lower efficacy rates of combined oral contraceptives. The Norplant device and the progestin-only pill should be avoided in those women on phenytoin or phenobarbital. The intrauterine device should be avoided in those women who are on immunosuppressants.

Migraine Headaches

While migraine headaches are not usually a serious neurological disease, they are extremely common, present in 17.6% of women,[96] and can be of concern to women of childbearing age who are considering using oral contraceptives. Pregnancy does not appear to be a problem in these women. Two reports demonstrated that the frequency and severity of migraine headaches decrease during pregnancy.[97,98] About 30% of women are free of attacks during pregnancy, with an additional 40% having only infrequent mild attacks. The ergot alkaloids and the beta-blockers are probably best avoided during pregnancy and instead the use of nonnarcotic analgesics is recommended.

Concern arises in whether to place women with headaches, especially migraine headaches, on oral contraceptives. There does not appear to be any causal relationship or interactions between oral contraceptives and nonmigraine headaches. Evidence exists that female hormones play a strong role in influencing migraine headaches.[99] Migraine headache frequency is equal in men and women before puberty, at which time migraine headaches become much more frequent in women. Sixty-eight percent of adults with migraine are women. Oral contraceptives may increase the severity and frequency of headaches in 15 to 50% of women with preexisting migraine headaches, especially during the drug-free period between cycles.[97,98,100] However, an additional one-third or more of women with migraine headaches may have improvement while on oral contraceptive pills.[1] Occasionally a woman will have the onset of migraine headaches after starting oral contraceptive pills, usually starting within the first several cycles. If migraine headaches significantly increase in frequency or severity after starting oral contraceptives, the pills should be stopped. However, it may take several months for the headache severity to return to baseline levels.

Another concern with oral contraceptive use in women with migraine headaches has been the question of stroke. The relationship between strokes, oral contraceptive use, and migraine headaches was first suggested in the Collaborative Group for the Study of Stroke in Young Women.[101] There was a twofold increase in the risk of strokes in women with migraine headaches and not on oral contraceptives compared with those women without migraine headaches. While the combination of migraine headaches and oral contraceptives did not increase the risk of hemorrhagic strokes, the risk of thrombotic strokes increased from 2.0 times normal to 5.7 times normal. This increase was not considered significant because of the small number of women and confounding factors involved. It is also important to consider that this study was conducted at a time when oral contraceptives contained estrogens at higher doses than what is used in current pills. There have been no prospective controlled studies examining the prevalence of stroke in women with migraine headaches who use oral contraceptives. Certainly women who develop either more severe headaches or focal neurological symptoms (i.e. visual disturbances, weakness or numbness) after starting oral contraceptives should be counseled to stop using the pills immediately.

Menstrual migraines are migraine attacks that occur regularly between 2 or 3 days before and after the start of the menstrual cycle and at no other time.[102] These headaches appear to be related to the fall in estrogen levels that occurs at that time.[102-104] Somerville demonstrated that estrogens given premenstrually delayed migraine headaches but did not alter menstruation.[105] Conversely, progesterone given premenstrually delayed menstruation but failed to alter migraine attacks.[105] Mechanisms for menstrual migraines related to estrogen withdrawal include a rise in prostaglandin and prolactin release as well as central nervous system opioid dysregulation.[104]

Using strict criteria, menstrual migraine may make up about 7 to 14% of women with migraine headaches.[102,106] Another 35% or more of women with migraine have an increased number of attacks at the time of menstruation with attacks at other times of the cycle.[102,106] These two groups, particularly the first, are most likely to respond to hormonal manipulation.[102]

Menstrual migraine may worsen during the first trimester of pregnancy but usually improves during the second and third trimesters.[104] This improvement may be a result of the sustained high levels of estrogen.

Hormonal manipulation has been demonstrated to alter menstrual migraines. DeLignieres et al., in a double-blind study, found that percutaneous estradiol effectively decreased menstrual migraine headaches when used perimenstrually.[106] Oral contraceptives may have several effects on menstrual migraines. The headaches may appear for the first time, or existing headaches may get worse, get better, or stay the same.[102] Menstrual migraines are not a contraindication to oral contraceptive therapy. The intensity of the headaches should be followed closely in each woman after starting oral contraceptives. In women with periovulatory headaches, suppression with combined oral contraceptives or DMPA may suppress the headaches.[107]

In summary, there is no contraindication to the use of oral or other hormonal contraceptives in women with tension/nonmigraine headaches. Hormonal contraceptives can also be used in women with a history of migraine headaches. However, if focal neurological symptoms are associated with the migraine headaches, an alternative contraceptive method is advised. When oral contraceptives are used, a low dose of estrogen or a progestin-only pill should be prescribed, and discontinued if there is an aggravation of the headaches. There would also appear to be no contraindication to the Norplant implant or DMPA. Since the Norplant device and DMPA are not readily reversible, it may be advisable to try several months of the progestin-only oral contraceptive pill before starting either of these methods, to evaluate whether there is an increase in frequency or severity of headaches.

Wilson's Disease

Pregnancy

No medical contraindications to pregnancy have been reported in the limited literature on Wilson's disease. However, affected women should receive preconception care to optimize their condition before pregnancy. Women should be stable on penicillamine and without active liver disease before pregnancy. Those symptomatic women with untreated disease have a higher-than-normal rate of spontaneous abortion and infertility. The side effects of penicillamine on the fetus have been controversial. Penicillamine has been reported to cause dose-related birth defects in rats and in humans.[108] Some individuals have recommended continuing its use during pregnancy while others have recommended that pregnant women avoid penicillamine during the first trimester but restart maintenance therapy at the start of the second trimester at the lowest possible dose required to stabilize the individual.[109] Chemin et al. reported on a case of one woman who stopped penicillamine during her pregnancy and developed fulminant hepatic failure during the perinatal period.[110] She previously had two uncomplicated pregnancies while taking penicillamine. It is also possible that triethylenetetramine dihydrochloride (trientine) may prove to be a safer chelating agent during pregnancy in these women.[111]

Contraception

Very little has been written about the interactions of Wilson's disease and contraception. However, in one report, Wilson's disease was found to be exacerbated by a combination oral contraceptive secondary to an increase in plasma ceruloplasmin level and consequently an increase of absorption of copper from the gastrointestinal tract.[112] Thus, combination oral contraceptives should be used only with extreme caution in these women. Copper intrauterine devices would be contraindicated because of possible absorption of copper. Progestin-only contraceptives should not induce ceruloplasmin production and would not be contraindicated.

Neurofibromatosis

Neurofibromatosis is an autosomal dominant disorder associated with café au lait spots and neurofibromas that can occur anywhere in the nervous system. Neurofibromas usually involve the skin but may involve deeper peripheral nerves and be present in locations innervated by the autonomic nervous system.

Fertility is unaffected by neurofibromatosis.[113] The lesions can first appear during puberty, and pregnancy may stimulate their growth.[114,115] Baker et al. reported one case of a sarcomatous degeneration of a pelvic neurofibroma associated with pregnancy.[116] Pregnancy has also been reported to cause the development of hypertension in these women.[115] Swapp and Main reported on 24 pregnancies in 11 women, with 10 developing hypertension.[114] Gulati and Malik reported on 10 pregnant women with neurofibromatosis, of whom 7 developed hypertensive disorders of pregnancy.[117] Neurofibromatosis has also been reported to be associated with a poor pregnancy outcome including spontaneous abortion, stillbirth, and a 50% chance of transmission of the disorder to the child.[115] Pre- and postconception genetic counseling is important, especially with prenatal diagnosis becoming available. Peripheral neurofibromatosis (NF1) has been localized to a gene on chromosome 17 and central neurofibromatosis (NF2), to a gene on chromosome 22.

There are no reports of trials of hormonal contraceptives in women with neurofibromatosis. Because of the potential negative effects, hormonal therapy should be used with extreme caution in these individuals. Progesterone therapy or low-dose combination pills should be considered if hormonal therapy is utilized. If a long-term delivery system of progestins is contemplated (DMPA or Norplant), a short-term trial with a progestin-only pill may be helpful in determining side effects. This formulation could more easily be stopped than DMPA or Norplant.

Myasthenia Gravis

Myasthenia gravis involves muscle weakness predominantly of oculomotor, facial, laryngeal, and respiratory muscles caused by a circulating antibody that decreases postjunctional acetylcholine receptors. This weakness is exacerbated by repetitive use of the affected muscles.

Most women with myasthenia gravis have no fertility problems. The effect myasthenia gravis has on pregnancy is unpredictable. Approximately one-third of women will become worse during pregnancy and two-thirds will remain the same or improved.[118] Plauche reviewed 322 pregnancies occurring in 225 women with myasthenia gravis.[119] Of these women, 41% had exacerbations during pregnancy, 28.6% had remissions during pregnancy, and 31.7% reported no change during pregnancy. Exacerbations have been noted to be most common in the first trimester and improvement has been noted more commonly in the second and third trimesters.[120] Maternal symptoms may worsen during the postpartum period. In the above-noted study, 29.8% experienced postpartum exacerbations including 9 women (4%) who died during or shortly following pregnancy. There is an associated 3% maternal mortality rate.[121] In contrast, Delmis et al. followed 29 women including 31 deliveries and 33 newborns.[122] They found that only 2 women experienced a significant exacerbation during pregnancy and there were no maternal and neonatal deaths.

Pregnant women with myasthenia gravis are at greater risk for respiratory problems because of the combination of underinflation of the basal segments of the lung during pregnancy and underlying weakness of the respiratory muscles. Another problem with pregnancy in these women can be the inability to retain medication because of the nausea and vomiting associated with pregnancy. Thus, parenteral medication should be available.

Labor can also enhance the muscle weakness in these women, leading to the potential of respiratory failure. Uterine muscle is not affected by myasthenia gravis; however, skeletal muscles used to perform the Valsalva maneuver in pushing the fetus during delivery can be affected. Forceps delivery may become necessary if the second stage of labor is prolonged due to muscle weakness. Magnesium sulfate should be avoided during labor as it can diminish the depolarizing action of acetylcholine and induce a myasthenic crisis. In addition, procaine and related anesthetics may be toxic since pyridostigmine and neostigmine may inhibit hydrolysis of these anesthetics.[123] Lidocaine used as a regional anesthetic is preferred.

In Plauche's review of 322 pregnancies in women with myasthenia gravis, 11.8% ended in spontaneous or induced abortion (14 spontaneous and 24 induced); 85.6%, in live births; and 6.8%, in perinatal death.[119] In addition, 14.9% developed neonatal myasthenia gravis. This occurs from passive transfer of acetylcholine receptor antibodies across the placenta and is a self-limiting disease resolving over several days or weeks.[124]

Congenital malformations have not been reported with cholinesterase inhibitors used for treatment.[119] Corticosteroids have been used with good success in pregnant women with myasthenia. After a steroid-induced remission appears to be a safer time for a woman to become pregnant. However, since withdrawal of steroids can exacerbate the disease, women who become pregnant should be continued on steroids but on the lowest dose possible to control the disease. Anticholinesterases and corticosteroids should be used as necessary during pregnancy. Plasmapheresis does not appear to be dangerous for either mother or fetus.[124] Thymectomy has also been performed before and during pregnancy either to reduce the risk of an exacerbation or to decrease an exacerbation in women with severe myasthenia.[125]

Interactions between myasthenia gravis and contraceptive devices have not been reported.

Spina Bifida

While spina bifida is one of the most common congenital abnormalities (1/1000 live births), little is known about the effects of this condition in the pregnant women. Only about 12 cases that discuss the effect of spina bifida on the course of a pregnancy have been reported.[126] Two recent studies demonstrated a 3% risk of spina bifida in offspring of spina bifida patients.[127,128] A similar risk was found in women who had delivered a previous infant with a neural tube defect. All women of childbearing age who are capable of becoming pregnant should consume 0.4 mg of folic acid per day to decrease the risk of pregnancy affected with spina bifida or other neural tube defects.[129] All women who had a previous neural tube defect-affected pregnancy should consume 4.0 mg of folic acid from at least 1 month before conception through the first 3 months of pregnancy.[130] This 4.0 mg dose should only be taken by prescription, under a physician's supervision.

Ideally, genetic counseling is offered before conception. Additionally, an obstetric evaluation is indicated to evaluate the pelvis, as well as a urological evaluation. As incontinence is a frequent problem as well as urinary tract infections, these women will have to be followed closely and treated for any infections. Women with prior urinary diversion procedures or bowel surgeries for fecal incontinence may have problems with obstruction. Ten of the 12 reported cases were able to deliver vaginally.

Problems with hormonal contraceptives have not been reported in women with spina bifida. Barrier methods can result in two problems. The diaphragm and sponge can increase the risk of urinary tract infection. If this is a problem in an affected woman, then these methods should be avoided. In addition, an affected woman may have difficulty manipulating a vaginal barrier device.

References

1. Mattson RH, Rebar RW. Contraceptive methods for women with neurologic disorders. Am J Obstet Gynecol 1993;168:2027–32.
2. Cramer JA, Jones EE. Reproductive function in epilepsy. Epilepsia 1991;32:S19–26.
3. Ziegelbaum MM. Hypogonadotropic hypogonadism and temporal lobe epilepsy. Urology 1991;38:235–6.
4. Falker G, Krause W. Oligoasthenoteratozoospermia in valproic acid therapy. Z Hautkrankheiten 1988;63:142–3.
5. Bardy AH. Epilepsy and pregnancy. A prospective study of 154 pregnancies of epileptic women. Academic dissertation. Pitajanmaki Epilepsy Research Centre and Department of Neurology, University of Helsinki, Helsink, Finland, 1982.
6. Bardy AH. Seizure frequency in epileptic women during pregnancy and puerperium: Results of the prospective Helsinki study. In Janz D, Bossi L, Dam M, eds. Epilepsy, Pregnancy, and the Child. New York, Raven Press, 1982, pp 85–99.
7. Bardy AH, Hiilesmaa VK, Teramo KA. Effect of pregnancy on the electroencephalogram of epileptic women. Acta Neurol Scand 1988;78:22–5.
8. Schmidt D, Canger R, Avanzini G, Battin, D, Cusi C, Beck-Mannagetta G, Koch S, Rating D, Janz D. Change of seizure frequency in pregnant epileptic women. J Neurol Neurosurg Psychiatry 1983;46:751–5.
9. Donaldson JO. Neurology of Pregnancy. 2nd ed. Philadelphia, WB Saunders, 1989, pp 229–65.
10. Canger R, Avanzini G, Battino D, Bossi L, Franceschetti S, Spina S. Modifications of seizure frequency in pregnant patients with epilepsy: A prospective study. In Janz D, Bossi L, Dam M, eds. Epilepsy, Pregnancy, and the Child. New York, Raven Press, 1982, pp 33–8.
11. Philbert A, Dam M. The epileptic mother and her child. Epilepsia 1982;247:331.
12. Patterson RM. Seizure disorders in pregnancy Med Clin North Am 1989;73:661–5.
13. Bag S, Behari M, Ahuja GK, Karmarker MG. Pregnancy and epilepsy. J Neurol 1989;236:311–3.
14. Lander CM, Edwards VE, Eadie MJ, Tyrer JH. Plasma anticonvulsant concentrations during pregnancy. Neurology (Minneap) 1977;27:128–31.
15. Dansky L, Andermann E, Sherwin AL, Andermann F. Plasma levels of phenytoin during pregnancy and the puerperium. In Janz D, Bossi L, Dam M, eds. Epilepsy, Pregnancy, and the Child. New York, Raven Press, 1982, pp 155–62.
16. Yerby MS. Problems and management of the pregnant woman with epilepsy. Epilepsia 1987;28(suppl 3):529–35.
17. Dam M, Christiansen J, Munck O, Mygind KI. Antiepileptic drugs: Metabolism in pregnancy. Clin Pharmacokinet 1979;4:53–62.
18. Ramsay RE, Strauss RG, Wilder BJ, Willmore L. Status epilepticus in pregnancy: Effect of phenytoin malabsorption on seizure control. Neurology (NY) 1978;28:85–9.
19. Suter C, Klingman WO. Seizure states and pregnancy. Neurology (Minneap) 1957;7:105–18.
20. Lander CM, Edwards VE, Eadie MJ, Tyrer JH. Plasma anticonvulsant concentrations during pregnancy. Neurology (Minneap) 1977;27:128–31.
21. Yerby MS. Risks of pregnancy in women with epilepsy. Epilepsia 1992;33:S26–7.
22. Buchanan N. Epilepsy and pregnancy: A review of 26 patients. N Z Med J 1988;101:509–10.
23. Huhmar E, Jarvinen PA. Relation of epileptic symptoms to pregnancy, delivery and puerperium. Ann Chir Gynaecol Fenn 1961;50:49–64.

24. Nelson KB, Ellenberg JH. Maternal seizure disorder, outcome of pregnancy and neurologic abnormalities in children. Neurology 1982;32:1247–54.
25. Andermann E, Dansky L, Kinch RA. Complications of pregnancy, labor and delivery in epileptic women. In Janz D, Dam M, Richens A, eds. Epilepsy, Pregnancy, and the Child. New York, Raven Press, 1982, pp 61–74.
26. Yerby MS. Problems and management of the pregnant woman with epilepsy. Epilepsia 1987;28(suppl 3):529–35.
27. Battino D, Bossi L, Canger R. Obstetrical monitoring of pregnancy in 59 patients with epilepsy. In Janz D, Dam M, Richens A, eds. Epilepsy, Pregnancy, and the Child. New York, Raven Press, 1982, pp 99–101.
28. Gaily E, Granstroem ML, Hiilesmaa V, Bardy A. Minor anomalies in offspring of epileptic mothers. J Pediatr 1988;112:520–9.
29. Hanson JW, Smith DW. The fetal hydantoin syndrome. J Pediatr 1975;87:285–90.
30. Hanson JW, Myrianthopoulos NC, Sedgwick Harvey MA, Smith DW. Risks to the offspring of women treated with hydantoin anticonvulsants, with emphasis on the fetal hydantoin syndrome. J Pediatr 1976;89:662–8.
31. Bossi L. Fetal effects of anticonvulsants. In: Morselli PL, Pippenger CE, Penry JK, eds. Antiepileptic Drug Therapy in Pediatrics. New York, Raven Press, 1983, pp 37–64.
32. Kelly TE. Teratogenicity of anticonvulsant drugs 1: Review of the literature. Am J Med Genet 1984;19:413–34.
33. Lindhout D, Schmidt D. In-utero exposure to valproate and neural tube defects. Lancet 1986;1:1392–3.
34. Lammer EJ, Sever LE, Oakley GP. Teratogen update: Valproic acid. Teratology 1987;35:465–73.
35. Dalessio DJ. Seizure disorders and pregnancy. N Engl J Med 1985;312:559–63.
36. Sowa MV. Use of antiepileptic drugs in pregnancy. West J Med 1991;155:64.
37. Vestermark V, Vestermark S. Teratogenic effect of carbamazepine. Arch Dis Child 1991;66:641–2.
38. Jones KL, Lacro RV, Johnson KA, Adams J. Pattern of malformations in the children of women treated with carbamazepine during pregnancy. N Engl J Med 1989;320:1661–6.
39. Guidelines for the care of epileptic women of childbearing age. Commission on Genetics, Pregnancy, and the Child, International League Against Epilepsy. Epilepsia 1989;30:409–10.
40. Bandler AA. Treatment of epileptic disorders of adults. Mayo Clin Proc 1953;28:39–44.
41. Gowers WR. Epilepsy and other chronic convulsive diseases: Their causes, symptoms, and treatment. London, 1881, p 197.
42. Lin TY, Greenblatt M, Solomon HC. A polygraphic study of one case of petit mal epilepsy: Effects of medication and menstruation. Electroencephalogr Clin Neurophysiol 1952;4:351–5.
43. Laidlaw J. Catamenial epilepsy. Lancet 1956;2:1235–7.
44. Livingston S. Comprehensive Management of Epilepsy in Infancy. Childhood, and Adolescence. Springfield, IL, Charles C Thomas, 1972.
45. Shavit G, Lerman P, Korczyn AD, Kivity S, Bechar M, Gitter S. Phenytoin pharmacokinetics in catamenial epilepsy. Neurology (Cleve) 1984;34:959–61.
46. Wooley DE, Timeras PS. Gonad brain relationship, effect of female sex hormone on electroshock convulsion in rat. Endocrinology 1962;70:196–209.
47. Logothetis J, Harner R. Electrocortical activation by estrogens. Arch Neurol 1960;3:290–7.
48. Julien RM, Fowler GW, Danielsonm MG. The effects of antiepileptic drugs on estrogen-induced electrographic spike-wave discharge. J Pharmacol Exp Ther 1975;193:647–56.
49. Gevorkyan ES, Nazaryan KB, Kostanyan AA. Modifying effect of estradiol and progesterone on epileptic activity of the rat brain. Neurosci Behav Physiol 1989;19:412–5.
50. Stitt SL, Kinnarch WJ. The effect of certain progestins and estrogens on the threshold of electrically induced sizure patterns. Neurology 1968;18:213–6.
51. Spiegel E, Wycis H. Anticonvulsant effects of steroids. J Lab Clin Med 1945;30:947–53.
52. Craig CR. Anticonvulsant activity of steroids: Separability of anticonvulsant from hormonal effects. J Pharmacol Exp Ther 1966;153:337–43.
53. Backstrom T, Zetterlund B, Blom S, Romano M. Effects of intravenous progesterone infusions on the epileptic discharge frequency in women with partial epilepsy. Acta Neurol Scand 1984;69:240–8.

54. Mattson RH, Cramer JA, Caldwell BV, Siconolfi BC. Treatment of seizures with medroxyprogesterone acetate: Preliminary report. Neurology 1984;34:1255–8.
55. Majewska MD, Harrison NL, Schwartz RD, Barker JL, Paul SM. Steroid hormone metabolites are barbiturate like modulators of the GABA receptor. Science 1986;232:1004–7.
56. Smith S, Waterhouse BDE, Chapin JK, Woodward DJ. Progesterone alters GABA and glutamate responsiveness: A possible mechanism for its anxiolytic action. Brain Res 1987;400:353–9.
57. Espir M, Walker ME, Lawson JP. Epilepsy and oral contraception. Br Med J 1969;1:294–5.
58. Toivakka E. Oral contraception in epileptics. Arzneimittelforschung 1967;17:1085.
59. Poser S. Oral contracepives—Indications and neurological complications. Fortschr Neurol Psychiatr 1977;45:412–9.
60. Diamond MP, Greene JW, Thompson JM, Vanhooydonk JE, Wentz AC. Interaction of anticonvulsants and oral contraceptives in epileptic adolescents. Contraception 1985;31:623–32.
61. Dana-Haeri J, Richens A. Effects of norethisterone on seizures associated with menstruation. Epilepsia 1983;24:377–81.
62. Mattson RH, Cramer JA, Caldwell BV, Siconolfi BC. Treatment of seizures with medroxyprogesterone acetate: Preliminary report. Neurology 1984;34:1255–8.
63. Kenyon IE. Unplanned pregnancy in an epileptic. Br Med J 1972;1:686–7.
64. Hempel E, Bohm W, Carol W. Medikamentose enzyminduktion und hormonale kontrazeption. Zentralbl Gynakol 1973;95:1451–7.
65. Janz D, Schmidt D. Antiepileptic drugs and failure of oral contraceptives. Lancet 1974;1:1113.
66. Belaisch J, Driguez P, Janaud A. Influence de certains medicaments sur l'action des pilules contraceptives. Nouv Presse Med 1976;5:1645–6.
67. Gagnaire JC, Tchertchian J, Revol A. Grossesses sous contraceplifs oraux chez les patientes recevant des barbituriques. Nouv Press Med 1975;4:3008.
68. Coulam CB, Annegers JF. Do anticonvulsants reduce the efficacy of oral contraceptives? Epilepsia 1979;20:519–25.
69. Sonnen AE. Sodium valproate and the contraceptive pill. Br J Clin Pract Symp Suppl 1983;27:31–6.
70. Back DJ, Grimmer SFM, Orme MLE, Proudlove C, Mann RD, Breckenridge AM. Evaluation of Committee on Safety of Medicines Yellow Card Reports on oral contraceptive-drug interactions with anticonvulsants and antibiotics. Br J Clin Pharmacol 1988;25:527–32.
71. Back DJ, Bates M, Bowden A, Breckenridge AH, Hall MJ, Jones H, MacIver M, Orme M, Perucca E, Richens A, Rowe PH, Smith E. The interaction of phenobarbital and other anticonvulsants with oral contraceptive steroid therapy. Contraception 1980;22:495–503.
72. Orme M. The clinical pharmacology of oral contraceptive steroids. Br J Clin Pharmacol 1982;14:31–42.
73. Haukkamaa M. Contraception by Norplant subdermal capsules is not reliable in epileptic patients on anticonvulsant treatment. Contraception 1986;33:559–65.
74. Odlind V, Olsson SE. Enhanced metabolism of levonorgestrel during phenytoin treatment in a woman with Norplant implants. Contraception 1986;33:257–61.
75. Back DJ, Breckenridge AM, MacIver M, Orme ML, Purbe H, Rowe PH. The interaction of ethinylestradiol with ascorbic acid in man. Br Med J 1981;282:1516.
76. Richardson J, Morrison J. Epileptiform convulsions during insertion of intrauterine device. Lancet 1977;2:148.
77. Conrad CC, Ghazi M, Kitay DZ. Acute neurovascular sequelae of intrauterine device insertion or removal. J Reprod Med 1973;2:211–2.
78. Birk K, Smeltzer SC, Rudick R. Pregnancy and multiple sclerosis. Semin Neurol 1988;18:205–13.
79. Dewis ME, Thornton NG. Sexual dysfunction in multiple sclerosis. J Neurosci Nurs 1989;21:175–9.
80. Valleroy ML, Kraft GH. Sexual dysfunction in multiple sclerosis. Arch Phys Med Rehabil 1984;65:125–8.
81. Vas CJ. Sexual impotence and some autonomic disturbances in men with multiple sclerosis. Acta Neurol Scand 1969;45:166–82.
82. Szasz G, Paty D, Lawton-Speert S, Eisen K. A sexual functioning scale in multiple sclerosis. Acta Neurol Scand 1984;70:37–43.

83. Minderhoud JM, Leemkius JG, Kremer J, Laban E, Smits PML. Sexual disturbances arising from multiple sclerosis. Acta Neurol Scand 1984;70:299–306.
84. Lilius HG, Valtonene EJ, Wikstrom J. Sexual problems in patients suffering from multiple sclerosis. Scand J Soc Med 1976;4:41–4.
85. Millar JHD, Allison RS, Cheeseman EA, Merrett JD. Pregnancy as a factor influencing relapse in disseminated sclerosis. Brain 1959;82:417–26.
86. Shapira K, Poskanzer DC, Newell DJ, Miller H. Marriage, pregnancy and multiple sclerosis. Brain 1966;89:419–28.
87. Ghezzi A, Caputo D. Pregnancy: A factor influencing the course of multiple sclerosis? Eur Neurol 1981;20:517–9.
88. Korn-Lubetzki I, Kahana E, Cooper G, Abramsky O. Activity of multiple sclerosis during pregnancy and puerperium. Ann Neurol 1984;16:229–31.
89. Birk K, Rudick R. Pregnancy and multiple sclerosis. Arch Neurol 1986;16:229–31.
90. Nelson LM, Franklin GM, Jones MC. Risk of multiple sclerosis exacerbation during pregnancy and breast-feeding. JAMA 1988;259:3441–3.
91. Birk K, Ford C, Smeltzer S, Ryan D, Miller R, Rudick RA. The clinical course of multiple sclerosis during pregnancy and the puerperium. Arch Neurol 1990;47:738–42.
92. Weinshenker BG, Hader W, Carriere W, Baskerville J, Ebers GC. The influence of pregnancy on disability from multiple sclerosis: A population-based study in Middlesex County, Ontario. Neurology 1989;39:1438–40.
93. Stenager EN, Stenager E, Jensen K. Pregnancy and disseminated sclerosis: A retrospective study. Ugeskr Laeger 1989;151:1744–6.
94. Royal College of General Practitioners. Oral Contraceptives and Health. New York, Pitman, 1974.
95. Poser S, Raun NE, Wikstrom J, Poser W. Pregnancy, oral contraceptives and multiple sclerosis. Acta Neurol Scand 1979;59:108.
96. Stewart WF, Lipton JRB, Celentano DD, Reed ML. Prevalence of migraine headache in the United States. Relation to age, income, race and other sociodemographic factors. JAMA 1992;267:64–9.
97. Callaghan N. The migraine syndrome in pregnancy. Neurology 1968;18:192–9.
98. Massey EW. Migraine during pregnancy. Obstet Gynecol Surv 1977;32:285.
99. Nattero G. Menstrual headache. Adv Neurol 1982;33:215–26.
100. Paulsen CA. The women with medical disease. In Current Concepts in Oral Contraceptive Treatment. Part 2. Bloomfield, IL, Health Learning System, 1976.
101. Collaborative Group for the Study of Stroke in Young Women. Oral contraception and increased risk of cerebral ischemia or thrombosis. N Engl J Med 1973;288:871–8.
102. MacGregor EA, Chia H, Vohrah RC, Wilkinson M. Migraine and menstruation: A pilot study. Cephalalgia 1990;10:305–10.
103. DeLignieres B. Menstrual migraine. Rev Prat 1990;40:395–8.
104. Silberstein SD. The role of sex hormones in headache. Neurology 1992;42:37–42.
105. Somerville BW. The role of estradiol withdrawal in the etiology of menstrual migraine. Neurology 1972;22:355–65.
106. DeLignieres B, Vincens M, Mauvais-Javis P, Mas JL, Touboul PJ, Bousser MG. Prevention of menstrual migraine by percutaneous oestradiol. Br Med J 1986;293:1540.
107. Rindt W. Treatment of menstrual cycle associated migraine. Methods and findings in experimental and clinical pharmacology. Methods Find Exp Clin Pharmacol 1982;4:521–3.
108. Dupont P, Irion O, Beguin F. Pregnancy in a patient with treated Wilson's disease: A case report. Am J Obstet Gynecol 1990;163:1527–8.
109. Klion FM. Liver in normal pregnancy. In Cherry SH, Merkatz IR, eds. Complications of Pregnancy: Medical, Surgical, Gynecologic, Psychosocial and Perinatal. 4th ed. Baltimore, Williams & Wilkins, 1991, pp 797–806.
110. Shimono N, Ishibashi H, Ikematsu H, Kudo J, Shirahama M, Inaba S, Maeda K, Yamasaki K, Niho Y. Fulminant hepatic failure during perinatal period in a pregnant woman with Wilson's disease. Gastroenterol Jpn 1991;26:69–73.
111. Walshe JM. The management of pregnancy in Wilson disease treated with trientine. Q J Med 1986;58:81–7.
112. Decherney AH. The use of birth control pills in women with medical disorders. Clin Obstet Gynecol 1981;24:965–75.

113. Meherzi F, Mintz P, Smadja S, Ferrand S, Ravina JH. Von Recklinghausen's disease and pregnancy. Rev Fr Gynecol Obstet 1991;86:592–5.
114. Swapp GH, Main RJA. Neurofibromatosis in pregnancy. Br J Dermatol 1973;80:431–5.
115. Ansari AH, Nagamani M. Pregnancy and neurofibromatosis. Obstet Gynecol 1976;47:25s–9s.
116. Baker VV, Hatch KD, Shingleton HM. Case report: Neurofibrosarcoma complicating pregnancy. Gynecol Oncol 1989;34:237–9.
117. Gulati N, Malik S. Maternal and perinatal complications in neurofibromatosis during pregnancy. Int J Gynaecol Obstet 1991;34:221–7.
118. Noble PW, Lavee AE, Jacobs MM. Respiratory diseases in pregnancy. Obstet Gynecol Clin North Am 1988;15:391–428.
119. Plauche WC. Myasthenia gravis in mothers and their newborns. Clin Obstet Gynecol 1991;34:82–99.
120. Giwa-Osagie OF, Newton JR, Larcher V. Obstetric performance of patients with myasthenia gravis. Int J Gynaecol Obstet 1981;19:267–70.
121. Plauche WC. Myasthenia gravis. Clin Obstet Gynecol 1983;26:592–604.
122. Delmis J, Drazancic A, Jusic A, Petric M. Myasthenia gravis in pregnancy (foreign). Lijec Vjesn 1990;112:9–10.
123. Donaldson JO. Neurologic emergencies in pregnancy. Obstet Gynecol Clin North Am 1991;18:199–211.
124. Fennell D, Ringel S. Myasthenia gravis and pregnancy. Obstet and Gynecol Surv 1987;42:414.
125. Fox MW, Harms RW, Davis DH. Selected neurologic complications of pregnancy. Mayo Clin Proc 1990;65:1595–618.
126. Farine D, Jackson U, Portale A, Baxi L, Fox HE. Pregnancy complicated by maternal spina bifida: A report of two cases. J Reprod Med 1988;33:323–6.
127. Carter CO, Evans KA: Children of adult survivors with spina bifida cystica. Lancet 1973;2:294–6.
128. Carter CO, Evans KS: Spina bifida and anencephalus in greater London. J Med Genet 1973;10:209–34.
129. Recommendations for the use of folic acid to reduce the number of cases of spina bifida and other neural tube defects. MMWR 1992;41:1–7.
130. Folic acid for prevention of neural tube defects. The Contraception Report 1993. Volume IV, No. 3, pp 11–13.

4

Dermatological Diseases

There is relatively little information in the medical literature on the interaction between skin diseases and pregnancy or contraception. Melanoma and acne have been the most frequently studied areas.

Melanoma

The prevalence of melanoma continues to rise, with a doubling in the incidence in the past decade.[1] Approximately 11,000 women develop melanoma yearly, with the highest rate in the 20- to 40-year-old age group,[2] making this problem of particular concern to childbearing women. Several recent studies examined the question of the effect of pregnancy on women with a malignant melanoma. Sutherland et al. reported on a small subgroup of melanoma patients whose pregnancy seemed to either initiate or stimulate melanoma. These women appeared to have a worse prognosis.[3] However, Sutherland et al. did not find that women without such a history had a worse prognosis with a pregnancy, and felt that pregnancy would not be contraindicated in such women. Reintgen and coworkers found a shorter disease-free interval in pregnant women with melanoma than in nonpregnant women with melanoma; however, the ultimate survival rates did not differ.[4] In three other retrospective studies, survival rates did not differ between pregnant and nonpregnant women with melanoma.[5-7] In another recent study, Slingluff et al. compared 100 pregnant women with melanoma with nonpregnant patients.[8] The pregnant women had an increased incidence of lymph node metastases, shorter disease-free interval, but similar survival rates. They reviewed another 11 recent studies and found that 10 of the 11 failed to show survival differences. Thus, there is little to suggest that pregnancy has a significant effect on survival of women with melanoma. There is a suggestion of a shorter disease-free interval but no effect on ultimate prognosis. It would appear prudent for women to wait 2 to 3 years after the diagnosis of melanoma before becoming pregnant. There does not seem to be any need, however, to abort a pregnancy in women in whom a diagnosis of melanoma is made.

Melanoma does not appear to have an effect on pregnancy other than that which chemotherapy and/or radiation may have. These effects are discussed in Chapter 13.

Melanoma and Contraception

There is a concern that exogenous estrogens or progesterones might influence melanoma. This dates back to work by Snell and Bischitz demonstrating that estrogens alone or in combination with progesterone cause an increase in the number of melanocytes and in their melanin content.[9] Both estrogen and progesterone receptors have been demonstrated on some melanoma cells.[1,10,11] Lopez et al. examined melanoma cells in rats treated with either estradiol, saline, or an antiestrogen.[12] Tumors grew fastest in the estradiol-treated group with more lung metastases. The slowest growth was in those rats treated with antiestrogens. Several studies examining rates of melanoma in long-term users of oral contraceptives also gave rise to some concern about the effect of estrogens on melanoma.[13-16] Lerner et al. reported on nine cases where melanoma either began or metastasized after estrogens, progesterones, or both were started.[17] Hartge et al. evaluated the risk of exogenous hormones in the development of intraocular malignant melanoma in a case-control study of 238 women with melanoma versus 223 controls with a detached retina.[18] The relative risk for melanoma in those taking estrogen replacement was 2.0 but there was no increased risk in those using oral contraceptives. The updated findings of the Walnut Creek Contraceptive Drug Study conducted in California demonstrated a threefold risk of melanoma among contraceptive users compared to nonusers.[19] However, there was no relationship between duration of use and risk and there were confounding factors including more sunbathing hours among pill users. This was not adjusted for in this study.

Hannaford et al. recently reviewed the latest findings regarding oral contraceptives and melanoma from the Royal College of General Practitioners (RCGP) Study and the Oxford Family Planning Association Contraceptive Study (Oxford/FPA).[20] The RCGP study involves 23,000 women using oral contraception compared to a similar number of controls never using oral contraception. The Oxford study is following over 17,000 white married women of whom 9654 are using oral contraceptives, 4217 are using the diaphragm, and 3162 are using an intrauterine device. In both of these studies there was little to suggest that oral contraceptives increased the risk of melanoma except in the RCGP study where there was a suggestion of an increased risk of melanoma in those using oral contraceptives for over 10 years, with a relative risk of 1.77 (95% confidence interval, 0.80–3.90). Similar findings of no association between melanoma and oral contraceptives were found by several other study groups.[21-26] Two other studies found an elevated risk of melanoma in certain subgroups of users. Holly et al. found an elevated risk of superficial spreading melanoma in oral contraceptive users of at least 5 years.[15] The amount of sun exposure was not controlled for in this study. Beral et al. did find an elevated risk in women using oral contraceptives over 5 years that was still present after adjusting for hair and skin color, level of outdoor activity, and history of sunburns.[16] Thus, the question concerning whether women with melanoma should use oral contraceptives is not satisfactorily answered. The studies done to date address the issue of birth control as a risk factor in developing melanoma but not the effects of exogenous estrogens or progestins on melanoma. There is no conclusive evidence that exogenous estrogen or progesterone positively or negatively affect a melanoma. However, it would seem prudent that an alternative contraceptive method be advised for a woman with the diagnosis of melanoma in recent years (1–5 years).

Acne

Pregnancy and Acne

While not a life-threatening problem, acne can be severely disfiguring in women, with consequent significant psychological sequelae. Pregnancy is known to exacerbate pregnancy in some women due to hormone fluctuations. While acne itself is not associated with effects on the fetus, antiacne medications may have negative effects. Information about antiacne medications is somewhat limited, as there are no published studies following women who took acne medications throughout pregnancy. Topical acne medications have not been reported to cause fetal deformities in human beings.[27] However, there have been reports in animals of fetal anomalies with the use of topical retinoic acid.[28,29] Oral tetracycline during pregnancy has been associated with deciduous tooth staining in the infant and other congenital anomalies.[27] The use of oral isotretinoin during pregnancy is associated with major craniofacial, cardiac, thymic, and central nervous system deformities.[27,30] The use of oral tetracycline and oral isotretinoin is contraindicated during pregnancy. During preconception care, women with acne need counseling regarding the dangers of these agents should they become pregnant. Before starting isotretinoin, women need pregnancy testing and the use of extremely reliable contraception. Isotretinoin has a short half-life and is eliminated from the body rapidly.[31]

As such, women could discontinue therapy 1 month before becoming pregnant without a risk of birth defects.[31] Erythromycin appears safe for use during pregnancy.

Contraception and Acne

Any estrogen in sufficient doses will decrease sebum production and improve acne. The majority of oral contraceptive users, particularly those who are using estrogen-dominant combination pills, have an improvement in acne. Some women, particularly those using progestin-only contraceptives or progestin-dominant combination pills, may notice a worsening of their acne. However, even women using norgestrel, a progestin with marked androgenic activity, may find that their acne improves when norgestrel is used in combination with estrogen. Lemay et al. reported on 41 women with acne using a triphasic combined pill with ethinyl estradiol and *dl*-norgestrel.[32] Acne significantly improved in this study, with a fall in all androgen precursors and a twofold increase in sex hormone–binding globulin (SHBG). In another study, Palatsi et al. compared combination pills containing 0.15 mg of desogestrel/0.03 mg of ethinyl estradiol, with pills containing 0.15 mg of levonorgestrel/0.03 mg of ethinyl estradiol.[33] After 6 months of treatment, a 250% increase in SHBG was seen in the desogestrel group and no significant change in the levonorgestrel group. However, serum free testosterone levels fell 60% in both groups and acne improved significantly in both groups. If acne worsens with oral contraceptive use, a combination pill with a higher dose of estrogen may be of benefit. Oral contraceptives should be used in women with acne only if there is a contraceptive need or for those women with recalcitrant acne.

There are potential interactions between antiacne medications and contraceptive devices. Tetracyclines have been reported to decrease the efficacy of oral contraceptives.[34] However, two recent studies did not confirm such an interaction.[35,36] Steroids used to treat acne can decrease the effectiveness of an intrauterine device.

Psoriasis

No significant relationship has been found between psoriasis and pregnancy.[37] In one survey, Dunna and Finlay found that of 112 pregnancies, psoriasis was unchanged in 42.9%, improved in 41.1%, and worsened in 14.3%.[38] However, during the 3 months postpartum there was no change in 36.6%, improvement in 10.7%, and worsening in 49.1%, suggesting that psoriasis improves during pregnancy but may worsen in the postpartum period.

A major consideration in individuals with severe psoriasis are the effects on pregnancy of methotrexate or methoxsalen photochemotherapy. At present, there are no reports of malformations in the offspring of fathers receiving methotrexate during the time of the child's conception. This is in contrast to abnormalities reported in mothers using methotrexate during the first trimester.[39]

Stern and Lange reported on the pregnancy outcomes among 1380 patients (892 men and 488 women) who had received methoxsalen photochemotherapy (psoralen long-wave ultraviolet light therapy, or PUVA).[40] There were 94 men reporting 167 pregnancies in their partners and 93 women with 159 pregnancies. In the men, 34% had received treatment near the time of conception and 19% of the women received PUVA at the time of conception or during pregnancy. Induced and spontaneous abortions occurred in 30% of the pregnancies reported by women and in 12% of the pregnancies reported by men. There were two congenital malformations and two stillbirths, an incidence similar to that in the general population. However, this study was limited by the number of patients exposed to PUVA and so caution is still indicated with use of PUVA during pregnancy because it is potentially mutagenic. It would be advisable for individuals with severe psoriasis on methotrexate to go off the medication for several months before conception is planned.

There has been little written on psoriasis and contraception except for two small studies reporting an exacerbation of psoriasis in women on oral contraceptives.[41,42]

Hereditary Hemorrhagic Telangiectasia

The major consideration written about this condition and contraception has been the possible positive effects of estrogens and progestogens on bleeding. Van Cutsem reported on a case of bleeding in a woman who did not respond to laser photocoagulation or surgery, but the problem responded to treatment with estrogens and progesterone.[43] A double-blind randomized trial of 17 individuals treated with estradiol and 14 individuals treated with placebo demonstrated a slight but not significant reduction in bleeding after 3 months of estradiol.[44] In another uncontrolled trial, estradiol and progesterone helped to stop gastrointestinal bleeding in telangiectasias associated with chronic renal failure.[45]

References

1. Schwartz BK, Zashin SJ, Spencer SK, Mills LE, Sober AJ. Pregnancy and hormonal influences on malignant melanoma. J Dermatol Surg Oncol 1987;13:276–81.
2. Silverberg E, Lubera J. Cancer statistics, 1986. CA 1986;36:9–25.
3. Sutherland CM, Loutfi A, Mather FJ, Carter RD, Krementz ET. Effect of pregnancy upon malignant melanoma. Surg Gynecol Obstet 1983;157:443–6.
4. Reintgen DS, McCarty KS, Vollmer R, Cox E, Seigler HF. Malignant melanoma and pregnancy. Cancer 1985;55:1340–4.

5. Wong JH, Sterns EE, Kopald KH, Nizze JA, Morton DL. Prognostic significance of pregnancy in stage I melanoma. Arch Surg 1989;124:1227–30.
6. Colbourn DS, Nathanson L, Belilos E. Pregnancy and malignant melanoma. Semin Oncol 1989;16:377–87.
7. McManamny DS, Moss AL, Pocock PV, Briggs JC. Melanoma and pregnancy: A long term follow-up. Br J Obstet Gynaecol 1989;96:1419–23.
8. Slingluff CL, Reintgen DS, Vollmer RT, Seigler HF. Malignant melanoma arising during pregnancy. Ann Surg 1990;211:552–9.
9. Snell RS, Bischitz PG. The effect of large doses of estrogen and estrogen and progesterone on melanin pigmentation. J Invest Dermatol 1960;35:73.
10. Fisher RI, Neifeld JP, Lippman ME. Estrogen receptors in human malignant melanoma. Lancet 1976;2:337–8.
11. Chaudhuri PK, Walker MJ, Briele HA, Beattie CW, Das Gupta TK. Incidence of estrogen receptor in benign nevi and human malignant melanoma. JAMA 1980;244:791–3.
12. Lopez RE, Bhakoo H, Paolini NS, Rosen F, Holyoke ED, Goldrosen MH. Effect of estrogen on the growth of B-16 melanoma. Surg Forum 1978;29:153–4.
13. Beral V, Ramcharan S, Faris R. Malignant melanoma and oral contraceptive use among women in California. Br J Cancer 1977;36:804–9.
14. Adam SA, Sheaves JK, Wright NH, Mosser G, Harris RW, Vessey MP. A case-control study of the possible association between oral contraceptives and malignant melanoma. Br J Cancer 1981;44:45–50.
15. Holly EA, Weiss NS, Liff JM. Cutaneous melanoma in relation to exogenous hormones and reproductive factors. J Natl Cancer Inst 1983;70:827–31.
16. Beral V, Evans S, Shaw H, Milton G. Oral contraceptive use and malignant melanoma in Australia. Br J Cancer 1984;50:681–5.
17. Lerner AB, Nordlund JJ, Kirkwood JM. Effects of oral contraceptives and pregnancy on melanoma. N Engl J Med 1979;310:47.
18. Hartge P, Tucker MA, Shields JA, Augsburger J, Hoover RN, Fraumeni JF Jr. Case control study of female hormones and eye melanoma. Cancer Res 1989;49:4622–5.
19. Ramcharan S, Pellegrin FA, Ray R, Hsu JP. The Walnut Creek Contraceptive Drug Study. A prospective study of the side effects of oral contraceptives. 1981. DHEW publication no. 74–562. Washington, DC.
20. Hannaford PC, Villard-Mackintosh LP, Vessey MP, Kay CR. Oral contraceptives and malignant melanoma. Br J Cancer 1991;63:430–3.
21. Bain C, Hennekin SC, Speizer FE, Rosner B, Willett W, Belanger W. Oral contraceptive use and malignant melanoma. J Natl Cancer Inst 1982;68:537–9.
22. Helmrich SP, Rosenberg L, Kaufman DW, Miller EDR, Schottenfeld D, Stolley PD, Shapiro S. Lack of an elevated risk of malignant melanoma in relation to oral contraceptive use. J Natl Cancer Inst 1984;72:617–20.
23. Holman CDJ, Armstrong BK, Heenan PJ. Cutaneous malignant melanoma in women: Exogenous sex hormones and reproductive factors. Br J Cancer 1984;50:673.
24. Gallagher RP, Elwood JM, Hill GB, Coldman AJ, Threlfall WJ, Spinelli JJ. Reproductive factors, oral contraceptives and risk of malignant melanoma. Western Canada melanoma study. Br J Cancer 1985;52:901–7.
25. Stevens RG, Lee JA, Moolgavkar SH. No association between oral contraceptives and malignant melanomas. N Engl J Med 1980;302:966.
26. Adam SA, Sheaves JK, Wright NH, Mosse G, Harris RW, Vessey MP. A case-control study of the possible association between oral contraceptives and malignant melanoma. Br J Cancer 1981;44:45–50.
27. Rothman KF, Pochi PE. Use of oral and topical agents for acne in pregnancy. J Am Acad Dermatol 1988;19:431–42.
28. Willhite CC, Sharma RP, Allen PV, Berry DL. Percutaneous retinoid absorption and embryotoxicity. J Invest Dermatol 1990;95:523–9.
29. Seegmiller RE, Carter MW, Ford WH, White RD. Induction of maternal toxicity in the rat by dermal application of retinoic acid and its effect on fetal outcome. Reprod Toxicol 1990;4:277–81.
30. Lammer EJ, Chen DT, Hoar RM, Agnish ND, Benke PJ, Braun JT, Curry CJ, Fernhoff PM, Grix AW Jr, Lott IT. Retinoic acid embryopathy. N Engl J Med 1985;313:837–41.
31. Shalita AR, Armstrong RB, Leyden JJ, Pochi PE, Strauss JS. Isotretinoin revisited. Cutis 1988;42:1–19.

32. Lemay A, Dewailly SD, Grenier R, Huard J. Attenuation of mild hyperandrogenic activity in postpubertal acne by a triphasic oral contraceptive containing low doses of ethynyl estradiol and d,l-norgestrel. J Clin Endocrinol Metab 1990;71:8–14.
33. Palatsi R, Hirvensalo E, Liukko P, Malmiharju T, Mattila L. Serum total and unbound testosterone and sex hormone binding globulin (SHBG) in female acne patients treated with two different oral contraceptives. Acta Dermatol Venereol Scand 1984;64:517–23.
34. de-Groot AC, Eshuis H, Stricker BH. Inefficacy of oral contraception during use of minocycline. Ned Tijdschr Geneeskd 1990;134:1227–9.
35. Murphy AA, Zacur HA, Charache P, Burkman RT. The effect of tetracycline on levels of oral contraceptives. Am J Obstet Gynecol 1991;164:28–33.
36. Neely JL, Abate M, Swinker M, D'Angio R. The effect of doxycycline of serum levels of ethinyl estradiol, norethindrone, and endogenous progesterone. Obstet Gynecol 1991;77:416–20.
37. Roberts MET, Wright V, Hill AGS, Mehra AC. Psoriatic arthritis. Follow up study. Ann Rheum Dis 1976;35:206–12.
38. Dunna SF, Finlay AY. Psoriasis: Improvement during and worsening after pregnancy. Br J Dermatol 1989;120:584.
39. Zachariae H. Methotrexate side-effects. Br J Dermatol 1990;122:127–33.
40. Stern RS, Lange R. Outcomes of pregnancies among women and partners of men with a history of exposure to methoxsalen photochemotherapy (PUVA) for the treatment of psoriasis. Arch Dermatol 1991;127:347–50.
41. Murphy FR, Stolman LP. Generalized pustular psoriasis. Arch Dermatol 1979;115:1215–6.
42. Shelley WB. Generalized pustular psoriasis induced by potassium iodide. JAMA 1967;201:1009–14.
43. Van Cutsem E, Rutgeerts P, Geboes K, Van Gompel F, Vantrappen G. Estrogen-progesterone treatment of Osler Weber Rendu disease. J Clin Gastroenterol 1988;10:676–9.
44. Vase P. Estrogen treatment of hereditary hemorrhagic telangiectasia. Acta Med Scand 1981;209:393–6.
45. Bronner MH, Pate MB, Cunningham JT, Marsh WH. Estrogen-progesterone therapy for bleeding gastrointestinal telangiectasias in chronic renal failure. Ann Intern Med 1986;105:371–4.

5

Disabled Individuals

Individuals with physical disabilities make up a highly heterogeneous group. Many of the problems in individuals with disabilities remove the person from social interactions, causing feelings of inadequacy and lack of attractiveness.[1] The disabled individual may also avoid sexual contact for fear of humiliation, resulting in further loneliness and social isolation. Cromer et al. compared a group of adolescents with myelomeningocele to controls.[2] In the control group, 60% had been sexually active and 100% planned on having a sexual relationship at some time. In the myelomeningocele group, only 28% had previous sexual intercourse and 73% planned on ever having a sexual relationship. In fact, only 60% of the parents thought their adolescent would ever be in a sexual relationship. However, each individual reacts differently to these stresses and would need to be responded to on his or her own terms.

Gynecological concerns are often a neglected area in women with physical disabilities. Beckmann et al. surveyed 55 women with acquired and congenital disabilities, 42% of whom became disabled after menarche.[3] Only 18.8% had been given sexuality counseling and 64%, information about contraception. While 55.5% indicated an interest in discussing their feelings about sexuality, only 25.5% had a sexual history taken after their disability. In particular, women with paralysis, impaired motor function, or obvious physical deformity were rarely given information about contraceptive methods. In Cromer's study of adolescents with myelomeningocele, only 23% of the teens had ever talked with a physician about sexual function[2] and despite the fact that 76% wanted children, only 24% had talked with a physician about the chances of spina bifida in their children. In addition, as compared to the 60% using any birth control in the control group, only 16% of the sexually active teens with myelomeningocele used any birth control.

The following items have been suggested to be included in a sexual history in disabled individuals[4]:

1. Information regarding the level of knowledge in the area of normal body anatomy and physiological function
2. Predisability experiences and perceptions about sexuality and sexual behaviors
3. Sexual preferences
4. The type of disability and its effects on motor and sensory function, cognition, fertility, and possible related conditions such as pain and bowel and bladder dysfunctions
5. Past medical history including other illnesses and surgery
6. Medications
7. Presence or absence and numbers of sexual partners
8. Other psychosocial factors that may enhance or interfere with sexual relations

Fertility

Fertility in women with disabilities is often unimpaired while fertility in males may or may not be affected, depending on the type of disability. In particular, male fertility depends on the ability to ejaculate in a predictable fashion.

Spinal cord injuries are a frequent cause of permanent disabilities in the reproductive age group. Menses has been reported to stop for several months following a spinal cord injury even if ovulation does occur.[4] Most of these women will resume menstruation by 6 months following their injury, regardless of the level of injury.[5] Fertility in these women as well as fetal development in their offspring appears unaltered, regardless of the presence of paraplegia or quadriplegia.[6]

In males with spinal cord injury, the effects depend on both the level of the lesion and whether the lesion is partial or complete. With upper motor neuron lesions above S2–4, reflex erections can occur.[1] However, if the upper motor neuron lesion is complete, psychogenically induced erections are not possible. Males with lower motor neuron lesions below or at the sacral segments cannot have reflex erections. However, psychogenic erections might be possible. If reflex erections are not of sufficient quality or duration for intercourse, alternatives include either injections with papaverine hydrochloride with or without phentolamine or a penile prosthesis.

Males with complete cord lesions above T11–12 are usually not able to ejaculate. With lower motor neuron lesions, ejaculation may be possible even without penile erections. However in these individuals, sperm quality may be decreased. Keeping the legs apart manually and having the individual wear loose clothing may help to increase sperm counts. If the problem involves retrograde ejaculation, then washing and sterilizing sperm from the bladder may be a possibility for use in artificial insemination.[4]

In women with complete upper motor neuron lesions, psychogenic stimuli will not lead to vaginal lubrication, but reflex lubrication is possible. With lower motor neuron lesions, psychogenic lubrication is possible.

Traumatic brain injury may lead to a combination of physical, cognitive, and psychological problems that can alter sexual function. Cognitive changes that can be of particular problem in these individuals include disturbances in attention and communication. Motor changes that can affect sexual function include a decrease in strength or lack of control over voluntary muscles, and a decrease in muscle tone or range of motion.

The sexual potential of individuals with myelomeningocele can be classified similar to those with spinal cord injury.[7] The presence of reflex activity of the external sphincter of the rectum suggests an upper motor neuron problem versus a lower motor neuron problem. Most of these individuals will have the ability for lower motor neuron sexual function. Women will generally be able to have sexual intercourse, whereas males with myelomeningocele may have problems with erection, ejaculation, and sterility. However, Comarr found that most of these individuals have had satisfactory sexual function with their partners.[7]

Pregnancy

Although larger numbers of physically disabled women are choosing to become pregnant, many of their needs are often neglected.[8] In a study of information given to expectant parents by the Nurses Association of the American College of Obstetricians and Gynecologists, special problems for the handicapped parent were ranked last among 94 topics.[9] Eighty-one percent of nurses, occupational therapists, and physical therapists surveyed felt that their training was inadequate to help disabled women with special postpartum needs.[10] In a study of disabled women both before or during pregnancy, Carty et al. found that the women had the following suggestions for improving education to disabled women considering childbirth[8]:

1. Provide health care and educational courses in accessible surroundings such as places without stairs.
2. Discuss pregnancy and family planning options without being judgmental or negative.
3. Develop and distribute to local libraries printed educational material on how to cope with pregnancy if disabled.
4. Discuss sexuality-related topics without being asked.

5. Include the partner in counseling and medical sessions.
6. Teach local health professionals to be able to answer questions of the disabled person regarding sexuality, pregnancy, and family planning. These women may have many questions regarding the effect of their disability on pregnancy and birth, the effect of medications on fetal development, the location of resources to help them through a pregnancy, and family planning options to help time their family.

The effect of pregnancy on a physical disability obviously depends greatly on the extent and type of disability. While many of these individuals can go through a pregnancy without significant problems, some women with spinal cord injuries may have exacerbations of skin problems, bladder and bowel function, and autonomic hyperreflexia during pregnancy. Autonomic hyperreflexia involves sudden sympathetic discharge at a level below the level of paralysis, and can be life-threatening. The individual may experience sudden hypertension, sweating, skin blotching, anxiety, and intense headache. These women are also at increased risk for anemia, deep venous thrombosis, and pulmonary complications. In addition, these women, who are already more susceptible to urinary tract infection because of intermittent catheterization or indwelling catheter, may be at greater risk due to the effect of progesterone on the ureters. Because existing orthostatic edema may be worsened by pregnancy, to prevent skin breakdown, more frequent position changing and additional padding for the wheelchair may be needed.[8] Women with spinal cord injuries can undergo vaginal delivery but labor may be sudden because of their inability to feel contractions.[11] Epidural anesthesia is indicated at times to prevent autonomic hyperreflexia.

Pregnancy and motherhood in these women may require special training and specially designed equipment and furniture for infant care. However, women with disabilities have the ability and right to become pregnant and have children, and their disability does not have to interfere with their ability to parent.[8]

Contraception

Family planning must be tailored to the individual's particular disability. Barrier methods, including condoms and spermicidal foams and jellies, can be used without deleterious side effects on physical disabilities. However, they require manual dexterity of at least one partner. This may or may not be a problem for the individuals involved. Likewise a diaphragm, sponge, or cervical cap would also require manual dexterity of at least one partner for both insertion and removal. In addition, a lack of vaginal muscle tone could possibly affect the position and retention of the diaphragm during its use. The two major considerations with the use of combination oral contraceptives would be the ability to physically take the pill and the possibility of increased risk of thromboembolic complications in a woman who has decreased mobility and use of her lower extremities. Combination oral contraceptives should be used only with caution in women in wheelchairs or with decreased mobility. In this regard, depomedroxyprogesterone acetate (DMPA) and the Norplant implant might be good possibilities as neither requires any manual dexterity and without any estrogen, neither is associated with a significant risk of thromboembolism. At present, there are no reports on the use of DMPA or Norplant in physically disabled women. DMPA has the advantage of being associated with amenorrhea in many women, which may be helpful in some physically disabled women. In distinction from DMPA, the Norplant may be associated with frequent spotting, presenting more of a hygienic challenge to the disabled women.

The intrauterine device has the advantages of high effectiveness and no need for frequent manual dexterity. However, someone would have to be able to check on the string at frequent intervals. In addition, in the woman with decreased pelvic sensation, there is the potential risk of the individual not being able to feel pain that would alert her to early symptoms of a pelvic infection. Permanent methods of sterilization could be considered for either partner if their planned family is complete or a child is not desired. Additional references regarding sexuality and the disabled are listed in the bibliography.

References

1. Glass DD, Padrone FJ. Sexual adjustment in the handicapped. J Rehabil 1978;44:43–7.
2. Cromer BA, Enrile B, McCoy K, Gerhardstein MJ, Fitzpatrick M, Judis J. Knowledge, attitudes and behavior related to sexuality in adolescents with chronic disability. Dev Med Child Neurol 1990;32:602–10.
3. Beckmann CR, Gittler M, Barzansky BM, Beckmann CA. Gynecologic health care of women with disabilities. Obstet Gynecol 1989;74:75–9.
4. Rieve JE. Sexuality and the adult with acquired physical disability. Nurse Clin North Am 1989;24:265–76.
5. Comarr AE. Observations on menstruation and pregnancy among female spinal cord injury patients. Paraplegia 1966;3:263–72.
6. Goller H, Paeslack V. Our experiences about pregnancy and delivery of the paraplegic woman. Paraplegia 1970;8:161–6.
7. Comarr AE. Neurological disturbance of sexual function among patients with myelodysplasia. In McLauren RL, ed. Myelomeningocele. New York, Grune & Stratton, 1976, pp 797–836.
8. Carty EM, Conine TA, Hall L. Comprehensive health promotion for the pregnant woman who is disabled: The role of the midwife. J Nurse Midwifery 1990;35:133–42.
9. Sasmor JL, Grossman E. Child-birth education in 1980. J Obstet Gynecol Neonatal Nurs 1981;10:155–60.
10. Conine TA, Christie GM, Hammond GK, Smith-Minton MF. Sexual rehabilitation of the handicapped: The roles and attitudes of health professionals. J Allied Health 1980;9:260–7.
11. Fox MW, Harms RW, Davis DH. Selected neurologic complications of pregnancy. Mayo Clin Proc 1990;65:1595–618.

Bibliography

An Easy Guide to Loving Carefully (for disabled individuals). Contra Costa, CA, Planned Parenthood, 1980.

Barret M, Case N. Sexuality and the Disabled. Toronto, Sex Information and Education Council of Canada, 1976.

Cass AS, Bloom BA, Luxenberg M. Sexual function in adults with myelomeningocele. J Urol 1986;136:425–6.

Chipouras S, Cornelius D, Daniels S, Makas E. Who Cares? A Handbook on Sex Education and Counseling Services for Disabled People. Washington, DC, Sex and Disability Project, 1979.

Eisenberg M. Sex and the Handicapped: A Selected Bibliography. Cleveland, Veterans Administration Hospital, 1975.

Mooney T, Cole T, Chilgren RA. Sexual Options for Paraplegics and Quadriplegics. New York, Little, Brown, 1975.

Planned Parenthood Federation of America, 810 Seventh Ave, New York, NY 10019. Bibliography entitled "Sexuality and the Disabled."

Walborehl GS. Sexuality in the handicapped. Am Fam Physician 1987;36:129–33.

6

Psychiatric Disease

Mental Illness

Overall, about 22% of individuals in the United States will have a psychiatric disorder during their life span, with anxiety disorders occurring in 14% of the population, depression in 8 to 10%, and schizophrenia in 1 to 2%.[1] More than 400,000 women of childbearing age are treated for significant mental illness in the United States each year. In addition, the prevalence of schizophrenia rises during the childbearing years starting with adolescence. There is less long-term institutionalization of mentally ill individuals, who are consequently increasingly exposed to the risk of pregnancy outside of a closed setting.[2] Those who are institutionalized are also at risk for pregnancy from sexual contact or abuse.

Institutionalized and mentally ill ambulatory women need effective and safe contraception but often have family planning needs and gynecological problems that are ignored by psychiatric and other health care professionals. These individuals are frequently socially disorganized, unable to communicate their needs, and unable to utilize community resources effectively.[3] This often leads to lack of compliance with prescribed contraceptives and places them at high risk for an unwanted pregnancy.[4] Coverdale and Aruffo interviewed 80 women with a chronic mental disorder.[5] Of these individuals, 73% had been pregnant at least once, with 31% having had at least one abortion. Of the 75 children, 60% were being cared for by others. Thirty-three percent had not used birth control at the time of last intercourse. Between the 1930s and the 1960s, the pregnancy rates in institutions for the mentally ill rose from 2.4 to 8.8 per 1000 women.[1] However, there is little in the medical literature that addresses family planning and pregnancy issues in this group of individuals.

Effect of Pregnancy on Mental Illness

Pregnancy may exacerbate underlying mental conditions. Postpartum psychosis is most commonly found in those women with a history of psychiatric illness. Approximately 20% of women with an affective disorder will have a puerperal psychosis.[6] Depression and mania occurring during pregnancy have a better prognosis than schizophrenia occurring during pregnancy.

Effect of Mental Illness on Pregnancy

While pregnancy, childbirth, and child care possibly may be exacerbated by mental problems, the literature on this issue is minimal. Some evidence exists that children born to schizophrenic or mentally disordered parents are at increased risk for social and emotional problems.[2,4,7] McNeil reviewed the literature regarding obstetric complications in schizophrenic parents,[8] and found that almost all studies found no significant difference in the birthweight of offspring of schizophrenics versus control parents. Most studies also showed no differences in pregnancy, birth, and neonatal complications. McNeil found that the few studies that found differences between controls and schizophrenic patients usually involved unusual samples or special analysis procedures. The conclusion was that while "pregnancies and birth of schizophrenics are more mentally, behaviorally and socially complicated, ... the pregnancies and deliveries of schizophrenics do not typically appear to be notably different from those of controls on a purely somatic basis."[8] McNeil did find some inconclusive evidence that schizophrenic patients as well as other mental patients, under some circumstances, have higher rates of perinatal deaths.

There are several other potential problem areas where pregnancy may be affected by mental illness.[1] If the mental illness has a genetic component, the child is at risk to inherit the problem. As many as 4 of 10 mentally ill patients have a substance abuse problem that can complicate pregnancy.[1] The interaction between substance abuse and pregnancy is discussed in Chapter 15. Lastly, a mentally ill women who is significantly handicapped may be unable to adequately care for the child.

Contraception and Mental Illness

Contraception in the mentally ill woman is often delayed by mental health care providers who may ignore family planning needs. In addition, psychiatrically impaired women have special problems in relation to contraception methods that require informed consent such as hormonal contraception and the intrauterine device. Informed consent requires the individual to have an adequate knowledge base on which to make a decision, and there must not be any coercion in the decision-making process.[3] However, in the psychiatrically impaired, judgment and reasoning may be impaired and it is difficult to ensure that these individuals fully comprehend the risks and benefits of various contraceptives.[2] It would thus be advisable, if possible, to have specially trained individuals involved in providing contraceptive services for the mentally ill. Another difficulty in prescribing contraceptive to these individuals is assessing sexual activity. Parental fears and anxieties often become highly involved in this decision process.

Mechanical methods have no adverse effects in the psychiatrically impaired but are often difficult to use by these individuals. These methods required decision-making skills every time they are used and psychiatrically impaired individuals may not be able to use them appropriately. Thus, they should only be used in selected individuals.

Oral contraceptives have no particular adverse effects in mentally ill women with the exception of the potential to worsen depression (see below). In fact, oral contraceptives may have an advantage in the woman who is hypoestrogenic related to hypothalamic-pituitary suppression of gonadotropins from phenothiazines or tricyclic antidepressants. Some mentally ill women are on anticonvulsants. The potential interaction causing a decrease in oral contraceptive and Norplant effectiveness in women on anticonvulsants is discussed in Chapter 3. One significant problem with oral contraceptives in mentally ill women is the possibility of poor compliance. This may not be a problem in institutionalized women where medication compliance is observed. Other hormonal contraceptive alternatives for these women are depomedroxyprogesterone acetate (DMPA) and the Norplant device. The role of DMPA and the Norplant implant has yet to be adequately studied in these individuals. The potential advantages include high efficacy and no need for daily involvement of the mentally ill individual. Potential problems include consent issues, exacerbation of depression with progestin-only contraceptives, and the high degree of breakthrough bleeding with the Norplant implant.

One subgroup of psychiatrically impaired individuals that requires special comment in regards to hormonal contraceptives are those who are depressed. In these individuals there is the concern that hormonal contraceptives may exacerbate depression. Reports in the literature primarily examine oral contraceptives and are contradictory as to whether oral contraceptives can worsen existing depression or cause depression. An excellent summary of recent studies was written by Slap.[9] Of the 12 studies reviewed, 9 found an association between oral contraceptive use and depression, with reports of depression ranging from 16 to 56% of the women using oral contraceptives. However, the 2 studies demonstrating the highest prevalence of depression used neither placebo trials nor control groups. In one randomized, double-blind study there was a 10 to 15%

increase in depression among oral contraceptive users as compared with nonusers.[10]

Several theories have been suggested to explain the relationship between oral contraceptives and depression:

1. Monoamine oxidase (MAO) activity may cause a decrease in catecholamines.
2. MAO activity may cause a decrease in serotonin.
3. Hydoxyindole-o-methyltransferase (HIOMT) inhibition causes decreased melatonin.[11]
4. There may be decreased conversion of tryptophan to serotonin.

With this last theory, it is suggested that oral contraceptives either increase hepatic metabolism, leading to a larger requirement of the cofactor pyridoxine (vitamin B_6),[11] or loosen the enzymatic binding of pyridoxine, leading to a functional pyridoxine deficiency. With inadequate pyridoxine there would be inadequate serotonin, resulting in depression. Estrogen and progesterone can also alter the biosynthesis, release, uptake, degradation, and receptor density of norepinephrine, dopamine, serotonin, and acetylcholine.[12,13]

These theories were studied in depressed women using oral contraceptives in a double-blind, crossover design to evaluate response to pyridoxine and to determine whether a vitamin B_6 deficiency actually was present.[14] The comparison groups included 22 depressed pill users, 31 nondepressed pill users, and 22 nondepressed nonpill users. Lower vitamin B_6 levels were found in pill users; however, there was no difference in the levels between depressed and nondepressed pill users. The investigators were unable to identify biochemically those individuals most susceptible for depression. However, 11 (50%) of the 22 depressed pill users had an absolute vitamin B_6 deficiency. This was the only group to respond to supplemental pyridoxine. There may be certain individuals who are more susceptible to developing this complication on oral contraceptives and this is probably of greater importance than the composition of the particular pill.[15] In addition, there may be a genetic predisposition to psychiatric side effects of depression with the use of oral contraceptives.[16]

Intrauterine devices are another method having the advantage of no regular user participation. However, this must be balanced with the risk of infection. Some of these women may be involved with multiple partners, increasing the risk of pelvic inflammatory disease.

Summary

Providing contraceptive services for psychiatrically impaired women is complex. It is helpful if contraceptive services for these individuals include the involvement of specially trained practitioners who are able to obtain informed consent, while taking into account the women's specific needs and problems. Barrier methods and oral contraceptives should only be used when it can be ensured that these methods will be used consistently and correctly. DMPA, the Norplant implant, and the intrauterine device may be good alternatives in these individuals. Further resources are given in the reference section.

Mental Retardation

The psychosexual development of mentally retarded individuals usually parallels that of normal individuals although it is somewhat delayed. Most of the mildly mentally retarded have similar interests in sex as the nonmentally retarded. These individuals often have gynecological concerns that are not dealt with, as they are often not able to verbalize their problems and both practitioners and staff are often not familiar with the best approach to their problems. Their vulnerability places them at high risk for an unwanted pregnancy.[4]

Chamberlain et al. reviewed their experience with mentally retarded teens with IQs of 69 or less in the areas of sexual activity and contraception.[17] Thirty-four percent had had sexual intercourse at least once, with 16% continuing to be sexually active. Forty-three percent (6/14) of the sexually active mentally retarded teens became pregnant. In fact, since the beginning of modern contraceptive methods in the mid 1950s, the birthrate of mentally retarded women has increased compared to a decrease among other women in western cultures.[18]

Contraception and Mental Retardation

Mentally retarded individuals have similar problems as the psychiatrically impaired in the area of informed consent. Mechanical methods have no adverse effects on women who are mentally retarded except that the individual may not be capable of understanding how to use the methods. Oral contraceptives have no particular adverse effects in mentally retarded women. However, in a study of mentally retarded female adolescents, there was only a 32% 1-year continuation rate.[17] In addition, use effectiveness and parental satisfaction were lower than with DMPA and the intrauterine device. Satisfaction was the lowest with the mothers of users. There were two pregnancies among the 18 teens using this method. The necessity of requiring the individual to be able to take the pill each day, unless provided by a care taker, can be a problem.

Another alternative used in many mentally retarded individuals has been DMPA. This has been used in these individuals for both menstrual control and contraception, although not without significant controversy. While DMPA has been used in mentally retarded teens for many years, until recently the US Food and Drug Administration had not approved it for this purpose. Since DMPA is now approved for contraceptive use, using this medication in mentally retarded individuals would seem appropriate.

Chamberlain et al. accumulated 594 women-months' experience in mentally retarded female adolescents with medroxyprogesterone acetate (Depo-Provera).[17] There were no reported pregnancies.

Norplant would also appear to be a contraceptive device providing excellent effectiveness with no need for compliance on the part of the mentally retarded individual. Potential problems include informed consent, a high degree of breakthrough bleeding, and the question of whether a general anesthetic would be required to put the implant in the severely retarded individual.

Intrauterine devices also require regular user compliance. However, this must be balanced with the risk of infection. In Chamberlain's study of mentally retarded female adolescents, seven used the intrauterine device, with a very high satisfaction rate among the mothers of users.[17] There was one pregnancy and one patient with recurrent infections. In addition, one teen removed the device. Regardless of the type of contraceptive prescribed, birth control is not a substitute for education, supervision, or protection of these individuals.

Another area of controversy regarding mentally retarded individuals is the issue of sterilization. On one side, the argument is made that the right to bear children is inviolable and cannot be taken away by anyone. Others feel that individuals have the equal right not to bear children. States differ on regulations regarding sterilization of mentally retarded individuals, with some allowing review of such requests and others prohibiting the procedure. Passer et al. examined parental views on the issue of sterilization of mentally retarded adolescents and found that 85% of parents of mentally retarded children were in favor of some sort of sterilization statute.[19] Most preferred a moderate position that would permit the procedure under certain circumstances and with specific safeguards. It has been suggested that the following formal requirements be met before such a procedure be permitted[20]:

1. That there is just cause
2. That the procedure be a last resort
3. That the process protect the rights of all involved

The issues of sterilization in mentally retarded individuals are examined in-depth elsewhere.[21–25]

Phenylketonuria

Phenylketonuria (PKU) involves an autosomal recessive inborn error of metabolism in which the lack of an enzyme hinders the metabolism of phenylalanine to tyrosine. Accumulation of phenylalanine and its metabolites leads to brain damage and mental retardation. In past decades, women with PKU were usually mentally retarded and few bore children.

However, since newborn screening began in the 1960s and phenylalanine-restricted diets were introduced, most of these individuals are mentally normal.[26] Currently there are approximately 4000 women of childbearing age with PKU in the United States, of whom most are at risk for pregnancies that could result in abnormal children.[27] While 99% of the offspring will be heterozygous carriers and 1% will have the disease, at the highest risk is the fetus of an affected mother who is not on a diet. Complications of pregnancy are quite high in the offspring of those women with the common, severe form of PKU who are not treated during pregnancy. Complications include a 92% rate of mental retardation, a 73% prevalence of microcephaly, a 12% prevalence of congenital heart disease, and a 40% prevalence of low birthweight.[28]

While dietary management can prevent complications in the fetus, this must be done prior to conception and continued throughout the pregnancy. Guettler et al. demonstrated normal offsprings from 26 pregnancies in women with PKU who were treated by diet before becoming pregnant.[29] In another study in Ireland, the outcome of 48 pregnancies in 18 women with PKU was studied.[30] In the nondiet group, there were three deaths and one stillbirth among the offspring. There were five miscarriages in the nondiet group and one in the diet group. Fetal growth appears best correlated to maternal phenylalanine levels, and optimal growth is only obtained in those women with near-normal levels at the time of conception.[31] However, treatment even in the first trimester may not prevent all of the complications of maternal PKU.[32,33] Strategies for these women must include careful family planning so that their diet can be identified and altered before conception, particularly since many young women discontinue their diet during childhood[34] and only seek treatment again after pregnancy.[33,35,36]

Waisbren et al. conducted a study to examine contraceptive use among women with PKU and their reasons for seeking treatment after pregnancy rather than before pregnancy.[37] The results demonstrated that these individuals were less sexually active than a comparison group of women with diabetes or healthy women (43% versus 71% versus 66%). Nineteen percent of the PKU individuals used no method of contraception and 35% either never used or only on occasion used contraception. It was not clear from the study why these individuals were less sexually active although most planned to marry and bear children. However, of concern was the fact that a significant number were sexually active and not using contraception, which could lead to a pregnancy when appropriate preconception dietary measures were not in place. Many of the women viewed the condition as a past, not a present problem. This might explain why their use of contraception was no higher than that in other groups. The best predictors of birth control use in the women with PKU were social support in using contraception ($r = 0.64$), positive attitudes about birth control ($r = 0.66$), and knowledge of family planning ($r = 0.43$). This was different when compared to women with diabetes where locus of control was the highest predictor (r = 0.39) and for acquaintances where social support was the most important (r = 0.46). The results did not indicate that these individuals were seeking out PKU diets before a pregnancy. Most did not consider that an unplanned pregnancy could occur. As more of these individuals are reproducing, it becomes important to be able to track these individuals into their adolescence and young adult years and provide complete family planning and pregnancy counseling. There are no reports of adverse reactions with any contraceptive method particular to individuals with PKU.

References

1. Hankoff LD, Darney PD. Contraceptive choices for behaviorally disordered individuals. Am J Obstet Gynecol 1993;168:1986–9.
2. Abernethy VD, Grunebausm H. Toward a family planning program in psychiatric hospitals. Am J Public Health 1972;62:1638–46.
3. Grunebaum H, Abernethy VD. Ethical issues in family planning for hospitalized psychiatric patients. Am J Psychiatry 1975;5:94–9.
4. Abernethy VD, Grunebaum H. Family planning in two psychiatric hospitals: A preliminary report. Fam Plann Perspect 1973;5:94–9.
5. Coverdale JH, Aruffo JA. Family planning needs of female chronic psychiatric outpatients. Am J Psychiatry 1989;146:1489–1.
6. Gitlin MJ, Pasnau RO. Psychiatric syndromes linked to reproductive function in women: A review of current knowledge. Am J Psychiatry 1989;146:1413–22.
7. Mednick SA. A longitudinal study of children with a high risk for schizophrenia. Ment Hyg 1966;50:522–32.
8. McNeil TF. Obstetric complications in schizophrenic parents. Schizophr Res 1991;5:89–101.
9. Slap GB. Oral contraceptives and depression. Impact, prevalence, and cause. J Adolesc Health Car, 1981;2:53–64.
10. Cullberg J. Mood changes and menstrual symptoms with different gestagen/estrogen combinations. Acta Psychiatr Scand Suppl 1972;236:1–86
11. Adams PW, Wynn V, Seed M, Folkard J. Vitamin B6, depression, and oral contraception. Lancet 1974;2:516–7.
12. McEwen BS, Parsons B. Gonadal steroid action on the brain: Neurochemistry and neuropharmacology. Annu Rev Pharmacol Toxicol 1982;22:555–98.
13. Oppenheim G. Estrogen in the treatment of depression: Neuropharmacological mechanisms. Biol Psychiatry 1983;18:721–5.
14. Adams PW, Rose DP, Folkard J, Wynn V, Seed M, Strong R. Effect of pyridoxine hydrochloride (vitamin B6) upon depression associated with oral contraception. Lancet 1973;1:897–904.
15. Winston F. Oral contraceptives, pyridoxine, and depression. Am J Psychiatry 1973;130:1217–21.
16. Kendler KS, Martin NG, Heath AC, Handelsman D, Eaves LJ. A twin study of the psychiatric side effects of oral contraceptives. J Nerv Ment Dis 1988;176:153–60.
17. Chamberlain A, Rauh J, Passer A, McGrath M, Burket R. Issues in fertility control for mentally retarded female adolescents. I. Sexual abuse and contraception. Pediatrics 1984;73:445–50.
18. David HP, Morgall JM. Family planning for the mentally disordered and retarded. J Nerv Ment Dis 1990;178:385–91.
19. Passer A, Rauh J, Chamberlain A, McGrath M, Burket R. Issues in fertility control for mentally retarded female adolescents: II. Parental attitudes toward sterilization. Pediatrics 1984;73:451–4.
20. Walters L. Sterilizing the retarded child. Hastings Cent Rep 1976;6:13–5.
21. Bernstein AH. Sterilization of incompetents. The quest for legal authority. Hospitals 1982;56:13–5.

22. Perrin JC, Sands CR, Tinker DS, Dominguez BC, Dingle JT, Thomas MJ. A considered approach to sterilization of mentally retarded youth. Am J Dis Child 1976;130:288–90.
23. Robinson FC, Robinson SW, Williams LJ. Eugenic sterilization: Medico-legal and sociologic aspects. J Natl Med Assoc 1979;71:593–8.
24. Wheeless CR. Abdominal hysterectomy for surgical sterilization of the mentally retarded. A review of parental opinion. Am J Obstet Gynecol 1975;122:872–5.
25. Whitcraft CJ, Jones JP. A survey of attitudes about sterilization of retardates. Ment Retard 1974;12:30–3.
26. Scriver CR, Clow CL. Phenylketonuria: Epitome of human biochemical genetics. N Engl J Med 1980;303:1336–42.
27. Waisbren SE, Doherty LB, Bailey IV, Rohr FJ, Levy HL. The New England maternal PKU project: Identification of at-risk women. Am J Public Health 1988;78:789–92.
28. Lenke RR, Levy HL. Maternal phenylketonuria and hyperphenylalaninemia: An international survey of the outcome of untreated and treated pregnancies. N Engl J Med 1980;303:1202–8.
29. Guettler F, Lou H, Andresen J, Kok K, Mikkelsen I, Nielsen KB, Nielsen JB. Cognitive development in offspring of untreated and preconceptionally treated maternal phenylketonuria. J Inherit Metab Dis 1990:13:665–71.
30. Naughten E, Saul IP. Maternal phenylketonuria—The Irish experience. J Inherit Metab Dis 1990;13:658–64.
31. Smith I, Glossop J, Beasley M. Fetal damage due to maternal phenylketonuria: Effects of dietary treatment and maternal phenylalanine concentrations around the time of conception. J Inherit Metab Dis 1990;13:651–7.
32. Lenke RR, Levy HL. Maternal phenylketonuria: Results of dietary therapy. Am J Obstet Gynecol 1982;142:548–53.
33. Drogari E, Smith I, Beasley M, Lloyd JK. Timing of strict diet in relation to fetal damage in maternal phenylketonuria. Lancet 1987;2:927–30.
34. Schuett VE, Brown ES. Diet policies of PKU clinics in the United States. Am J Public Health 1984;74:501–3.
35. Rohr FJ, Doherty LB, Waisbren SE, Bailey IV, Ampola MG, Benacerraf B, Levy HL. New England Maternal PKU Project: Prospective study of untreated pregnancies and their outcomes. J Pediatr 1987;110:391–8.
36. Hanley WB, Clarke JTR, Schoonheyt W. Maternal phenylketonuria (PKU)—A review. Clin Biochem 1987;20:149–56.
37. Waisbren SE, Shiloh S, St. James P, Levy HL. Psychosocial factors in maternal phenylketonuria: Prevention of unplanned pregnancies. Am J Public Health 1991;81:299–304.

Bibliography

A Resource Guide in Sex Education for the Mentally Retarded. New York, AAHPER Publications, 1971.
David HP, Smith MA, Freedman E. Family planning services for person handicapped by mental retardation. Am J Public Health 1976;66:1053–7.
Edwards J, Wapnick S. Being Me: A Social/Sexual Training Guide for Those Who Work with the Developmentally Disabled. Portland, OR, Ednick Communications, 1981.
Hammer SL, Wright LS, Jasen DL. Sex education for the retarded adolescent. A survey of parental attitudes and methods of management in fifty adolescent retardates. Clin Pediatr 1967;6:621–7.
Haavik SF, Menninger KA. Sexuality, Law and the Developmentally Disabled: Legal and Clinical Aspects of Marriage, Parenthood and Sterilization. Baltimore, MD, Paul H. Brookes, 1981.
Hein K, Coupey SM, Cohen MI. Special considerations in pregnancy prevention for the mentally subnormal adolescent female. J Adolesc Health Care 1980;1:46–9.
Kempton W, Foreman R. Guidelines for Training in Sexuality and the Mentally Handicapped. 2nd ed. Philadelphia, Planned Parenthood of Southeastern Pennsylvania, 1976.
Kempton W. Love, Sex and Birth Control for Mentally Handicapped People (A Guide for Parents). Publication no. 1272. New York, Planned Parenthood Federation, 1985.
Schultz JB, Adams DU. Family life education needs of mentally disabled adolescents. Adolescence 1987;22:221–30.
Simons JF. Sexual behaviors in retarded children and adolescents. JDBP 1980;1:173–9.

7

Renal Disease

Chronic renal disease and renal failure may occur secondary to many different underlying diseases. Obviously the underlying disease process itself may interact with pregnancy in other ways than just those secondary to kidney disease. This section focuses primarily on the profound effects that pregnancy and the kidney disease may have on each other, particularly in women with chronic renal failure, women on dialysis, and women who have had a renal transplantation.

Fertility

Most women who have chronic renal failure and are on hemodialysis are either hypomenorrheic or amenorrheic and infertile secondary to hypothalamic-pituitary dysfunction.[1-13] However, because of anovulatory cycles and qualitative platelet abnormalities, some of these women also have episodes of abnormal uterine bleeding. Hypomenorrhea or amenorrhea is more likely to occur if the creatinine concentration is above 3 mg/dL and the blood urea nitrogen (BUN) is greater than 30 to 40 mg/dL.[2,4] As the parenchymal disease increases, fertility decreases.[2-5,14,15] On dialysis, some women have a return of menstrual function, with some women having ovulatory cycles.[3,16] In one study, 40% of investigated cycles in five uremic women on hemodialysis were ovulatory although the hormonal patterns were atypical.[9] In another study of women on hemodialysis, two of four were anovulatory and two of four had ovulatory cycles but with a luteal phase deficiency.[11] Despite some ovulatory cycles, conception is not common in women on long-term hemodialysis, with an incidence of about 1 per 200 patients.[1] The true incidence is not known since many of these pregnancies probably end in an early spontaneous abortion.[17] There is also a large number of therapeutic abortions, suggesting that some of these women become pregnant not realizing that it is possible. However, some individuals on dialysis and most women after renal transplantation have their fertility restored, with numerous pregnancies reported.[1,5,18–21]

In those women who undergo renal transplantation, ovulation and menstruation usually return within 6 months of a successful transplantation.[21] More than 2000 pregnancies have been recorded in women with renal transplants.[22–24] It is estimated that about 1 of 50 women of reproductive age with a functioning graft will become pregnant each year.[22] Slavis et al. reported on six pregnant women who had a prior renal transplant.[25] All of these women had regular cycles while only one had menses before the transplantation. Two of the women had a total of five pregnancies and children after transplantation. One woman did not want any further children and three had had families and underwent either tubal ligation or hysterectomy.

Renal disease can also affect testicular function. Dialysis can be associated with a reduction in testosterone production and defective spermatogenesis.[8] A decrease in libido and impotence are also common. Many factors may be involved in uremic impotence including a neuropathy, vascular insufficiency, medication side effects, nutritional deficiencies, and stress. Lim also suggested that there may be a hypothalamic disorder involving luteinizing hormone–releasing hormone (LH-RH) secretion leading to hypogonadism.[8] Slavis et al. reported on seven males who had had a renal transplantation.[25] All seven males reported having an excellent libido after transplantation and were sexually active. Three have fathered children, while two had not wanted any children and two tried unsuccessfully following the transplantation.

Effect of Pregnancy on Renal Disease

Pregnancy involves several physiological changes that place women with renal disease at additional risk. Renal blood flow is increased as a result of increased cardiac output and decreased renal vascular resistance.[18,26] In addition, the glomerular filtration rate (GFR) increases by 50% from an average of 96 mL/min to 146 mL/min during pregnancy, and the creatinine clearance rate increases from an average of 70 to 125 mL/min before pregnancy to about 175 mL/min in the third trimester.[18] Changes also occur in the anatomy of the urinary tract. The capacity of the bladder increases and the bladder becomes an abdominal organ.[18] The kidneys increase in size by about 1.0 to 1.5 cm. The collecting system also undergoes changes including dilatation of the renal calices, pelves, and ureters. These changes begin in the first trimester but are most marked in the third trimester and continue until 12 weeks postpartum.[23] The peristaltic activity of the ureters declines under the influence of progesterone and prostaglandin E_2,[18] and also as a result of mechanical obstruction caused by the enlarging uterus.

Effect of Pregnancy on Chronic Renal Disease

The effect of pregnancy on chronic renal disease is somewhat controversial. Cunningham et al. reviewed the course over an 18-year period of 37 pregnant women with moderate or severe renal insufficiency.[19] Six (16%) of the 37 had worsening of their renal disease but it was not clear that this was related to their pregnancy. Common maternal complications included preeclampsia, anemia, and chronic hypertension. There were also another 6 women who had stable renal function during pregnancy which deteriorated later on. Individuals with only moderate renal insufficiency had a normal blood volume expansion, whereas in those with severe renal insufficiency this was significantly decreased. In prior studies, worsening of renal function with pregnancy occurred in 8 to 50% of women.[19,27] In one study, over 50% of women with underlying proteinuria had a worsening during pregnancy and hypertension developed or worsened in 25 to 75% of these women.[28] Overall, if renal function is mild with a creatinine concentration less than 1.4 to 1.5 mg/dL, pregnancy tends to have little adverse effect on renal function. However, with more severe renal dysfunction, pregnancy can accelerate the renal damage.[22] In general, women with chronic renal disease have most of their adverse reactions either if hypertension is poorly controlled or if lupus nephritis is present. If the function of either kidney markedly deteriorates or blood pressure becomes uncontrollable, a therapeutic abortion or early delivery should be contemplated.[2]

The reason for possible advancement of renal damage with pregnancy is unknown but may be related to the hyperfiltration associated normally with pregnancy.[22] Baylis and Wilson examined the effect of pregnancy on underlying renal disease in rats.[26] Their presumption was that the chronic vasodilation of pregnancy might prove damaging to glomeruli, especially if there was an underlying renal disease. Their study of female rats failed to confirm such a hypothesis.

Effect of Pregnancy on Hemodialysis Patients

While conception is not common in women on long-term hemodialysis, it does occur. Women on hemodialysis and chronic peritoneal dialysis who become pregnant are at risk of volume overload and severe exacerbations of hypertension with superimposed preeclampsia.[1] However, a few successful pregnancies have been reported both with hemodialysis and with chronic ambulatory peritoneal dialysis (CAPD).[17,29–31] Close attention must be paid to controlling anemia, fluid balance, and blood pressure. Considerations include increasing the frequency of dialysis, minimizing heparin doses, and switching to a high-calcium/bicarbonate bath.[29] Another occasional problem reported with pregnancy is a clotted access site.[1] Redrow et al. recommended that if dialysis is attempted in a pregnant women, CAPD is the preferred method.[29]

Effect of Pregnancy on Renal Transplant Patients

Renal transplantation has now been performed for over two decades, with almost 10,000 transplantations performed a year.[25] With longer survival of renal transplant recipients, more and more pregnancies are occurring, with over 2000 pregnancies reported.[1] There have not been any well-matched prospective studies examining the effects of pregnancy on transplant recipients. In addition, most of the reported pregnancies in renal transplant recipients occurred in women on prednisone and azathioprine, while most women are currently on cyclosporine as part of their posttransplantation medication. However, in general, these women do not have significant problems with their renal disease if their underlying renal function is good and their blood pressure is controlled.[18] Complications may include hypertension, proteinuria, infections from immunosuppression, and deterioration of graft function from either obstruction of the ureter, rejection, or a recurrence of an underlying renal disease.[32]

Hypertension is a frequent problem in pregnant women with renal transplants. In one series, preeclampsia occurred in 30% of renal transplant recipients.[33] It may be difficult to differentiate preeclampsia from the usual problems of renal disease including hypertension, edema, and proteinuria.

Rudolf et al. surveyed 440 pregnancies in women who had a renal transplant, and reported a rejection rate of 9%.[33] It was not clear whether these rejections were due to the pregnancy or would have occurred regardless. Whetham et al. reported on a small number of women who had received cadaveric transplants and became pregnant, and compared them to women who were not pregnant.[34] In this study two of the five patients who became pregnant lost their grafts 7.7 and 18 months postpartum while 2 of 10 women in the comparison group lost their grafts. There was no statistical difference, but the number of subjects was small.

In women with a renal transplant, a 30% reduction in GFR is normal during the third trimester and without any other suggestions of a problem, need not be extensively evaluated. However, if the GFR reduction occurs in the first two trimesters or is greater than 30% in the third trimester, a careful evaluation is recommended to examine for problems including change in volume status, nephrotoxins, renal obstruction, and renal infections. It may be particularly difficult to distinguish between acute rejection, cyclosporine toxicity, preeclampsia, and the progression of underlying renal disease during pregnancy. The diagnosis of rejection cannot be made with certainty without a renal biopsy.

Effects of Renal Disease on Pregnancy

Renal dysfunction, even mild degrees, can affect pregnancy. Ferris found that while the rate of fetal loss was 1.2% in women without renal disease, it was 4.1% in those with renal disease with a creatinine concentration of less than 1.5 mg/dL.[28] The effects of various degrees of chronic renal insufficiency on pregnancy (moderate: creatinine level of 1.4–2.5 mg/dL; severe: level > 2.5 mg/dL) were evaluated in another study.[19] The perinatal complications studied included midpregnancy losses, low birthweight, and fetal growth retardation. In the 26 women with moderate disease, 85% had a live-born infant. There was one stillbirth and no neonatal deaths. Of the 11 women with severe renal insufficiency, seven had live-born infants after 26 weeks' gestation. Fetal growth retardation and preterm delivery were associated more with chronic hypertension than with severe renal insufficiency. However, birthweight correlated well with creatinine concentration. Abe et al. found a correlation of pregnancy outcome to both blood pressure and renal function.[27] The percentage of women with normal deliveries was 77% for those with a blood pressure less than 140/90 mm Hg and 50% for those with a blood pressure above 140/90 mm Hg. Normal deliveries occurred in 76% of women with a GFR higher than 70 mL/min and only 36% with a GFR below 70 mL/min. In the group with impaired renal function, only 50% had pregnancies that resulted in live births. In another study, a 17% prematurity rate and 20% rate of spontaneous or therapeutic abortion were found compared with 8% and 12% in the normal population.[32] These rates rose to 64% for women with preexisting hypertension and 70% for those with preexisting renal impairment.

Effect of Dialysis on Pregnancy

There is a high prevalence of complications including spontaneous abortion and stillbirths associated with a pregnancy while a women is on hemodialysis, even though normal outcomes have been reported.[1,3,5,20,30,35–38] There is a high number of fetal losses during all stages of pregnancy, with a live birthrate of only 19%.[1] These women are prone to volume overload, hypertension, and superimposed preeclampsia and so close attention must be paid to their fluid balance, dialysis, and blood pressure control. Dialysis strategies for these women are found in reviews by Davison[1] and by Hou.[17] Most authorities do not advise attempts at pregnancy or its continuation in women on hemodialysis. A few successful pregnancies in women on CAPD have also been reported.[17,29,30] Most of these pregnancies have been associated with premature labor and hypertension.

Effect of Renal Transplants on Pregnancy

Gaudier et al. surveyed 2309 pregnancies in 1594 women with a renal transplant.[24] Forty percent ended in a spontaneous or therapeutic abortion in the first trimester. However, over 90% of those pregnancies going beyond the first trimester ended successfully. In a more negative report, O'Connell et al. evaluated the problem of prematurity in these pregnancies.[32] In this study of 15 pregnancies in eight renal transplant recipients, only 1 of 10 (including one set of twins) live births reached 38 weeks' gestation and 4 (40%) were small for gestational age. There were five intrauterine deaths and one spontaneous abortion. One of the infants died early from an intraventricular hemorrhage and hyaline membrane disease and another had hydrocephalus. In this small study, no pregnancy was uncomplicated and only 53% ended with a live healthy baby. Factors in O'Connell's study that related to poor fetal outcome included deterioration in graft function, preexisting hypertension, and development of hypertension before the third trimester. In comparison, the survey by Rudolf et al. of 440 pregnancies revealed a 20% prevalence of prematurity and a 44% rate of low birthweight.[33] In the largest single series of 56 pregnancies in 37 women, Penn and Makowski reported a 45% rate of premature delivery and a 14% prevalence of low birthweight.[39] O'Connell's results suggest more problems than these other two studies, which may relate to the fact that the women in O'Connell's study had multiple pregnancies and few women electively terminated their pregnancy. Hou reviewed data from six studies of transplant recipients and found that the prevalence of fetal losses from spontaneous abortion or stillbirths ranged from 0 to 26.3%.[22] Overall, transplant recipients with excellent renal function and normal blood pressure are probably at low risk of maternal and fetal morbidity.[40]

All women with a renal transplant should be counseled about the potential complications both in the mother and in the fetus. Those women with lower renal function or hypertension are more likely to encounter problems. Overall, about 49% of these women will have problems during pregnancy, 92% will have a successful obstetric outcome, but 12% will have long-term problems. Those women who have had a transplantation are advised to wait approximately 2 years after the transplantation to ensure that graft function is well stabilized and that immunosuppressive therapy is at maintenance levels. Davison listed guidelines for women with a renal transplant considering a pregnancy[1,23]:

- Good general health for about 2 years after transplantation
- Stature compatible with good obstetric outcome

- No or minimal proteinuria
- No hypertension
- No evidence of graft rejection
- No pelvicalyceal distension on a recent intravenous urogram
- Stable renal function with plasma creatinine concentration of 180 μmol/L (2.0 mg/dL) or less, preferably less than 130 μmol/L (1.5 mg/dL)
- Drug therapy reduced to maintenance levels (prednisone, 15 mg/day or less, and azathioprine, 2 mg/kg of body weight/day or less)

While limited experience precluded Davison from recommending a safe dose of cyclosporine, anecdotally 5 mg/kg/day is listed.

One other consideration for women with renal failure is that with either dialysis or renal transplantation, there is a considerable shortening of maternal life span. This may play a role in family planning when considering who will be available to care for the child.

Renal Medications and Pregnancy

Another risk to the infant in mothers with renal disease involves the possible effects on the pregnancy and fetus of multiple medications, including antihypertensives, diuretics, and immunosuppressive therapy. Diuretics could be used if necessary. Thiazide diuretics have not been reported to cause congenital malformations.[41] Thiazide diuretics have been reported to cause neonatal hemolysis and thrombocytopenia while furosemide can cause hyponatremia.[42] There is no evidence that methyldopa, hydralazine, or beta-blockers cause congenital malformations. Beta-blockers have been associated with neonatal respiratory depression, bradycardia, hypoglycemia, and rarely, intrauterine growth retardation.[41] Angiotensin-converting enzyme inhibitors have become popular antihypertensive medications for nonpregnant women. However, seven cases of neonatal renal failure have been reported in women with exposure to these medications that continued to the time of delivery.[43] Two of the newborns died. It is recommended to avoid angiotensin-converting enzyme inhibitors in the third trimester.

Perhaps of most concern is the possible effects of immunosuppressive therapy used in renal transplant patients. Overall, the incidence of congenital anomalies appears to be small but reports have been made of congenital abnormalities in women using prednisone and azathioprine.[32,39] More women are now exposed to cyclosporine but this drug has been used for a shorter period of time. Early reports seem encouraging, with cyclosporine seemingly no worse than azathioprine. However, few reports are available and most of these are usually limited to case reports.[32,40,44] Sandoz Pharmaceuticals collected information on 51 pregnancies in 48 women treated with cyclosporine through 1988.[17] There were 43 live births, one spontaneous abortion, one missed abortion, and six therapeutic abortions. There were congenital anomalies in two live-born infants and one aborted fetus. As cyclosporine is nephrotoxic, it could potentially lead to higher fetal morbidity and mortality. Further studies will be helpful in this regards. Unpublished reports from Sandoz indicate potential complications of jaundice, thrombocytopenia, leukopenia, hypoglycemia, and cataracts.[40] The drug has not been found to be teratogenic in animal studies.

Another potential risk of immunosuppressive therapy is infection in the newborn. Exposed neonates have been reported to be more prone to serious infections in the first 8 days of life.[32,39] Azathioprine can cross the placenta and correlations have been reported between maternal and fetal cord blood leukocyte count.[32,45] Women with a renal transplant are at risk for cytomegalovirus, herpes hominis virus, and infectious hepatitis, all of which can be transmitted to the infant. The risks of maternal immunosuppression in the infant, however, are limited to case reports and the long-term complications are unknown. Animal studies evaluating the effects of mercaptopurine in offspring have demonstrated reproductive defects when the offspring mature.[46]

Contraception and Renal Disease

Because the possible significant impact of pregnancy in women with renal disease and on the course of their illness, adequate and safe contraception becomes a very important consideration. While these women might assume they are infertile, in fact, this may not be the case—those women with a transplant have a significant chance of becoming pregnant. Contraception is also important so that women with a transplant can delay a potential pregnancy for 1 to 2 years after transplantation. Unfortunately, no studies that directly address the risks and prevalence of different contraceptive agents in these women have been performed.

There are some reports on the use of hormonal contraceptives in controlling hypermenorrhea, a problem in some women with chronic renal disease or on dialysis. In one report of a woman on hemodialysis, oral contraceptives were found to be helpful in controlling hypermenorrhea without an adverse outcome on cannula function.[16] In another report, intramuscular progestins were used to successfully control hypermenorrhea.[21] In other reports, estrogens were also used to control bleeding, such as epistaxis, purpura, and gastrointestinal bleeding, associated with uremia.[47] Shemin et al. found that oral conjugated estrogens improved prolonged bleeding times and stopped clinical bleeding in four of four patients.[47]

However, at present, experience in using hormonal contraceptives in women with renal disease is limited. An obvious contraindication to hormonal therapy, particularly with combination hormonal therapy, would be the presence of hypertension. Another contraindication to hormonal therapy with estrogen-containing compounds would be in those women with a history of thrombophlebitis. An additional potential problem relates to the report from the Royal College of General Practitioners demonstrating a greater risk of urinary tract infection in women on oral contraceptives. If a woman with renal disease were placed on oral contraceptives, this potential complication would have to be watched for, with discontinuation of the pill if it is present. Recommendations on the use of oral contraceptives in women on hemodialysis and after transplantation have been mixed.[48,49] However, in those women without other medical contraindications and with no significant hypertension or history of thromboembolic complications, low-dose combination oral contraceptives or the progestin-only pill could be considered. One other possible problem would be that contraceptive steroids may inhibit hepatic microsomal enzyme metabolism and increase the concentration and effect of some beta-blocking drugs and cyclosporine, so doses of these drugs might have to be altered.[50] Other progestin contraceptives including depomedroxyprogesterone acetate (DMPA) and the Norplant implant can also be considered for these women. Since DMPA usually causes a reduction in overall menstrual bleeding, this form of contraception might be beneficial in helping with any associated abnormal uterine bleeding, especially in women with chronic anemia. There are no reports available about the use of the Norplant implant in women with renal disease. The location of the implant would have to be selected carefully to avoid the risk of infection at the implant site, with the possible loss of a shunt site. There are no studies available that have examined the levels of estrogen and progesterone before and after dialysis. However, there have been no reported failures in women using hormonal contraception related to oral contraception associated with hemodialysis.

The intrauterine device would probably not be a sensible choice in these women who are at greater risk of infection and usually have an underlying anemia. In addition, those women on steroids would have the problem of a potentially lower effectiveness rate. Most barrier methods would have no major contraindications although because of their lower effectiveness, they might be problematic should the contraception fail and pregnancy pose a significant medical risk to a woman who would not allow a therapeutic abortion. The diaphragm could be a problem if it led to an increase in a woman's frequency of urinary tract infection. This has been previously reported with the diaphragm.[51]

Pregnancy and Augmentation Cystoplasty

In the past 10 to 15 years many children with congenital anomalies of the lower urinary tract have undergone reconstruction with augmentation cystoplasty. These women are now in their reproductive years. Little is known about the effects of pregnancy on these women. However, Hill et al. summarized two cases pointing to potential problems.[52] These two pregnancies were complicated by multiple infections of the urinary tract, urinary calculi, and incontinence. Thus the potential exists in these women to have problems with infections, renal deterioration, and premature labor. Follow-up should be performed in conjunction with both an obstetrician and a urologist.

Summary

1. Adequate contraceptive counseling is important, as many women with renal disease may assume they are infertile. Pregnancy timing is also important in women who have had a renal transplantation.
2. Fertility declines with worsening renal function. Although most cycles are anovulatory in women on hemodialysis, ovulatory cycles can occur and women on hemodialysis can get pregnant. Fertility rises in women after transplantation.
3. Pregnancy can worsen chronic renal disease and the condition of those on hemodialysis and with a transplant. Those with preexisting hypertension or poorly functioning kidneys are more likely to have a problem.
4. The effect of a pregnancy on renal disease is related to the degree of hypertension and renal function. Women with a creatinine concentration over 2.5 mg/dL in particular do more poorly. Women on hemodialysis have an extremely high rate of fetal losses. Women with a renal transplant have higher-than-normal rates of premature delivery and low-birthweight infants. However, if blood pressure is controlled and renal function is good, most women will have an uncomplicated pregnancy and delivery.
5. Immunosuppressive therapy in renal transplant recipients can be associated with congenital malformations in newborns, although the risk is relatively small. In addition, there can be a risk of infections in the newborn.
6. Barrier methods are a reasonable alternative for women with significant renal disease, with the exception of the diaphragm in individuals who are at risk of recurrent urinary tract infections.
7. Hormonal contraceptives, especially low-dose pills and progestin-only contraceptives, could be considered in those women without significant hypertension or thrombosis problems.
8. The intrauterine device would not be recommended because of the risk of infection in an already immunocompromised group of individuals. In addition, in those women on immunosuppressives, the intrauterine device may be less effective.

References

1. Davison JM. Dialysis, transplantation and pregnancy. Am J Kidney Dis 1991;17:127–32.
2. Zacur HA, Mitch WE. Renal disease in pregnancy. Med Clin North Am 1977;61:89–109.
3. Ackrill P, Goodwin FJ, Marsh FP, Stratton D, Wagman H. Successful pregnancy in a patient on regular dialysis. Br Med J 1975;2:1172–4.
4. Coward RA, Mallick NP, Warrell DW, Grimes D, Kirkpatrick H. Successful pregnancy in severe chronic renal failure not requiring dialysis. Br Med J 1980;2:830–40.
5. Trebbin WM. Hemodialysis and pregnancy. JAMA 1979;241:1811–2.
6. Johnson TR, Lorenz RP, Menon KMJ, Nolan GH. Successful outcome of a pregnancy requiring dialysis. Effects on serum progesterone and estrogens. J Reprod Med 1979;22:217–8.
7. Lim VS, Auletta F, Kathpalia S, Frohman LA. Gonadal function in women with chronic renal failure: A study of the hypothalamopituitary ovarian axis. Proc Clin Dial Transplant Forum 1977;7:39–47.
8. Lim VS. Reproductive endocrinology in uremia. Baillieres Clin Obstet Gynaecol 1987;1:997–1007.
9. Espersen T, Schmitz O, Hansen HE, Moller J, Klebe JG. Ovulation in uremic women: The reproductive cycle in women on chronic hemodialysis. Int J Fertil 1988;33:103–6.
10. Chisvert LJ, Valderrabano QF. Alterations of the hypophyseal-gonadal axis in chronic renal insufficiency and after renal transplantation. Anal Med Intern 1991;8:587–94.
11. Phocas I, Sarandakou A, Kassanos D, Rizos D, Tserkezis G, Koutsikos D. Hormonal and ultrasound characteristics of menstrual function during chronic hemodialysis and after successful renal transplantation. Int J Gynaecol Obstet 1992;37:19–28.
12. Mantouvalos H, Metallinos C, Makrygiannakis A, Gouskos A. Sex hormones in women on hemodialysis. Int J Gynaecol Obstet 1984;22:367–70.
13. Ferraris JR, Domene HM, Escobar ME, Caletti MG, Ramirez JA, Rivarola MA. Hormonal profile in pubertal females with chronic renal failure: Before and under haemodialysis and after renal transplantation. Acta Endocrinol (Copenh) 1987;115:289–96.
14. Oken DE. Chronic renal disease and pregnancy. A review. Am J Obstet Gynecol 1966;94:1023–43.
15. Leppert P, Tisher CC, Cheng SC. Antecedent renal disease and the outcome of pregnancy. Ann Intern Med 1979;90:747–51.
16. Rice GG. Hypermenorrhea in the young hemodialysis patient. Am J Obstet Gynecol 1973;116:539–43.
17. Hou S. Peritoneal dialysis and haemodialysis in pregnancy. Baillieres Clin Obstet Gynaecol 1987;1:1009–25.
18. Rosenfeld JA. Renal disease and pregnancy. Am Fam Physician 1989;39:209–12.
19. Cunningham FG, Cox SM, Harstad TW, Mason RA, Pritchard JA. Chronic renal disease and pregnancy outcome. Am J Obstet Gynecol 1990;163:453–9.
20. Wing AJ, Brunner FP, Brynger H. Successful pregnancies in women treated by dialysis and kidney transplantation. Br J Obstet Gynaecol 1980;87:839–45.
21. Merkatz IR, Schwartz GH, David DS, Stenzel KH, Riggio RR, Whitsell JC. Resumption of female reproductive function following renal transplantation. JAMA 1971;216:1749–54.
22. Hou S. Pregnancy in organ transplant recipients. Med Clin North Am 1989;73:667–83.
23. Davison JM. Pregnancy in renal allograft recipients. Prognosis and management. Baillieres Clin Obstet Gynaecol 1987;1:1027–45.
24. Gaudier FL, Santiago-Delpin E, Rivera J. Pregnancy after renal transplantation. Surg Gynecol Obstet 1988;167:533–43.
25. Slavis SA, Novick AC, Steinmuller DR, Streem ST, Braun WE, Straffon RA, Mastroianni B, Graneto D. Outcome of renal transplantation in patients with a functioning graft for 20 years or more. J Urol 1990;144:20–2.
26. Baylis C, Wilson CB. Sex and the single kidney. Am J Kidney Dis 1989;13:290–8.
27. Abe S, Amagasaki Y, Konishi K, Kato E, Sakaguchi H, Iyori S. The influence of antecedent renal disease on pregnancy. Am J Obstet Gynecol 1985;153:508–14.
28. Ferris TF. Renal diseases. In Burrow GN, Ferris TF, eds. Medical Complications during Pregnancy. 3rd ed. Philadelphia, WB Saunders, 1988, pp 277–99.
29. Redrow M, Cherem L, Elliott J, Mangalat J, Mishler RE, Bennett WM, Lutz M, Sigala J, Byrnes J, Phillipe M, Hou S, Schon D. Dialysis in the management of pregnant patients

with renal insufficiency. Medicine (Baltimore) 1983;67:199–208.
30. Kioko M, Shaw KM, Clarke AD, Warren DJ. Successful pregnancy in a diabetic patient treated with continuous ambulatory peritoneal dialysis. Diabetes Care 1983;6:298–300.
31. Nageotte MP, Grundy HO. Pregnancy outcome in women requiring chronic hemodialysis. Obstet Gynecol 1988;72:456–9.
32. O'Connell PJ, Caterson RJ, Steart JH, Mahony JF. Problems associated with pregnancy in renal allograft recipients. Int J Artif Organs 1989;12:147–52.
33. Rudolf JE, Schweizer RT, Bartus SA. Pregnancy in renal transplant patients. Transplant Proc 1979;27:26–9.
34. Whetham JC, Cardella C, Harding M. Effect of pregnancy on graft function and graft survival in renal cadaver transplant patients. Am J Obstet Gynecol 1983;145:193–7.
35. Jungers P, Forget D, Henry-Amar M, Albouze G, Fournier P, Vischer V, Droz D, Noeel LH, Grunfeld JP. Chronic kidney disease and pregnancy. In Grunfeld J, Maxwell M, Bach J, eds. Advances in Nephrology. Vol 15. Chicago, Year Book Medical Publishers, 1986, pp 103–41.
36. Yasin SY, Beydown SN. Hemodialysis in pregnancy. Obstet Gynecol Surv 1988;43:655–68.
37. Gaucherand P, Chalabreysse JP, Audra P, Clement HJ, Laurent G, Dargent D, Rudigoz RC. Pregnancy in women undergoing dialysis in chronic renal insufficiency. J Gynecol Obstet Biol Reprod 1988;7:889–95.
38. Nageotte MP, Grundy HO. Pregnancy outcome in women requiring chronic hemodialysis. Obstet Gynecol 1988;72:456–9.
39. Penn I, Makowski EL. Parenthood in kidney and liver transplant recipients. Transplant Proc 1981;13:36–9.
40. Mallat SG, Brensilver JM, McCabe R, Nurse HM. Successful pregnancy in a cyclosporine-treated renal transplant recipient with sickle cell disease. Transplantation 1988;45:660–1.
41. Cefalo RC. Drugs in pregnancy: Which to use and which to avoid. Drug Ther 1983;13:167–75.
42. Blake JP, Collinge DA, McNulty H, Leach FN, Grant EJ. Drugs in pregnancy: Weighing the risks. Patient Care 1980;14:22–106.
43. Rosa FW, Bosco LA, Graham CF, Milstien JB. Neonatal anuria with maternal angiotensin-converting enzyme inhibition. Obstet Gynecol 1989;74:371–4.
44. Lewis GJ, Lamont CAR, Lee HA, Slapak M. Successful pregnancy in a renal transplant recipient taking Cyclosporin A. Br Med J 1983;286:603.
45. Davison JM, Dellagrammatikas H, Partkin JM. Maternal azathioprine therapy and depressed haemopoieses in the babies of renal allograft patients. Br J Obstet Gynaecol 1985;92:233–9.
46. Reimers TJ, Sluss PM. 6-Mercaptopurine treatment of pregnant mice: Effects on second and third generations. Science 1978;201:65–7.
47. Shemin D, Elnour M, Amarantes B, Abuelo JG, Chazan JA. Oral estrogens decrease bleeding time and improve clinical bleeding in patients with renal failure. Am J Med 1990;89:436–40.
48. Golby M. Fertility after renal transplantation. Transplantation 1970;10:201–7.
49. Sciarra JJ, Toledo-Pereyra LH, Bendel RP, Simmons RL. Pregnancy following renal transplantation. Am J Obstet Gynecol 1975;123:411–25.
50. Shenfield GM, Griffin JM. Clinical pharmacokinetics of contraceptive steroids. An update. Clin Pharmacokin 1991;20:15–37.
51. Fihn SD, Latha NRH, Roberts P, Running K, Stamm WE. Association between diaphragm use and urinary tract infection. JAMA 1985;254:240–5.
52. Hill DE, Chantigian PM, Kramer SA. Pregnancy after augmentation cystoplasty. Surg Gynecol Obstet 1990;170:485–7.

8

Gastrointestinal Diseases

Inflammatory Bowel Disease

There are between 1 and 2 million individuals with inflammatory bowel in the United States.[1] Both ulcerative colitis and Crohn's disease are most common in young individuals, especially during the childbearing years. Thus, it is fairly common to find a young adult with inflammatory bowel disease (IBD) who is either contemplating a pregnancy or is pregnant.

Fertility

Early studies suggested a reduction in fertility in women with IBD.[2,3] However, these studies did not account for the fact that these women were often advised not to get pregnant by their health care providers. More recent data suggest that fertility in women, especially with ulcerative colitis, is not affected.[4-8] In the study by Baird et al. of fertility in women with IBD, 177 women with Crohn's and 84 with ulcerative colitis were compared with healthy controls.[7] When the rates of childlessness, fecundability, and fertility and methods of birth control were evaluated, the results suggested that the decrease in birthrate was secondary to the women's choice rather than an effect of the disease process. Thus, fear of getting pregnant from warnings by physicians or others may be a factor. A small percentage of women with Crohn's disease will be infertile secondary to fistulization to fallopian tubes with resultant tuboovarian abscesses.[9] In addition, perineal or labial abscesses and fistulas, if associated with pain, may discourage intercourse.[1] Another group at risk for infertility are those who have undergone surgery. Wikland et al. reported on 71 women who underwent a proctocolectomy for either ulcerative colitis or Crohn's disease.[10] Fertility was significantly reduced after surgery such that only 37% who attempted to become pregnant succeeded within 5 years, compared to 72% before surgery.

Narendranathan et al. studied fertility in males with IBD, comparing 106 males with Crohn's disease and 62 with ulcerative colitis with 140 normal controls.[11] The mean number of pregnancies for the males with Crohn's disease was significantly lower than that for the controls (2.14 versus 1.75). There was no difference between controls and those with ulcerative colitis. However, overall fertility was not markedly diminished. Several other studies have shown reduced fertility in men with IBD secondary to sulfasalazine. Although sulfasalazine has been used for treating IBD since the 1940s, this problem was first reported in 1979.[12–16] Since then, many cases of male infertility associated with sulfasalazine have been reported.[17,18] Within 2 months of starting sulfasalazine, abnormalities detected by semen analysis have been described and include oligospermia, reduced sperm motility, and an increased proportion of abnormal forms of sperm.[18] Birnie et al. demonstrated abnormal findings on semen analysis in 86% of 21 males taking sulfasalazine for IBD.[19] The problem seems to be a common phenomenon in males using sulfasalazine and seems not related to an idiosyncratic reaction.[20] Sulfasalazine is split by colonic bacteria into sulfapyridine and 5-aminosalicylic acid (5-ASA). While the latter is thought to be the active therapeutic component, the sulfapyridine carrier is probably responsible for many of the toxic side effects including sperm dysfunction and infertility.[21,22]

The infertility problems caused by sulfasalazine seem to be reversible by discontinuation of the drug or replacing sulfasalazine with oral 5-ASA preparations or 5-ASA enemas.[14,18,20,23,24] Chatzinoff et al. reported on an infertile male using sulfasalazine who was found to have an abnormal sperm penetration, as determined by assay, but it returned to normal after discontinuation of sulfasalazine and starting 5-ASA enemas.[18] His wife conceived after his stopping the drug. Reintroduction of sulfasalazine has also been reported to cause deterioration again in sperm quality and quantity.[14]

Another potential fertility problem in males with IBD is associated with surgery. However, in contrast to total colectomy for cancer in males, proctocolectomy for ulcerative colitis rarely results in permanent impotence. Bauer found a rate of 1.5% in a series of 130 patients.[25] There is nothing reported to suggest that IBD by itself is associated with infertility in males.

Effect of Pregnancy on Inflammatory Bowel Disease

Many studies have examined the possibility of exacerbation of IBD with pregnancy.[3,5,9,26–31] Recent reports appear encouraging compared to earlier reports. Hopefully, this represents improved treatment and not only the exclusion of more severe cases. IBD includes both ulcerative colitis and Crohn's disease and these are discussed separately.

ULCERATIVE COLITIS

In most studies, pregnancy has not been shown to significantly alter the course of ulcerative colitis.[3,9,26,27] In a study involving 97 women with ulcerative colitis, the spontaneous rate of exacerbation in nonpregnant women was 32% per year while in the pregnant women the rate was 34%.[26] If exacerbations occurred, they were most likely in the first and second trimesters. In the study by Nielsen et al., three of the women had colectomies without an effect on the pregnancy. Those women with active disease at the beginning of pregnancy tended to have a similar or worse course throughout pregnancy.[26] There has been no evidence of an initial attack of colitis during pregnancy being more severe than in nonpregnant women.[9] A therapeutic abortion also does not affect the course of disease.

Another concern in pregnant women with ulcerative colitis is the effect of an ileostomy following a proctocolectomy. While ileostomies do not seem to have an adverse effect on pregnancy,[26,28,29] potential problems do exist. These include stomal ileal prolapses and intestinal obstructions, which developed in 10% of women during pregnancy in one study.[29] Overall, even women with a total colectomy and ileal pouch–anal anastomosis seem to tolerate pregnancy, with six of six in one study doing well.[30] Three of the six women did develop transient deterioration of anorectal function during the third trimester that resolved after delivery. Thus, pregnancy is not contraindicated in women with ulcerative colitis, but it would be advisable for women to wait until their disease is in a quiescent state.[4]

CROHN'S DISEASE

Similar to ulcerative colitis, pregnancy does not seem to increase the risk of an exacerbation of Crohn's disease. In a study of 59 women with Crohn's disease, Nielsen and coworkers found a 44% risk of an exacerbation when these women were not pregnant and a 38% risk in the same women when they were pregnant or in the postpartum period.[31] The course tended to correlate with the activity state at the beginning of the pregnancy. Those who had inactive disease at the beginning of pregnancy had about a 60% chance of their disease remaining inactive during the pregnancy. In over 50% of those with active disease, the course either continued with the same activity or worsened throughout the pregnancy. Another study, evaluating postpartum exacerbations found that of 145 women with Crohn's disease, 62% had no change, 23% had a decrease in disease activity, and 15% became worse.[27] In contrast to first- and second-trimester exacerbations with ulcerative colitis, those women with Crohn's disease are more likely to experience an exacerbation in the third trimester.[1]

Effect of Inflammatory Bowel Disease on Pregnancy

ULCERATIVE COLITIS

Most reviews indicate that the outcomes of pregnancy in the majority of women with ulcerative colitis will be similar to those in the general population.[5,9,32–35] Jaernerot reviewed 18 reports of 1155 pregnancies and found an overall good outcome.[33] There has been no evidence in the literature of increased rates of stillbirths, spontaneous abortions, or fetal malformations. Most studies have indicated that births are of normal weight and full term.[26,32,34] However, Baird et al. found a 2.7 times risk of preterm birth in those with ulcerative colitis.[7] Most studies suggest that those with more active or severe disease during pregnancy are more likely to have a preterm infant. Those women who require surgical intervention are at high risk for fetal loss.[28,36,37] In one series of nine women having surgery during pregnancy, only five delivered a live infant and three of the women died during pregnancy or soon after.[28]

CROHN'S DISEASE

Problems during pregnancy in women with Crohn's disease including spontaneous abortion, prematurity, and low-birthweight infants are related to the activity of their disease at the time of conception.[2,3,8] However, even with severe disease, women have been able to have normal pregnancies utilizing long-term management with total parenteral nutrition.[31,38–40] The risk of a preterm birth has been reported to be about 16%, about double that of control groups.[32,34] Baird et al. found the risk to be 3.1 times normal.[7] Site of involvement does not seem to affect pregnancy. However, similar to ulcerative colitis, surgical intervention for Crohn's disease is associated with a high risk of fetal loss.[2]

Medications and Pregnancy

Another major concern for many of these women is the potential effect of medication on the fetus. These women may be confused by advice, on the one hand, from obstetricians that their medications may not be safe during pregnancy and to stop or decrease their use, while on the other hand, from their gastroenterologist who may advise continuation.

Sulfasalazine and its metabolite sulfapyridine cross the placenta and inhibit the metabolism of folic acid, so there is concern about its use in pregnancy. However, in reports on its usage in pregnant women, sulfasalazine does not seem to be associated with harmful side effects, including fetal loss, congenital abnormalities, and neonatal jaundice even when used at any stage during pregnancy and lactation.[26,27,33,41] Thus, while sulfasalazine is indicated when needed during pregnancy, it is not recommended to continue its use during pregnancy in women who are in remission.

Most studies have not shown a significant risk with the use of steroids. The studies involving steroids during pregnancy included mostly women with diseases other than IBD. In a study of pregnant women with IBD, 287 women were treated with either sulfasalazine or prednisone or both, and 244 received neither. The rate of fetal complications was lower in both groups than in the general population.[27] However, there has been the suggestion that steroids at a dose of 10 mg/day during the entire course of pregnancy can lead to low birthweights.[42] In mice, steroids can increase the rate of fetal loss and problems with cleft palate and exophthalmos but this does not appear to be a significant problem in humans.[1] Both sulfasalazine and steroids could be used during pregnancy and should not be avoided to control an exacerbation.

Of possibly even greater concern to women and physicians have been the possible side effects of azathioprine and mercaptopurine when used during conception and pregnancy. While there have been reports of teratogenicity in animals, this has not been well demonstrated in humans.[43,44] While women have been advised to avoid azathioprine during pregnancy, many normal pregnancies have been reported among women on azathioprine.[6,45–51] Alstead et al. evaluated 16 pregnancies in 14 women using azathioprine for IBD. In this report, there were no congenital abnormalities or health problems in the offspring.[52] However, problems have occurred in infants of mothers who took azathioprine, and included lymphopenia, leukopenia, thrombocytopenia, hypogammaglobulinemia, and thymic hypoplasia.[53–56] In one study of 103 births in women with renal transplants who were taking azathioprine, 7 infants had birth defects.[55] Thus, while it would not be advisable to start azathioprine in a pregnant woman with IBD, it should not necessarily be stopped if the drug has been helpful in putting the patient into remission. The use of azathioprine during pregnancy would also not be an absolute indication for a therapeutic abortion, although some researchers have made this recommendation.[57,58] This decision would have to made through an informed discussion between the physician and the individual or couple involved.

Mercaptopurine has been reported to cause significant disorders in fetuses in animal models including lymphopenia, thymic hypoplasia, immunoglobulin deficiency, low cortisol levels, and chromosomal abnormalities.[28] While some researchers advise weaning the medication before pregnancy, and therapeutic abortion if pregnancy occurs while on the medication, many successful pregnancies have been reported in women receiving renal transplants who became pregnant while on the medication. Termination of a pregnancy should be elective rather than mandatory.

Metronidazole has been associated with fetal loss, congenital defects, and cancer in mice. However, in humans it would appear that very large doses over a long period of time would be needed to cause cancer.[1] However, it would be advisable to avoid this antibiotic, if possible, during pregnancy and especially during the first trimester.

Contraception and Inflammatory Bowel Disease

Most of the results of studies on contraception and IBD are from several large cohort studies and several smaller case-control studies. These have mainly examined the associations between oral contraceptives and IBD. There is little information in these studies to implicate oral contraceptives as a major risk factor for causing IBD. In addition, the incidence of IBD is similar in men and women, which is not suggestive of a hormonal effect. However, no studies have directly examined the effects of oral contraceptives on the course of women with IBD. Thus, one must extrapolate conclusions from the results of these other studies.

Three large cohort studies showed a modest elevation in relative risk of developing IBD with oral contraceptive use.[59-61] However, the studies had low statistical power because of the extremely small number of inflammatory bowel cases. The Royal College of General Practitioners (RCGP) study demonstrated a risk ratio of 2.06 for ulcerative colitis for current users and 0.43 for former users and 1.41 for risk of Crohn's disease but neither was statistically significant.[59] In addition, no adjustment was made for cigarette smoking. The Walnut Creek Contraceptive Drug Study examined 17,939 women from 1968, followed for an average of 6.5 years.[60] The relative risk of developing IBD was 3.4 for current and 2.5 for former users. These results were also of low statistical power because of the small numbers of cases. The third large study, the Oxford Family Planning Association Contraceptive Study, followed 17,032 women from 1968 to 1974 in 17 family planning clinics in England and Scotland, of which 56% of women were oral contraceptive users. For Crohn's disease, there was no increase in risk for those using contraceptives for less than 2 years and for former users. Current users for more than 2 years had a risk ratio of 2.0. For ulcerative colitis the risk ratio was 2.4 for current users and 2.6 for former users. However, again the effect was of low statistical power because of the rarity of IBD.

Several case-control studies have also examined this question. One case-control study involving community controls showed oral contraceptives to have a protective effect against Crohn's disease.[62] Another demonstrated a weak association between Crohn's disease and oral contraceptive use but did not adjust for smoking.[63] Lashner et al. carried out two case-control studies examining the effects of oral contraceptives in Crohn's disease and ulcerative colitis.[64,65] Both studies failed to show an association with oral contraceptives. Stratifying by disease location also failed to demonstrate an association. These two studies controlled for the effects of cigarette smoking, which did not alter their results. The results of all of these studies seem to be somewhat conflicting, although there is no overall strong association between IBD and use of oral contraceptives. One reason for some confusion may be that certain cases of mesenteric vascular ischemia are being confused with IBD. Several cases of mesenteric vascular ischemia have been reported to be induced by oral contraceptives.[66–72] At present, there does not seem to be any strong evidence that hormonal contraceptives will cause a flare in women with IBD. However, disease activity should be monitored closely and if a flare seems temporally associated with the pill, then it should be discontinued. No side effects of barrier methods have been reported in women who have IBD. The intrauterine device would not be recommended in a woman with Crohn's disease who has had problems with abdominal or pelvic fistulas.

There are potential interactions between IBD and medications that are used by women with IBD that could potentially lead to a decrease in efficacy of a contraceptive device. Many of these women are on chronic antibiotics which may interact with oral contraceptives. This is probably not a major problem and is discussed further in Chapter 16. In addition, many of these women have either diarrhea or a loss of their colon secondary to prior surgery, which theoretically could cause contraceptive failure secondary to malabsorption of the oral contraceptive. However, in a study evaluating women with a prior ileostomy for ulcerative colitis involving only the colon who were on oral contraceptives, there was no change in bioavailability of ethinyl estradiol and levonorgestrel.[73] Similar results have been found in women with unoperated ulcerative colitis.[74] However, levonorgestrel levels were demonstrated to be reduced in women after either a conventional ileostomy or proctocolectomy with construction of a continent ileostomy.[74] It was thought that this might be related to the loss of absorptive capacity secondary to the loss of part of the terminal ileum used in construction of the pouch. However, studies have shown that the pouch maintains its absorptive capacity in spite of morphological changes and bacterial overgrowth, so the mechanism for the reduced hormone levels has not been explained.[75,76] Reduced bioavailability of both norethisterone and levonorgestrel has been demonstrated in morbidly obese women having a jejunoileostomy that significantly decreased their small-bowel absorptive surface.[77] Thus, if the small-bowel absorbing surface is significantly reduced via surgery or diarrhea, there is the potential for contraceptive failure. In these individuals, parenteral administration of contraceptive hormones via depomedroxyprogesterone acetate (DMPA) or the Norplant implant would be preferred to oral contraceptives.

Summary

1. Pregnancy in most women does not exacerbate IBD.
2. IBD has only minor effects on pregnancy except for those with severe, active Crohn's disease or those requiring surgery during pregnancy.
3. Use of sulfasalazine and steroids in pregnancy is unlikely to increase fetal morbidity or mortality.
4. Women with stable quiescent IBD could use either a barrier method or hormonal contraceptives. If oral contraceptives are used, a low-dose

combination pill or progestin-only contraceptive should be recommend-ed with close monitoring of disease activity. If there is evidence of mal-absorption, women should be advised that oral contraceptives may be ineffective and DMPA or Norplant would be preferred. If the disease is very active, women should be advised that hormonal contraceptives might complicate the disease, although good evidence for this is lacking, and a barrier method recommended.

Gallbladder

Pregnancy

Gallbladder function may change with pregnancy. Studies have shown an increase in fasting gallbladder volume, an increase in residual volume, and a decrease in the rate of emptying, as well as development of sludge during pregnancy.[78–80] While there may be a slight increase in the risk of gallstone formation during pregnancy,[81] the risk appears to be minimal and in some studies to not be present at all.[82,83]

Contraception

There are no contraindications for women with a history of gallstones in utilizing barrier methods. Several studies indicate that hormonal contra-ceptives might be a problem in women with a history of gallstones. Petitti et al. conducted a prospective cohort study of women to evaluate the asso-ciation between cholecystectomy and use of supplemental estrogens. After adjusting for age, the relative risk in those women who had ever used oral contraceptives was 2.1 (1.5–3.0).[84] In current users the relative risk was 2.7 (1.8–4.0) and for past users it was 1.6 (1.1–2.5). The RCGP study also exam-ined the association between gallstones and oral contraceptives and found that women on oral contraceptives seem to be operated on earlier if not more frequently.[85] The results of this latter study suggest that perhaps oral contraceptives alter gallstone formation by changing gallbladder motility. An increased risk for cholecystectomy has been noted for individuals who use exogenous estrogens.[86–88] Two other studies, one prospective and one retrospective, found no association between oral contraceptive use and cholelithiasis.[81,83]

Estrogen and progesterone receptors have been found in the gallbladder and can affect motility. Hould et al. studied progesterone receptors in gall-bladders of female guinea pigs.[89] Gallbladders from oophorectomized women demonstrated minimal progesterone receptor activity and maximal gallbladder motility to cholecystokinin. Oophorectomized women who had been treated with estrogen and progesterone for 14 days had high levels of progesterone receptor activity but minimal gallbladder motility response to cholecystokinin. These results suggest that the gallbladder may contain progesterone receptors susceptible to motility changes dependent on circulating hormonal conditions. Other studies have suggested that estrogen may increase the lithogenicity of bile.[90-93] If hormonal contraceptives were to be a problem, it seems most likely that it would be in women with a history of gallbladder disease. It is not entirely clear whether the estrogen component alone or both estrogen and progesterone may affect gallbladder disease in these individuals. Combined oral contraceptives would have to be used with caution in those with gallbladder disease and would be contraindicated in those with prior cholestasis during pregnancy. Most likely, similar recommendations would have to be made about progestin-only contraceptives including the Norplant implant, but no studies that specifically address this question are available. There is nothing reported in the literature to suggest that women who have had cholecystectomy are at higher risk when using hormonal contraceptives.

Liver Disorders

Hepatitis

PREGNANCY

Jaundice during pregnancy is not common, with a prevalence of 1 in 1500 pregnancies.[94] Liver diseases occurring during pregnancy may be related or unrelated to pregnancy. The most common cause of jaundice in pregnancy is viral hepatitis, which is no more frequent in the pregnant population than in the general population. Cholestatic jaundice of pregnancy is another common cause of jaundice occurring during pregnancy.

Results of some laboratory tests used to measure liver status are altered during pregnancy. Total bilirubin levels do not change but the conjugated fraction increases.[95] Alkaline phosphatase is usually elevated up to two to four times normal.[96] Transaminases also remain unchanged throughout a normal pregnancy.[97] Fibrinogen, transferrin, and ceruloplasmin may also increase along with alpha- and beta-globulins. Gamma-globulins and albumin often decrease.

There is no definitive evidence of transmission of type A viral hepatitis from mother to fetus. However, if transmission occurs, it is most likely primarily at the time the mother is viremic or during delivery. Treatment with 0.02 mL/kg of immune globulin is recommended for the infant if hepatitis antigen is present in the mother's stools at the time of delivery.

Viral B hepatitis is the most common form of viral hepatitis during pregnancy. Women who are chronic hepatitis B surface antigen (HBsAg) and e antigen (HBeAg) positive have more than a 90% rate of transmission to their infants, with 80 to 90% of these infected infants becoming chronic carriers. The risk of infection to those infants whose mother is HBsAg positive but HBeAg negative is about 31%.[98] Vertical transmission from mother to infant is most likely when the infection occurs during the last trimester or in the immediate postpartum period. In one series the risk of vertical transmission was 0% with acute infections in the first trimester, 6% in second trimester cases, 67% in third trimester cases, and 100% in immediate postpartum cases.[99] Since transmission probably occurs primarily during birth or soon thereafter, infants born to carrier mothers should be treated with both hepatitis B immune globulin, 0.5 mL intramuscularly at birth, followed by hepatitis B virus vaccine, 0.5 mL intramuscularly within 7 days of birth and 1 and 6 months later. While screening has been recommended for mothers in high-risk areas, the Advisory Committee on Immunization Practices of the Centers for Disease Control now recommends that all pregnant women be screened for HBsAg early in pregnancy. Some authorities recommend universal immunization in the newborn. High-risk groups include Asian Americans, Alaska Eskimos, sub-Saharan Africans, Pacific Islanders, Haitians, intravenous drug users, institutionalized individuals, women with a history of liver disease, women working in a hemodialysis unit, women with prior blood transfusions, and women with a history of multiple sexually transmitted diseases. Type B viral hepatitis does not appear to be more severe during pregnancy than in the nonpregnant women.

It is not clear whether hepatitis C and other non-A, non-B, non-C viruses are transmitted during pregnancy or whether they have an effect on the pregnancy. Inoue et al. reported on a case of probable transmission of hepatitis C during birth from grandmother to mother to child.[100] It does appear that epidemic non-A, non-B hepatitis in Asia and the Middle East is more frequent and severe in pregnant women.[95]

Viral hepatitis does not appear to be teratogenic during pregnancy.[95] However, prematurity may be a sequela of viral hepatitis during pregnancy.[101]

Intrahepatic cholestasis may occur during pregnancy. At least half of these women have a family history of jaundice during pregnancy. Usually the cholestasis occurs during the last trimester, although it can occur during the first trimester. Pruritus is one of the major symptoms and usually precedes jaundice by about 1 to 2 weeks. Maternal health is usually not affected but there is an increased prevalence of fetal distress, prematurity, and stillbirths.[95]

Liver transplants are not common at present but are occurring with an increasing frequency. Experience with pregnant women who have had a liver transplantation is very limited. However, Sims et al. reported one case of a successful pregnancy in a 26-year-old woman following a liver transplantation, and reviewed four other similar cases.[102]

Contraception

The ingestion of contraceptive steroids, both estrogens and 19-norprogestins, can alter hepatocellular function similar to changes that occur during pregnancy. These changes include alterations in the composition of bile, reduced volume of biliary secretion, a rise in cholesterol concentration, and a fall in the bile acid level.[103,104] These changes are related to dose and are reversible.[105] Hormonal contraceptives should thus be avoided during active liver disease or cirrhosis. However, after recovery from hepatitis, when liver function returns to normal, hormonal contraceptives could be restarted. Liver function tests should again be done in 1 to 2 months after starting. If the test results become abnormal, hormonal contraceptives should be discontinued. Progestin-only contraceptives including DMPA and the Norplant implant should probably have the same precautions. Patients with chronic liver disease can use a barrier method or an intrauterine device. In fact, condoms should be used if one partner is a hepatitis B carrier.

Liver tumors are another problem that would contraindicate the use of hormonal contraceptions. Long-term use of oral contraceptives has been reported to be associated with hepatic adenomas.[106] Oral contraceptive use has also been implicated as a possible risk factor in the development of hepatic carcinoma, although this association is controversial.[107–109] Some case-control studies that did not control for hepatitis B infection indicated an increased risk, particularly with use over 5 years.[107] However, prospective studies and a large international World Health Organization case-control study did not show such a risk.[108,109]

One group of women predisposed to benign liver tumors are those with autosomal dominant polycystic kidney disease (ADPKD). Extrarenal manifestations of this disease include hepatic cysts, mitral valve prolapse, cerebral aneurysms, and possible diverticular disease of the colon. Hepatic cysts are the most frequent associated nonrenal problem. In one survey of these women, it was found that hepatic cysts developed only in those women with ADPKD who had used exogenous hormones or had been pregnant.[110] The highest risk was to those women who had been pregnant in the past and had used exogenous hormones (65% prevalence). This compared to a prevalence of 26% in women who had used exogenous steroids but had not been pregnant, 46% in women who had been pregnant but never used steroids, and 0% in those who had never been pregnant or used steroids. These results suggest that steroid hormones regulate the degree of hepatic cyst formation. Hormonal contraceptives should be avoided in women with ADPKD or in those women with a history of a benign liver cyst.

References

1. Korelitz BI. Pregnancy, fertility, and inflammatory bowel diseae. Am J Gastroenterol 1985;80:365–70.
2. De Dombal FT, Burton IL, Goligher JC. Crohn's disease and pregnancy. Br Med J 1972;3:550–3.
3. Fielding JF, Cooke WT. Pregnancy and Crohn's disease. Br Med J 1970;2:76–7.
4. Webb MJ, Sedlack RE. Ulcerative colitis in pregnancy. Med Clin North Am 1974;58:823–7.
5. Willoughby CP, Truelove SC. Ulcerative colitis and pregnancy. Gut 1980;21:469–74.

6. Sorokin JJ, Levine SM. Pregnancy and inflammatory bowel disease: A review of the literature. Obstet Gynecol 1983;62:247–52.
7. Baird DD, Narendranathan M, Sandler RS. Increased risk of preterm birth for women with inflammatory bowel disease. Gastroenterology 1990;99:987–94.
8. Khosla R, Willoughby CP, Jewell DP. Crohn's disease and pregnancy. Gut 1984;25:52–6.
9. Zeldis JB. Pregnancy and inflammatory bowel disease. West J Med 1989;151:168–71.
10. Wikland M, Jansson I, Asztely M, Palselius I, Svaninger G, Magnusson O, Hulten L. Gynaecological problems related to anatomical changes after conventional proctocolectomy and ileostomy. Int J Colorectal Dis 1990;5:49–52.
11. Narendranathan M, Sandler RS, Suchindran CM, Savitz DA. Male infertility in inflammatory bowel disease J Clin Gastroenterol 1989;11:403–6.
12. Toth A. Male infertility due to sulphasalazine. Lancet 1979;1:538–40.
13. Toth A. Reversible toxic effect of salicylazosulfapyridine on semen quality. Fertil Steril 1979;1:538–540.
14. Levi AJ, Fisher AM, Huges L, Hendry WF. Male infertility due to sulphasalazine. Lancet 1979;2:276–8.
15. Grieve J. Male infertility due to sulphasalazine. Lancet 1979;2:464.
16. Traub AI, Thompson W, Carville J. Male infertility due to sulphasalazine. Lancet 1979;2:639–40.
17. Collen MJ. Azulfidine–induced oligospermia. Am J Gastroenterol 1980;74:441–2.
18. Chatzinoff M, Guarino JM, Corson SL, Batzer FR, Friedman LS. Sulfasalazine induced abnormal sperm penetration assay reversed on changing to 5-aminosalicylic acid enemas. Dig Dis Sci 1988;33:108–10.
19. Birnie GG, McLeod TIF, Watkinson G. Incidence of sulphasalazine-induced male infertility. Gut 1981;22:452–5.
20. Toovey S, Hudson E, Hendry WF, Levi AJ. Sulphasalazine and male infertility. Reversibility and possible mechanism. Gut 1981;22:445–51.
21. Hudson E, Dore C, Sowter C, Toovey S, Levi AH. Sperm size in patients with inflammatory bowel disease on sulfasalazine therapy. Fertil Steril 1982;38:77–84.
22. Taffet SL, Das KM. Sulfasalazine—Adverse effects and densensitization. Dig Dis Sci 1983;28:833–42.
23. Cann PA, Holdsworth CD. Reversal of male infertility on changing treatment from sulphasalazine to 5-aminosalicylic acid. Lancet 1984;1:1119.
24. Shaffer JL, Kershaw A, Berrisford MH. Sulphasalazine-induced infertility reversed on transfer to 5-aminosalicylic acid. Lancet 1984;1:1984.
25. Bauer JJ. Sexual dysfunction after colectomy. Mt Sinai J Med 1983;50:187–9.
26. Nielsen OH, Andreasson B, Bondesen S, Jarnum S. Pregnancy in ulcerative colitis. Scand J Gastroenterol 1983;18:735–42.
27. Mogadam M, Korelitz BI, Ahmed SW, Dobbins WO III. The course of inflammatory bowel disease during pregnancy and postpartum. Am J Gastroenterol 1981;75:265–9.
28. McEwan HP. Ulcerative colitis in pregnancy. Proc R Soc Med 1972;65:279–81.
29. Hudson CN. Ileostomy in pregnancy. Proc R Soc Med 1972;65:281–3.
30. Metcalf A, Dozois RR, Beart RW Jr, Wolff BG. Pregnancy following ileal pouch-anal anastomosis. Dis Colon Rectum 1985;28:859–61.
31. Nielsen OH, Andreasson B, Bondesen S, Jacobsen O, Jarnum S. Pregnancy in Crohn's disease. Scand J Gastroenterol 1984;19:724–32.
32. Porter RJ, Stirrat GM. The effects of inflammatory bowel disease on pregnancy: A case-controlled retrospective analysis. Br J Obstet Gynaecol 1986;93:1124–31.
33. Jaernerot G. Fertility, sterility, and pregnancy in chronic inflammatory bowel disease, review. Scand J Gastroenterol 1982;17:1–4.
34. Mayberry JF, Weterman IT. European survey of fertility and pregnancy in women with Crohn's disease: A case control study by European collaborative group. Gut 1986;27:821–5.
35. Fedorkow DM, Persaud D, Nimrod CA. Inflammatory bowel disease: A controlled study of late pregnancy outcome. Am J Obstet Gynecol 1989;160:998–1001.
36. Anderson JB, Turner GM, Williamson RCN. Fulminant ulcerative colitis in pregnancy and the puerperium. J R Soc Med 1987;80:492–4.
37. Bohe MG, Ekelund GR, Genell SN, Gennser GM, Joborn HA, Leandoer LJ, Lindstrom CG, Svanberg LK. Surgery for fulminating colitis during pregnancy. Dis Colon Rectum 1983;26:119–22.

38. Tresadern JC, Falconer GF, Turnberg LA, Irving MH. Successful completed pregnancy in a patient maintained on home parenteral nutrition. Br Med J (Clin Res) 1983;286:602–3.
39. Jacobson LB, Clapp DH. Total parenteral nutrition in pregnancy complicated by Crohn's disease. J Parenter Enter Nutr 1987;11:93–6.
40. Rivera-Alsina ME, Saldanaa LR, Stringer CA. Fetal growth sustained by parenteral nutrition in pregnancy. Obstet Gynecol 1985;64:138–141.
41. Brostrom O. Prognosis in ulcerative colitis. Med Clin North Am 1990;74:201–18.
42. Reinisch J, Simon NG, Karow WG, Gandelman R. Prenatal exposure to prednisone in humans and animals retards intrauterine growth. Science 1978;202:436–8.
43. Tuchmann-Duplessis H, Mercier-Parot L. Production in rabbits of malformations of the limbs by azathioprine and 6-mercaptopurine. C R Soc Biol 1966;166:501–6.
44. Rosenkrantz JG, Githens JH, Cos SM, Kellum DL. Azathioprine (Imuran) in pregnancy. Am J Obstet Gynecol 1967;97:387.
45. Erkman J, Blyth JG. Azathioprine therapy complicated by pregnancy. Obstet Gynecol 1972;40:708–10.
46. Farber M, Kennison RD, Jackson HT. Successful pregnancy after renal transplantation. Obstet Gynecol 1976;48(suppl 1):25–45.
47. Registration Committee of the European Dialysis and Transplant Association. Successful pregnancies in women treated by dialysis and kidney transplantation. Br J Obstet Gynaecol 1980;87:839–45.
48. Davidson AM, Guillon PJ. Successful pregnancies reported to the registry up to the end of 1982. Proc Eur Dialysis Transplant Assoc London 1984;21:54–5.
49. Meehan RT, Dorsey JK. Pregnancy among patients with systemic lupus erythematosus receiving immunosuppressive therapy. J Rheumatol 1987;14:252–9.
50. Gaudier FL, Santiago-Delphin E, Rivera J, Gonzales Z. Pregnancy after renal transplantation. Surg Gynecol Obstet 1988;167:533–43.
51. Hou S. Pregnancy in organ transplant recipients. Med Clin North Am 1989;734:667–83.
52. Alstead EM, Ritchie JK, Lennard-Jones JE, Farthing MJ, Clark ML. Safety of azathioprine in pregnancy in inflammatory bowel disease. Gastroenterology 1990;99:443–6.
53. Cote CJ, Meuwissen HJ, Pickering RJ. Effects on the neonate of prednisone and azathioprine administered to the mother during pregnancy. J Pediatr 1974;85:324–8.
54. Dewitte DB, Buick MK, Cyran SE, Maisells MJ. Neonatal pancytopenia and severe combined immunodeficiency associated with antenatal administration of azathioprine and prednisone. J Pediatr 1984;105:625–8.
55. Davison JM, Dellagrammatikas H, Partkin JM. Maternal azathioprine therapy and depressed haemopoieses in the babies of renal allograft patients. Br J Obstet Gynaecol 1985;92:233–9.
56. Lawson DH, Lovatt GE, Gurton CS, Hennings RC. Adverse effects of azathioprine. Adverse Drug React Acute Poisoning Rev 1984;3:161-74.
57. Present DH, Meltzer SJ, Krumholz MP, Wolke A, Korelitz BI. 6-Mercaptopurine in the management of inflammatory bowel disease: Short- and long-term toxicity. Ann Intern Med 1989;111:641–9.
58. Vender RJ, Spiro HM. Inflammatory bowel disease and pregnancy. J Clin Gastroenterol 1982;4:231–49.
59. Royal College of General Practitioners. Oral Contraceptives and Health. New York, Pitman, 1974.
60. Ramcharan S, Pellegrin FA, Ray R, Hsu JP. The Walnut Creek Contraceptive Drug Study. A Prospective Study of the Side Effects of Oral Contraceptives. 1981. DHEW publication no. 74–562. Washington, DC.
61. Vessey M, Jewell D, Smith A, Yeates D, McPherson K. Chronic inflammatory bowel disease, cigarette smoking and use of oral contraceptives: Findings in a large cohort study of women of childbearing age. Br Med J (Clin Res) 1986;292:1101–3.
62. Calkins BM, Mendeloff AI, Garland C. Inflammatory bowel disease in oral contraceptive users (letter). Gastroenterology 1986;91:523–4.
63. Lesko S, Kaufman D, Rosenberg L, Helmrich SP, Miller DR, Stolley PD, Shapiro S. Evidence for an increased risk of Crohn's disease in oral contraceptive users. Gastroenterology 1985;89:1046–9.
64. Lashner BA, Kane SV, Hanauer SB. Lack of association between oral contraceptive use and Crohn's disease: A community based matched case control study. Gastroenterology 1989;97:1442–7.

65. Lashner BA, Kane SV, Hanauer SB. Lack of association between oral contraceptive use and ulcerative colitis. Gastroenterology 1990;99:1032–6.
66. Hurwitz RL, Martin AJ, Grossman BE, Waddell WR. Oral contraceptives and gastrointestinal disorders. Ann Surg 1970;172:892–6.
67. Morowitz DA, Epstein BH. Spectrum of bowel disease associated with use of oral contraceptives. Med Ann DC 1973;42:6–10.
68. Bonfils S, Hervoir P, Girodet J, LeQuintrec Y, Bader JP, Gastard J. Acute spontaneously recovering ulcerative colitis: Report of 6 cases. Am J Dig Dis 1977;22:429–36.
69. Simon L, Figus AI. Colite ulcereuse spontaneous regressive: Consequence des anti conceptionnels. Gastroenterol Clin Biol 1978;2:422–3.
70. Camelleri M, Schafler K, Chadwick VS, Hodgeson HJ, Weinbren K. Periportal sinusoidal dilatation, inflammatory bowel disease and the contraceptive pill. Gastroenterology 1981;80:810–5.
71. Tedesco FJ, Volpicelli NA, Moore FS. Estrogen and progesterone associated colitis: A disorder with clinical and endoscopic features mimicking Crohn's colitis. Gastrointest Endosc 1982;28:247–9.
72. Woermann B, Hoechter W, Ottenjann R. Drug-induced colitis. Dtsch Med Wochenschr 1985;110:1504-9.
73. Grimmer SFM, Back DJ, Orme J L'E, Cowie A, Gilmore I, Tijia J. The bioavailability of ethinyloestradiol and levonorgestrel in patients with an ileostomy. Contraception 1986;33:51–9.
74. Nilsson LO, Victor A, Kral JG, Johansson EDB, Kock NG. Absorption of an oral contraceptive gestagen in ulcerative colitis before and after proctocolectomy and construction of a continent ileostomy. Contraception 1985;31:195–204.
75. Philipson BM, Brandberg A, Jagenburg R, Kock NG, Lager I, Ahren C. Mucosal morphology, bacteriology, and absorption in intraabdominal ileostomy reservoir. Scand J Gastroenterol 1975;10:145–53.
76. Kay RM, Cohen Z, Siu KP, Petrunka CN, Strasberg SM. Ileal excretion and bacterial modification of bile acids and cholesterol in patients with continent ileostomy. Gut 1979;21:128–32.
77. Victor A, Odlind V, Kral JG. Oral contraceptive absorption and sex hormone binding globulins in obese women: Effects of jejunoileal bypass. Gastroenterol Clin North Am 1987;16:483–91.
78. Braverman DZ, Johnson ML, Kern F Jr. Effects of pregnancy and contraceptive steroids on gallbladder function. N Engl J Med 1980;302:362–4.
79. Lee SP, Maher K, Nicholls JF. Origin and fate of biliary sludge. Gastroenterology 1988;94:170–6.
80. Maringhini A, Ciambra M, Baccelliere P, Raimondo M, Pagliaro L. Sludge, stones and pregnancy. Gastroenterology 1988;95:1160–1.
81. Van-Beek EJ, Farmer KC, Millar DM, Brummelkamp WH. Gallstone disease in women younger than 30 years. Neth J Surg 1991;43:60–2.
82. Sali A, Oates JN, Acton CM, Elzarka A, Vitetta L. Effect of pregnancy on gallstone formation. Aust N Z J Obstet Gynaecol 1989;29:386–9.
83. Basso L, McCollum PT, Darling MR, Tocchi A, Tanner WA. A study of cholelithiasis during pregnancy and its relationship with age, parity, menarche, breast-feeding, dysmenorrhea, oral contraception and a maternal history of cholelithiasis. Surg Gynecol Obstet 1992;175:41–6.
84. Petitti DB, Sidney S, Perlman JA. Increased risk of cholecystectomy in users of supplemental estrogen. Gastroenterology 1988;94:91–5.
85. Gallstones: Epidemiological adverse versus preventive stalemate (editorial). Lancet 1990;335:21–2.
86. Boston Collaborative Drug Surveillance Program. Surgically confirmed gallbladder disease, venous thromboembolism, and breast tumors in relation to post-menopausal estrogen therapy. N Engl J Med 1974;290:15–9.
87. Everson RB, Byar DP, Bischoff AJ. Estrogen predisposes to cholecystectomy but not to stones. Gastroenterolgoy 1982;82:4–8.
88. The Coronary Drug Project Research Group. Gallbladder disease as a side effect of drugs influencing lipid metabolism: Experience in the Coronary Drug Project. N Engl J Med 1977;296:1185–90.
89. Hould FS, Fried GM, Fazekas AG, Tremblay S, Mersereau WA. Progesterone receptors regulate gallbladder motility. J Surg Res 1988;45:505–12.

90. Anderson JB, Turner GM, Williamson RCN. Fulminant ulcerative colitis in late pregnancy and the puerperium. J R Soc Med 1987;80:492–4.
91. Heuman R, Larsson-Cohn ELF, Hammar M, Tiselius H. Effects of postmenopausal ethinyl estradiol treatment on gallbladder bile. Maturitas 1980;2:69–72.
92. Tritapepe R, DiPadova C, Zuin R, Bellomi M, Podda M. Lithogenic bile after conjugated estrogen. N Engl J Med 1976;295:961–2.
93. Everson GT, Fennessey P, Kern F Jr. Contraceptive steroids alter the steady-state kinetics of bile acids. J Lipid Res 1988;29:68–76.
94. Haemmerli UP. Jaundice during pregnancy. Acta Med Scand Suppl 1966;444:7–99.
95. Rustgi VK. Liver disease in pregnancy. Med Clin North Am 1989;73:1041–6.
96. Adeniyi FA, Olatunbosun DA. Origins and significance of the increased plasma alkaline phosphatase during normal pregnancy and pre-eclampsia. Br J Obstet Gynaecol 1984;91:857–62.
97. Carter J. Liver function in normal pregnancy. Aust N Z J Obstet Gynaecol 1990;30:296–302.
98. Arevalo JA. Hepatitis B in pregnancy. West J Med 1989;150:668–74.
99. Schweitzer I, Dunn A, Peters R, Spears R. Viral hepatitis B in neonates and infants. Am J Med 1973;55:762–71.
100. Inoue Y, Miyamura T, Unayama T, Takahashi K, Saito I. Maternal transfer of HCV. Nature 1991;353:609.
101. Smithwick EM, Pascual E, Go SC. Hepatitis-associated antigen. A possible relationship to premature delivery. J Pediatr 1972;81:537–40.
102. Sims CJ, Porter KB, Knuppel RA. Successful pregnancy after a liver transplant. Am J Obstet Gynecol 1989;161:532–3.
103. Mishell DR, Davajan V. Reproductive Endocrinology, Infertility and Contraception. Philadelphia, FA Davis, 1979, p 505.
104. Howat JMT, Jones CB, Schofield PF. Gallstones and oral contraceptives. J Int Med Res 1975;3:59.
105. Khoo SK, Correy J. Contraception and the "high-risk" woman. Med J Aust 1981;1:60–8.
106. Shortell CK, Schwartz SI. Hepatic adenoma and focal nodular hyperplasia. Surg Gynecol Obstet 1991;173:426–31.
107. Rosenberg L. The risk of liver neoplasia in relation to combined oral contraceptive use. Contraception 1991;43:643–52.
108. The WHO Collaborative Study on Neoplasia and Steroid Contraceptives. Combined oral contraceptives and liver cancer. Int J Cancer 1989;43:254–9.
109. Grimes DA, ed. The Contraception Report: Highlights from the 1991 AAFP Symposium. Vol II, No. 5. 1991, pp 7–8.
110. Everson GT. Hepatic cysts in autosomal dominant polycystic kidney disease. May Clin Proc 1990;65:1020–5.

Bibliography

Donaldson RM Jr. Management of medical problems in pregnancy—Inflammatory bowel disease. N Engl J Med 1985;312:1616–9.
Fielding JF. Pregnancy and inflammatory bowel disease. Ir J Med Sci 1982;151:194–202.
Hanan IM, Kirsner JB. Inflammatory bowel disease in the pregnant woman. Clin Perinatol 1985;12:669–82.
Miller JP. Inflammatory bowel disease in pregnancy. A review. J R Soc Med 1986;76:221–5.
Questions and Answers about Pregnancy in Ileitis and Colitis. National Foundation for Ileitis and Colitis, 295 Madison Avenue, New York, NY 10017 (212-685-3440).
Warsof SL. Medical and surgical treatment of inflammatory bowel disease in pregnancy. Clin Obstet Gynecol 1983;26:826–31.

9

Endocrine Diseases

Diabetes Mellitus

Diabetes mellitus affects some 5.5 to 12 million individuals in the United States,[1,2] with insulin-dependent diabetes mellitus making up about 10% of this number.[3] In addition to those individuals with diabetes, depending on the diagnostic criteria, about 2.4 to 5.0% of all pregnancies are associated with gestational diabetes.[4,5] Women with gestational diabetes have diabetes during pregnancy, with abnormal glucose tolerance returning to normal postpartum. Many women with gestational diabetes develop clinical diabetes and diabetic complications as they get older. Another 8 to 10% of women of reproductive age have impaired glucose tolerance without clinical diabetes mellitus.[6] Prepregnancy medical care and contraceptive counseling are important, as women with diabetes mellitus are at increased risk for both maternal morbidity during pregnancy and fetal morbidity and mortality.[7,8] They may also have a higher rate of congenital abnormalities in offspring, possibly from poor diabetic control at the time of conception.[8,9]

Fertility and Diabetes Mellitus

Diabetes that is uncontrolled can affect fertility in both men and women.[10–13] Studies in women have shown that diabetes can delay the onset of menarche and increase the prevalence of primary amenorrhea, secondary amenorrhea, and oligomenorrhea.[11] Studies in rats have demonstrated a decrease in testicular function and fertility potential associated with diabetes.[12,13] However, fertility rates and the length of the fertile period have risen significantly among diabetic individuals during the past 20 years, secondary to improved metabolic control.[10]

Effects of Pregnancy on Diabetes Mellitus

Prior to the insulin era, 65% of pregnancies ended in perinatal death and the maternal death rate was 30%.[14] This has been markedly reduced with extensive medical care during pregnancy.

Concerns exist regarding pregnancy and possible microvascular complications, particularly diabetic retinopathy and nephropathy. Retinopathy is an extremely common complication in individuals with insulin-dependent diabetes, occurring in almost 100% of those who have had diabetes for over 15 years. Some of these individuals will have a more severe, progressive form of retinopathy called proliferative retinopathy. The progression of retinopathy appears to be worse in those individuals who have poor glycemic control, proteinuria, and high blood pressure and who smoke. In addition, pregnancy may lead to a progression in diabetic retinopathy. Carstensen et al. compared 44 insulin-dependent diabetic women who had one or two complete pregnancies with matched diabetic women who had never been pregnant.[15] No differences were found between the two groups in complication rates including eye, renal, or neuropathy problems. However, women with preexisting renal or eye problems in whom complications with pregnancy may have been the most severe were excluded. Klein et al. prospectively followed diabetic retinopathy in a group of diabetic women who were pregnant compared to a control group of diabetic women who were not pregnant.[16] After adjustments for glycosylated hemoglobin, those women with a current pregnancy had an elevated risk of progression of their retinopathy of 2.3.

In past years, women with severe proliferative retinopathy were advised to terminate a pregnancy.[17] However, it is important to evaluate studies performed since the advent of laser photocoagulation and better measurement and control of diabetes. Berk et al. reviewed seven studies of retinopathy in pregnant diabetic women.[18] Overall, the results suggest that women with no preexisting retinopathy before pregnancy appear at low risk of developing retinopathy during pregnancy. Of those with background retinopathy, progression may occur in a small group of women but with frequent regression following pregnancy. However, only one of the studies included a control group of nonpregnant diabetic women so it is difficult to assess whether the effects were from pregnancy or from the natural course of diabetes. Proliferative retinopathy is a much less frequent event in these studies, as it takes longer to develop in individuals with diabetes. Of the 505 pregnancies evaluated in this review, only 39 women had proliferative retinopathy, of which 19 had progression during pregnancy. Photocoagulation before pregnancy seemed to have a favorable effect on the progression of retinopathy during pregnancy. Ophthalmologic evaluation before pregnancy may be of significant benefit in preventing the progression of proliferative disease. It would seem that termination of pregnancy would only be needed in those women with the more severe cases of proliferative retinopathy unresponsive to photocoagulation.

Another major complication of diabetes is nephropathy, occurring in about 20 to 25% of individuals with diabetes. Few large studies have examined the long-term effects of pregnancy on diabetic nephropathy, particularly studies that include long-term follow-up and nonpregnant controls. However, there have been several small studies evaluating the effect of pregnancy on nephropathy.[18–23] These studies indicated that pregnancy with preexisting nephropathy leads to an increase in proteinuria in many women that resolves in 50% or more of cases. Creatinine clearance and serum creatinine levels do not appear to be adversely affected. In addition, the long-term progression to end-stage renal disease does not seem to be different from that in historic controls. These individuals do seem at increased risk of anemia, hypertension, and preeclampsia during pregnancy.[23]

The impact of pregnancy on other complications such as cardiac disease, peripheral vascular disease, and neuropathy is limited to findings in case reports without providing any definite conclusions. While pregnancy is not a contraindication in women with diabetes, the long-term prognosis needs to be discussed with these individuals and their partners, preferably before a pregnancy. In addition, a thorough medical evaluation should be performed before pregnancy to assess the extent of diabetic complications. A complete physical examination evaluating the degree of diabetic complications should be done at that time. Also, laboratory studies should be ordered and include hemoglobin A_{1c}, creatinine clearance, thyroxine (T_4) and thyroid-stimulating hormone (TSH), urinary protein, and serum lipids. Thyroid function tests are most important in those women with insulin-dependent diabetes mellitus, since this group has a high association with autoimmune thyroid disease. Those women with diabetes for over 10 years and in particular those with renal dysfunction should have an evaluation of cardiac function.

Effect of Diabetes Mellitus on Pregnancy

Women with diabetes mellitus are at greater risk of maternal morbidity and fetal mortality and morbidity including congenital malformations.[24–30] It is thought that there is a toxic effect of abnormal glucose metabolism on the developing embryo leading to teratogenicity, including spontaneous abortions and congenital malformations. In one study the relative risk for major malformation among infants of mothers with insulin-dependent diabetes mellitus was 7.9, compared to infants of nondiabetic mothers.[31] Types of defects include central nervous system defects, cleft palate and lip, anophthalmia and microphthalmia, cataracts, congenital heart lesions, tracheoesophageal fistula, pyloric stenosis, small-intestine atresia, limb defects, and anomalies of the spine. However, with tighter metabolic control, particularly during the first trimester, the risk of these complications is diminished. Rosenn et al. studied the effect of preconception counseling and tighter control before pregnancy in insulin-dependent diabetics.[32] In the study group, who had significantly lower glycohemoglobin values, the rate of spontaneous abortion was 7%, compared to 24% in the control group. There was one major congenital malformation in the control group and none in the study group. Steel et al.[33] and Kitzmiller et al.[34] found similar effectiveness in prepregnancy counseling in reducing the incidence of major congenital malformations. Oral hypoglycemic agents have also been reported to be associated with congenital malformations.[35] In one study, congenital malformations were found in 20 of 40 women on hypoglycemic agents compared to only 6 of 40 non–insulin-dependent pregnant diabetic women not exposed to oral hypoglycemic drugs. The exposed group also had infants with ear anomalies not commonly seen in diabetic embryopathy.

Diabetic ketoacidosis is a serious complication during pregnancy but seems to be declining in prevalence in recent years.[18] Potential problems of ketoacidosis during pregnancy include fetal hypoxemia and severe electrolyte deficits.[18,36,37] However, with the institution of more strict glycemic control in these women, the risk of insulin-induced hypoglycemia becomes more significant. While minor episodes are not a major problem, prolonged, untreated episodes, particularly if seizures occur, could be a threat to the health of the fetus. Effects to the fetus include decreased fetal heart rate and an association with infant respiratory distress syndrome.[38,39] Berk et al. reported that over 50% of their pregnant women with diabetes experienced during pregnancy more than 10 episodes of significant hypoglycemia requiring help from others.[38]

Women with diabetes mellitus and renal involvement may be at greater risk during pregnancy. Reece et al. reported on 31 pregnancies complicated by diabetic nephropathy.[22] Live births occurred in 29 of the pregnancies at a mean gestational age of 36 weeks, with stillbirths occurring in two women. Seventy percent of the infants were appropriate for gestational age while 16% were small and 13% were large. Other complications included respiratory distress syndrome in 19%, hyperbilirubinemia in 26%, and congenital malformations in 10%. This group of authors felt that the risks and outcomes were similar to those of other insulin-dependent diabetics without renal involvement, and with good prenatal and neonatal care, pregnancies should not be contraindicated in this group of women.[22] Combs and Kitzmiller, in their review of 100 cases of pregnant women with diabetic nephropathy, found a significant number of cases of preeclampsia, cesarean sections, and preterm delivery.[23]

Diabetes Mellitus and Contraception

Contraceptive counseling is essential in any individual. However, contraception counseling becomes even more critical in diabetic women to prevent fetal problems, including congenital malformations, associated with a pregnancy where diabetes is out of control. Good metabolic control becomes essential before women with diabetes become pregnant. As women with diabetes have underlying metabolic problems including hyperglycemia and hyperlipidemia, contraceptive counseling should include explaining the risks of the various alternative methods on their underlying health. The need for contraceptive counseling in these women is demonstrated by a report showing that 40% of the diabetic women studied failed to use any contraception and 16% used the rhythm method.[40] Unfortunately, while there are many contraceptive choices for these women, none is entirely satisfactory. In any patient with diabetes, the physician must consider

- The severity and duration of the diabetes
- The number of diabetic complications or other associated medical problems
- The risk of pregnancy to the individual
- The individual's and partner's compliance, motivation, and preference of contraception

Compliance issues may be of particular concern in adolescents with diabetes. These individuals often are poorly compliant with their insulin, often have diabetes out of control, and are at high risk for pregnancy. Thus, teens with diabetes need highly effective contraceptive methods.

Hopefully, the chosen method will be as reliable as possible without hindering metabolic control. Fontbonne et al. studied 209 women with diabetes in France and found that the most common forms chosen in these women were the intrauterine device (IUD) (32% of users), hormonal contraceptives (27%), barrier and natural methods (27%), and tubal ligation (14%).[41] Most of the women using hormonal contraceptives used progestin-only methods.

Hormonal contraceptives in women with diabetes mellitus usually raise the most concern among these individuals and their physicians. The major concerns involve the possibility of a decrease in glycemic control and an increase in the risk of vascular complications.

The effect of contraceptives on carbohydrate metabolism has been most intensively researched in nondiabetic women using oral contraception. Since the early 1960s, at least 200 reports have been published on this topic. In evaluating these studies, it is important to consider that many of the studies were done in the 1960s and early 1970s when oral contraceptives contained estrogen doses significantly larger (> 50 µg of ethinyl estradiol) than pills used today.

The results of some of these studies demonstrate a decrease in glucose tolerance in women on oral contraceptives.[42–50] These women have a response similar to that of women with type II diabetes (non–insulin-dependent diabetes) with a blunting of the initial rise in insulin followed by hyperinsulinemia. The decrease in glucose tolerance is more common in those individuals with gestational diabetes mellitus, obesity, or a family history of diabetes. Gaspard and Lefebvre reviewed 22 studies of 867 women with normal glucose tolerance and found that 3.9% developed glucose intolerance after 1 to 48 months of use of high-dose oral contraceptives.[50] However, the latest findings from the Royal College of General Practitioners, with data available up to May 1989, demonstrate no evidence of an increased risk of glucose intolerance among current users, even for those on oral contraceptives over 10 years, or for former users.[51] Similar negative results have also been found in other studies.[52,53]

Both estrogens and progestins have been implicated in possible alterations of glucose metabolism. Estrogen-induced changes have been thought to result from either insulin resistance as a result of increases in growth hormone or cortisol, or a reduction in insulin receptors.[42,54] With lower doses of estrogen, the progestins have been under scrutiny in influencing glucose tolerance. Hyperinsulinemia and reduced insulin receptors have been reported in women using oral contraceptives containing levonorgestrel independent of estrogen dose.[55] In a study by Spellacy et al., results demonstrated a 5- to 10-mg/dL increase in serum glucose per milligram of estrane progestins in a 1- and 2-hour glucose tolerance test compared to an 18- to 35-mg/dL increase per milligram of norgestrel.[56] However, as norgestrel is used in lower amounts, its effect on carbohydrate metabolism may be comparable. Both the dose of progestin and the type are important in carbohydrate metabolism. Several studies have demonstrated that the largest effect on glucose tolerance is with the gonane derivative norgestrel, while estrane derivatives, such as norethindrone or ethynodiol diacetate, moderately affect them, and megestrol acetate, a 17-acetoxyprogesterone derivative, does not affect glucose tolerance.[56–58] The newest progestins include three gonane progestins (desogestrel, gestodene, and norgestimate). Combination pills with either desogestrel and norgestimate are currently available in the United States. These progestins appear to have minimal effect on carbohydrate metabolism.[59–61] Overall, most studies using lower-dose pills with reduced progestin content demonstrate a low risk, if any, of impaired glucose tolerance.[7,10,50,57]

Another group studied have been those women with gestational diabetes. Some studies have suggested that combined oral contraceptives might negatively impact on glucose tolerance in women with prior gestational diabetes.[62,63] For example, Kung et al. found that 27% of women with gestational diabetes developed glucose intolerance while on a low-dose triphasic oral contraceptive while no women in the group with gestational diabetes using an IUD developed glucose intolerance.[63] However, numerous other recent studies did not find significant problems with glucose tolerance in this group of women while on oral contraceptives.[64–69] Skouby et al. evaluated a low-dose triphasic oral contraceptive (ethinyl estradiol/levonorgestrel) in 16 women with previous gestational diabetes.[65] There were no changes in glucose, insulin, and glucagon responses to oral glucose as compared to measurements before the start of the oral contraceptives. There were also no changes in lipoproteins and high-density-lipoprotein (HDL) cholesterol–total cholesterol ratios. Kjos et al. found no difference in glucose tolerance between women with recent gestational diabetes mellitus who were randomly assigned to either ethinyl estradiol/norethindrone, ethinyl estradiol/levonorgestrel, or a nonoral contraceptive method.[66] The prevalence of diabetes at 6 to 13 months was also similar between the groups: 17% in the nonoral contraceptive group, 15% in the ethinyl estradiol/norethindrone group, and 20% in the ethinyl estradiol/levonorgestrel group. Skouby et al. also evaluated glucose tolerance in gestational diabetics on oral contraceptives, using the euglycemic clamp technique.[67] In this technique the amount of glucose needed to maintain a predetermined serum glucose level is determined while insulin is infused at a steady rate. In the Skouby study, six nondiabetic women were compared to six women with gestational diabetes before and after use of triphasic oral contraceptives containing ethinyl estradiol and levonorgestrel for 6 months. While there was a decrease in insulin sensitivity in those women with gestational diabetes, this was not sufficient to alter glucose tolerance as measured by serum glucose and insulin levels. Overall, while there may be subtle changes in glucose metabolism in women on oral contraceptives who have a history of gestational diabetes, low-dose oral contraceptives appear safe in these women for at least limited periods of time.

Of major concern has been the effect of oral contraceptives in those women with already existing diabetes mellitus. Several studies have examined directly the effect of oral contraceptives on glycemic control in women with diabetes. Skouby et al. compared the metabolic effects of four oral contraceptives (monophasic nonalkylated estrogen/norethindrone, low-dose monophasic ethinyl estradiol/norethindrone, progestin-only using norethindrone, and triphasic ethinyl estradiol/levonorgestrel) in insulin-dependent diabetic women.[70] During the 6-month study, there were no differences in fasting glucose, 24-hour insulin requirements, glycosylated hemoglobin, low-density-lipoprotein (LDL) cholesterol levels or HDL cholesterol–total cholesterol ratio between each treatment group. There was a slight increase in triglycerides and very-low-density-lipoprotein (VLDL) cholesterol in the monophasic ethinyl estradiol/norethindrone group. In a study of insulin requirements among 50 women with insulin-dependent diabetes who took oral contraceptives for 1 year, there were no significant changes in insulin requirements, hemoglobin A_{1c} levels and no difficulties in diabetic control.[10] The oral contraceptive used in this study, however, contained 1 mg of norethindrone and a nonalkylated estrogen not used in the United States. It was felt by Skouby et al. that the nonalkylated natural estrogens may have less adverse metabolic effects than the artificial 17-c alkylated estrogens like ethinyl estradiol and mestranol. In another study, Steel and Duncan evaluated 88 insulin-dependent women taking a combination low-dose oral contraceptive.[71] There were no changes in insulin requirements in 81% of the women, with 17% requiring an increase of 8 to 20 units/day and 2% requiring an increase of 20 to 40 units/day. There were no problems in maintaining control of their glucose levels. Similar findings were demonstrated in another study of 38 insulin-dependent diabetic women on either combined pills or progestin-only pills, in which the average increase in insulin dose was 7%.[72] Thus, glycemic control does not seem to be a major problem in insulin-dependent diabetic women on oral contraceptives.

The other major concern in prescribing oral contraceptives for women with diabetes is the potential effect on vascular disease, especially since these women are already atherosclerotic prone. This is a more difficult question to answer since the number of women with insulin-dependent diabetes on oral contraceptives who have been followed for long periods of time in controlled studies is relatively small.

Current researchers argue that oral contraceptives' potential negative impact on vascular disease is secondary to their impact on the lipoprotein profile. Evidence suggests that the risk of coronary heart disease is correlated to the level of LDL cholesterol and inversely related to HDL cholesterol.[73–75] The HDL_2 subfraction is felt to be particularly protective. Of greatest concern in recent years has been the reported decrease in HDL cholesterol by progestins, seemingly in proportion to their degree of androgenicity.[76–78] In fact, the Royal College of General Practitioners study demonstrated a direct relationship between the amount of progestins in oral contraceptives and the incidence of major vascular disease.[79]

Two studies evaluating women with insulin-dependent diabetes taking oral contraceptives failed to find changes in lipoproteins or HDL fractions.[72,80] These researchers felt that oral contraceptives could be used in women with diabetes but that pills with a low dose of progestin (< 1 mg of norethindrone or 150 µg of levonorgestrel) should be used. Skouby and coworkers, using norethisterone alone or with either a nonalkylated estrogen or levonorgestrel, found no adverse effects on lipid metabolism.[69] However, in this study, the monophasic combination of ethinyl estradiol and norethisterone had a small but significant negative change in lipoprotein levels. Godsland et al. examined the correlation between various types of oral contraceptives and effect on lipids in nondiabetic women.[58,81] These two studies indicate that oral contraceptives containing levonorgestrel and high-dose norethindrone (1000 µg) had the most negative impact on LDL and HDL cholesterol, while either combination pills containing low-dose norethindrone (500 µg) or desogestrel (150 µg), or progestin-only pills had the most favorable metabolic profile.

There are no prospective studies showing a significant increase in cardiac and cerebrovascular complications in women with diabetes using oral contraceptives. In one retrospective study of women with diabetes, there was no association between current or past use or number of years of use of oral contraceptives with severity of retinopathy or hypertension.[82] The one other retrospective study examining vascular side effects in insulin-dependent diabetics women on oral contraceptives was done in the 1970s.[83] In this study, 120 insulin-dependent diabetic patients taking oral contraceptives were compared with 156 diabetic patients who had never been on an oral contraceptive agent.[83] Five women in the first group who were less than 30 years old had a major vascular event, including three with cerebral thrombosis, one with a myocardial infarction, and one with an axillary vein thrombosis, compared with one myocardial infarction in a woman aged 43 in the nonuser group. The estrogen content in the five users with complications was 30 µg of ethinyl estradiol in three women and 50 µg in two of the women. The prevalence of proliferative retinopathy in both groups was the same, but there was a suggestion that the patients using the pill had a more accelerated course. One patient had rapidly progressive retinopathy and nephropathy 3 months after starting oral contraceptives. However, it is difficult to draw conclusions from this isolated study involving pills available in the 1970s.

A last potential minor complication in using oral contraceptives in women with diabetes mellitus is the potential of monilial vaginitis. Monilial vaginitis is a known complication of diabetes mellitus. While oral contraceptives have been associated with recurrent yeast infections, the relationship between low-dose oral contraceptive use and this problem is not clear. In women with diabetes who have a history of recurrent monilial vaginitis, an alternative contraceptive method might be considered, particularly if the problem worsened or became uncontrollable on oral contraceptives.

The progestin-only pills are potential good contraceptives for women with diabetes and are preferred by some practitioners for this group of women.[7,71] Progestin-only pills do not seem to increase the prevalence of coronary or cerebrovascular disease.[84] Steel and Duncan evaluated 45 insulin-dependent diabetic women taking norethisterone, 0.35 mg/day.[71] They found no changes in insulin requirement, blood pressure, and retinopathy. Plasma lipoprotein levels were also normal in the 20 patients in whom they were measured. No pregnancies occurred in their study group. A disadvantage with progestin-only oral contraceptives is their higher failure rate (6/100 compared with 3.5/100 for combined oral contraceptives) and a high incidence of irregular bleeding. Depomedroxyprogesterone acetate (DMPA) and the Norplant implant have very low failure rates and minimal metabolic side effects, providing other reasonable alternatives for these women. There are no studies available that have examined the use of either DMPA or the Norplant in women with diabetes. Since progestins may have minor alterations on glucose and lipid metabolism, these women would have to be monitored during use.

Adolescents with diabetes mellitus are of special concern. Fennoy found that this group was at higher risk than expected to become pregnant at a time when their diabetic control was often at its worse.[85] This population also usually has fewer vascular complications than the adult population. Thus, hormonal preparations may be even more appropriate in this population than in adult women with diabetes. In particular, with noncompliant adolescents with diabetes mellitus, DMPA or the Norplant implant may be a good alternative. However, more research is needed in adolescents with diabetes mellitus to determine the safest contraceptive in this population at high risk for pregnancy.

Because of the limited amount of information available from well-controlled prospective studies, recommendations regarding hormonal contraceptive use in women with either a family history of diabetes, gestational diabetes, or insulin-dependent diabetes vary. Contraceptive Technology lists these three conditions as considerations "that may suggest that pills are not the ideal contraception."[84] In his book on contraceptive care, Dickey recommended that for women with a family history of diabetes, a normal 2-hour postprandial blood glucose level of under 105 mg/dL be obtained and that the glucose measurement be repeated after 3, 6, and 12 months and yearly thereafter when oral contraceptives are used.[86] He advised against oral contraceptives in women with either gestational or insulin-dependent diabetes. Derman advised extreme caution in using oral contraceptives in women with diabetes, but that low-dose pills could be used in women in whom the risk of pregnancy outweighs the risk of the oral contraceptives.[87] In their review, Breckwoldt et al. felt that low-dose oral contraceptives could be used for a limited duration in healthy young women with diabetes with careful monitoring. In those women with vascular lesions, oral contraceptives would be contraindicated.[88] The Medical Task Force of the Family Planning Federation of Australia developed guidelines for contraceptive use in women with diabetes.[8] Its conclusion was that the benefits of combined low-dose oral contraceptives outweigh the potential risks of impairment to glycemic control or of vascular disease. The Task Force recommended low-dose oral contraceptives as the method of choice for most women with diabetes. However, oral contraceptives were not favored if a woman had an additional risk factor such as smoking, hypertension, or obesity or was over the age of 35. The Task Force also felt there was uncertainty about the use of oral contraceptives for over 10 years in these women. The Task Force believed that progestin-only pills had no special advantage in women with diabetes and were associated with a higher failure rate. The Task Force did not address the use of DMPA or the Norplant implant.

The IUD has been considered as an alternative to oral contraceptives. The major risk of the IUD is the potential for pelvic inflammatory disease (PID). The risk for PID is particularly elevated in adolescents and in those women with multiple partners.[89,90] There is no evidence to suggest that women with diabetes are at a higher risk for PID than nondiabetic women; however, PID could cause a significant worsening in diabetic control or cause an episode of diabetic ketoacidosis. Because of the risk of PID, the IUD is primarily useful in women in a stable monogamous relationship.

Some researchers have reported higher failure rates of the IUD in women with diabetes.[90,91] In the study by Gosden et al., 11 (36%) of 30 women with insulin-dependent diabetes became pregnant within 1 year of being fitted with an IUD. The pregnancy rate for nondiabetic women treated by the same consultant was 4% (4/100). They examined IUDs removed from diabetic and nondiabetic women. They found that 40% of IUDs removed from diabetic women had sulfur and chloride deposits, compared with 15.3% of IUDs from nondiabetic women. Also, fewer IUDs from diabetic women had calcareous deposits. IUDs from nondiabetic women who became pregnant with the IUD also had depositions similar to those of diabetic women. The outcome of pregnancies in the women having an IUD in situ was poor. Of the 11 diabetic women becoming pregnant with an IUD, 6 requested termination, 1 had a spontaneous abortion at 12 weeks, another aborted an abnormal fetus at 24 weeks, and 2 had a successful outcome.[91] However, other studies have not demonstrated any difference in pregnancy rates in diabetic women with an IUD.[92–94] Skouby et al., in a study of 103 women with insulin-dependent diabetes and 199 women without diabetes, found no difference in pregnancy rate, IUD removal rate, PID rate, and discontinuation rate between the two groups.[94] After 12 months there were no differences between IUDs removed from the diabetic women and those from nondiabetic women in regards to the biochemical composition of the corrosion products or the maximum depth of corrosion.[94] The Medical Advisory Panel of the Family Planning Association (UK) concluded that insufficient evidence exists to condemn use of the IUD in diabetic women.[95] However, the IUD cannot be recommended for diabetic women if the individual is nulliparous or not involved in a stable monogamous relationship.

Barrier methods are without significant side effects in women with diabetes, although they do have higher failure rates than hormonal contraceptives or the IUD. Some barrier methods, particularly the diaphragm, may increase the risk of urinary tract infection, which could be a problem in women with diabetes. Steel reported on 69 women with insulin-dependent diabetes using either the condom, diaphragm, or both.[71] There were three pregnancies in the group using condoms alone and three in the group using the diaphragm alone. No failures occurred in those women using both. Barrier methods are an alternative in the well-motivated individual. In addition to their lack of side effects, they also help to lower the risk of sexually transmitted diseases.

Another contraceptive alternative is sterilization in couples who have completed their family. In couples in which the female partner is diabetic, vasectomy may be the sterilization method of choice as it is a minor surgical procedure and thus avoids a surgical procedure in the diabetic woman.

Summary

1. Vascular complications of women with diabetes increase with age so these individuals should plan to have their families at a relatively early age.

2. Fertility can be decreased in men and women whose diabetes is not well controlled.

3. Pregnancy carries a greater risk in women with diabetes including problems of ketoacidosis and hypoglycemia on the fetus and potential progression of retinopathy and nephropathy. Women with proliferative retinopathy seem to have more progression than women with background retinopathy. Ophthalmologic evaluation is important before pregnancy. Pregnancy leads to an increase in proteinuria in many women, which resolves in about 50% or more. Creatinine clearance and the long-term progression to end-stage renal disease do not appear to be adversely affected.

4. Women with diabetes are at greater risk for fetal morbidity and mortality. This risk is greatly reduced with close management before and during pregnancy. Congenital malformations are also increased in these women, and seem related to poor glycemic control during conception and during pregnancy.

5. Women with diabetes should have close preconception care so as to optimize glycemic control and diabetic complications before pregnancy.

6. Women with insulin-dependent diabetes who have completed their families or those with significant vascular complications should consider sterilization in themselves or their partners.

7. Contraception counseling is essential in these women because of the significant complications associated with pregnancy and poor diabetic control. Adolescents with diabetes may be at particular high risk to become pregnant and to have poorly controlled diabetes. Thus, there is a special need for effective contraception in teens.

8. Combination oral contraceptive pills potentially decrease glucose tolerance, increase insulin requirements, and alter lipoproteins. However, the effects with low-dose combination pills or progestin-only pills appear minimal. A low-dose combination oral contraceptive pill could be recommended to a healthy women with either a family history of diabetes or gestational diabetes. A low-dose combination pill or a progestin-only pill could be used for limited periods of time in women with diabetes. These women will need monitoring of both their glucose and lipoprotein levels. In women with diabetes, the presence of a vascular complication or other risk factors such as hypertension, smoking, or obesity would contraindicate the use of oral contraceptives. If a combination pill is used, the pill should contain no more than 35 µg of estrogen and preferably 1 mg or less of norethindrone. Norethindrone would be preferred to norgestrel as it generally has less effects on the

lipoprotein panel. New pills with either norgestimate or desogestrel are also a reasonable choice. The progestin-only pill is another alternative, although the associated menstrual problems and lower effectiveness are disadvantages.

9. DMPA and the Norplant implant are reasonable alternatives although experience with these methods in women with diabetes is limited.

10. The IUD is another good alternative in women with diabetes who are in a stable monogamous relationship and are not nulliparous. Early studies indicated a decreased effectiveness in women with diabetes but this was not confirmed in more recent studies.

11. Barrier methods usually have no adverse effects in women with diabetes or gestational diabetes and they also lower the risk of sexually transmitted diseases. However, they are less effective then the IUD and hormonal contraceptives. The diaphragm may increase the risk of urinary tract infection. Barrier methods are worth considering in the well-motivated individual.

Thyroid Disease

Thyroid dysfunction is a relatively common disorder in women of reproductive age. The prevalence of thyroid disease during pregnancy is between 0.05 and 3% of pregnancies.[96,97] Autoimmune thyroid disease may be present in as much as 5 to 15% of women in the reproductive age group.[98]

Fertility

Thyroid disorders may have an effect on menses and fertility. Hypothyroidism can be associated with amenorrhea and anovulation in severe cases and menorrhagia in more mild cases.[99] Associated infertility may also be related to a luteal phase defect caused by hyperprolactinemia that is found with hypothyroidism. Mild to moderate thyrotoxicosis does not usually affect fertility; however, severe thyrotoxicosis is more likely associated with menstrual irregularities, anovulation, and infertility.[99] These women often have oligomenorrhea or scanty menstrual flow. Treatment of thyroid disorders can lead to a rebound in fertility and so women should be warned of the increased possibility of pregnancy when treatment is started.

Effect of Pregnancy on Thyroid Disorders

Pregnancy alters the normal physiology of the thyroid and interpretation of laboratory test results. Total serum T_4, triiodothyronine (T_3), and reverse T_3 rise because of elevations in thyroid-binding globulin (TBG) secondary to estrogen. The levels return to normal by about 6 weeks after delivery. However, free T_4 and free T_3 are usually within the normal range to slightly elevated during the first trimester, becoming low normal by the third trimester.[99] The rise in early pregnancy is secondary to the TSH activity of human chorionic gonadotropin (hCG). Thyroid gland size may increase about 20% during pregnancy.

Pregnancy may have an effect on thyroid disorders. Glinoer et al. examined prospectively 120 women with mild thyroid abnormalities including a goiter, thyroid nodules, and thyroid autoantibodies.[100] Those women who were pregnant had either an increase in goiter size, an increase in number or size of thyroid nodules, or indirect evidence of partial thyroidal autonomy. Pregnancy may have a beneficial effect on the course of thyroid diseases that are immune mediated. Thyroid antibody titers may decline during pregnancy and rise postpartum.[101] There has been at least one case reported of hypothyroidism that went into remission during pregnancy, with a postpartum relapse.[102]

In women with mild hyperthyroidism secondary to Graves' disease, pregnancy may lead to an exacerbation of hyperthyroidism at about 10 to 15 weeks of pregnancy.[103,104] However, this may only be a result of higher T_4 levels induced by the TSH effects of hCG in early pregnancy. This is often followed by a remission in late pregnancy which continues until after delivery when most women will again become thyrotoxic. The remission may be due to the general immunosuppressive changes of pregnancy. If autoimmune thyroid disease severity is decreased during pregnancy, treatment may need to be altered. Conversely, a rebound may occur postpartum, with transient or permanent alterations of thyroid function. Thus, women with thyroid abnormalities should be closely monitored during pregnancy.

Pregnancy in most reports appears to have no effect on the course of thyroid cancer and vice versa.[105] However, Fukuda et al. reported on one case of a papillary carcinoma of the thyroid that enlarged during pregnancy.[106]

Effect of Thyroid Disease on Pregnancy

Hyperthyroidism during pregnancy, if left untreated, can have fetal morbidity and mortality rates as high as 50%.[97] The fetus is least likely to be affected in mothers with only moderate hyperthyroidism because the placenta is impermeable to maternal thyroid hormone until moderately high levels are reached.[107] At very high levels, thyroid hormone will cross the placenta and if uncontrolled cause a high rate of premature delivery, fetal demise, and low birthweight.[103,108] In one study of fetal anomalies in pregnant women with Graves' disease, those women treated with methimazole and who became euthyroid had the same prevalence (< 1%) of fetal anomalies as euthyroid untreated mothers.[109] On the other hand, those hyperthyroid mothers who were untreated had a 6% prevalence of fetal anomalies, while partially treated mothers had a prevalence in between that for treated and the rate for untreated women. In another study of thyrotoxicosis in pregnancy, metabolic status at delivery was directly correlated with pregnancy outcome.[110] Women who were treated earlier in pregnancy and who became euthyroid were more likely to have a good pregnancy outcome. Preterm delivery, perinatal mortality, and maternal heart failure occurred mainly in those women who were thyrotoxic despite therapy or who were never treated.

Untreated hypothyroidism is unlikely to lead to a successful pregnancy and is most often associated with anovulation.[111–113] If conception occurs, the prevalence of spontaneous abortion is about 30 to 50% during the first trimester.[111,113] In one study, hypothyroid women had a 20 to 40% prevalence of maternal complications, including anemia, preeclampsia, placental abruptio, and postpartum hemorrhage.[114] In addition, there was a 30% prevalence of low birthweight and 12% prevalence of fetal death. Even in those women with subclinical hypothyroidism, these problems occurred at about one-third the rate of those in women with clinical hypothyroidism.

Medications and Pregnancy

Replacement thyroid hormone during pregnancy, if thyroid levels are kept in normal ranges, is not associated with toxicity during pregnancy and is important to prevent complications related to hypothyroidism. Women with hyperthyroidism have been treated with various modalities including antithyroid medications, surgery, and iodine-131 that could potentially complicate a pregnancy. Antithyroid medications can be used during pregnancy but since they readily cross the placenta, they have the potential to cause fetal hypothyroidism with resulting mental retardation.[115] With antithyroid medications, the practitioner needs to balance the dose needed to avoid significant maternal hyperthyroidism with an amount that will not cause hypothyroidism in the fetus.[116] Uncontrolled maternal hyperthyroidism can be associated with a greater risk than the possible teratogenic effects of methimazole. Iodine-131 is contraindicated during pregnancy because of the possibility of congenital anomalies or ablation of fetal thyroid tissue. Surgery is another option, most often performed during the second trimester. At present, antithyroid medication with either methimazole or propylthiouracil appears to be the treatment of choice.

Thyroid Disease and Contraception

There are few reports on the effects of contraceptives on thyroid disease. No contraindications exist for the use of barrier methods. Decherney, in a review, concluded that there was no evidence that oral contraceptives influence thyroid disease.[117] Phillips et al. found no association between thyroid disease and oral contraceptives or exogenous estrogens when they compared 89 patients with Hashimoto's thyroiditis with controls.[118] However, only a small number of those with thyroid disease were exposed to the hormones. Reports from the Royal College of General Practitioners study and the Walnut Creek study also did not demonstrate an association between oral contraceptives and thyroid disease.[119,120] In fact, the former study demonstrated a lower incidence of thyroid disease in oral contraceptive users, with relative rates of thyrotoxicosis and myxedema in users of 0.71 and 0.57, compared to nonusers. Oral contraceptives were speculated to possibly have an effect on preventing or retarding autoimmune processes.[119] Thus, there appears to be no contraindication to hormonal contraceptives in women with hyperthyroidism or hypothyroidism. While the effect on thyroid disease has not been specifically studied in women using the Norplant implant or DMPA, the same conclusion is likely to be found. Diaz et al. evaluated the effect of Norplant implants and copper T IUDs on thyroid hormones, and found no alterations.[121]

Hormonal contraceptives also may alter thyroid laboratory test results. Oral contraceptives increase TBG, and thus increase total T_4; however, adjusted T_4 levels and free T_4 do not significantly change.[122] Olsson et al. found a decrease in T_4 levels, an increase in T_3 uptake with the Norplant implant, indicating a decrease in TBG.[123] However, the free T_4 index remained unchanged, indicating that free T_4 was not altered.

The possible effects of hormonal contraceptives on thyroid cancer are less clear. In the Walnut Creek study, there was a weakly positive association between hormonal contraceptive use and thyroid cancer.[120] Estrogen and progesterone receptors have been found in both normal thyroid tissue and neoplastic tissue[124,125]; however, differentiated carcinomas and adenomas have a much higher prevalence of estrogen receptors compared with goiters and normal thyroid tissue.[124] One would have to be very cautious in the use of estrogens in a woman with a history of thyroid carcinoma.

Oligomenorrhea and Amenorrhea

Although oligomenorrhea and amenorrhea are symptoms and not chronic illnesses per se, concerns have been expressed regarding the use of hormonal contraception in these conditions. The concerns include the difficulty in diagnosis of pregnancy, the possibility of infertility once hormonal contraceptives are stopped, and the possibility of worsening an underlying pituitary adenoma.

In women with secondary amenorrhea, the underlying etiology should be evaluated before starting hormonal contraceptives, including evaluating for pregnancy. In women with oligomenorrhea without an underlying organic abnormality, menses and fertility usually return after discontinuing oral contraceptives, but at a slightly prolonged time interval as compared to women using other methods of contraception. The average delay in return of ovulation in all women after stopping oral contraceptives is 2 weeks, with a normal range of up to 6 months. Ninety percent of prior pill users conceive by 24 months, compared to 14 months for prior IUD users, 10 months for prior diaphragm users, and 13 months for previous users of "other" methods.[126] The average time to ovulation following the last DMPA injection and ovulation is 4.5 to 5.8 months.[127,128] The median time to conception is 9 to 10 months after the last injection, with a range from 4 to 31 months.[127,128] Women with prolonged posthormonal contraceptive amenorrhea are usually those women with amenorrhea or oligomenorrhea before starting hormonal contraceptives. Before hormonal contraceptives are started in women with either secondary amenorrhea or oligomenorrhea, they should be counseled that after stopping their contraceptive, there may be a delay in return of menstrual cycles.

Pituitary Adenomas

While most young women with oligomenorrhea or secondary amenorrhea will have hypothalamic-pituitary dysfunction, some women will have a pituitary microadenoma. Pituitary tumors are common, with a prevalence of 10 to 25% in autopsy patients.[129–131] The most common pituitary tumors are prolactinomas, with amenorrhea and galactorrhea being the most frequent clinical manifestations.

Pituitary adenomas are associated with a decrease in fertility. In one review of 73 women with pituitary adenomas who desired to become pregnant, only 9% had spontaneous ovulation and 91% needed bromocriptine to conceive.[132]

It is known that pregnancy increases the size of these tumors.[133,134] Magyar and Marshall compared the outcome of pregnancy to whether the patient was untreated or treated before pregnancy or during pregnancy.[135] There were no significant differences in perinatal mortality except that the group treated before pregnancy had a higher risk of prematurity. Patients with adenomas greater than 1.0 cm have as high as a 30% chance of requiring therapy during pregnancy compared to a 3 to 5% risk for women with adenomas less than 1.0 cm. Thus, adenomas greater than 1.0 cm should be treated before pregnancy while adenomas smaller than 1.0 cm could be either followed or treated with medical therapy.

Samaan et al. compared the effects of surgical versus bromocriptine therapy for prolactin-secreting pituitary adenomas diagnosed before pregnancy.[136] Similar rates of complications were found with both modalities. None of the women treated with either method had headaches or visual field changes during subsequent pregnancies.

Bromocriptine is usually the treatment of choice in women with prolactinomas. Because of the anovulatory, amenorrheic state, these women are often estrogen deficient and potentially have an abnormal loss of bone mineralization. Bromocriptine usually lowers prolactin levels to normal, restores ovulatory cycles and fertility, eliminates the estrogen-deficient state, and often reduces tumor size. If possible, bromocriptine should be discontinued before conception or during pregnancy. However, there is no evidence to date that bromocriptine is teratogenic or related to other obstetric complications. Bromocriptine has been continued by some centers throughout pregnancy.[131]

Loriaux and Wild suggested combination oral contraceptives as an alternative treatment to regulate menses and prevent osteoporosis in these women.[131] The question has also been raised regarding the safety of using oral contraceptives to prevent pregnancy in women who become ovulatory after treatment with bromocriptine. In women with a prolactinoma, concern has been expressed as to whether hormonal contraceptives might increase the size of these tumors.[137] Badawy et al. found a relative risk of developing hyperprolactinemia of 2.64 in oral contraceptive users compared to nonusers and a 6.25 relative risk if use started before the age of 25.[137] However, several other studies did not show an association between prolactinomas and oral contraceptive use.[138–140] Voelker et al. did not find evidence that existing adenomas deteriorated during use of oral contraception.[139] However, prospective randomized studies examining the influence of hormonal contraceptives have not been done in women with prolactinomas. In women with microadenomas, hormonal contraceptives could be used with caution and with close monitoring of prolactin levels. The use of hormonal contraceptives would not be recommended in those women with macroadenomas.

Hirsutism

Hirsutism is a frequent problem in women of reproductive age, with a prevalence of about 5%.[141] Hirsutism implies an increased growth of terminal (long, coarse, and pigmented) hair in a degree greater than cosmetically acceptable in a particular culture. Virilism implies the development of male secondary sex characteristics in a women. There are numerous conditions causing hirsutism or virilism that could affect fertility, pregnancy, and contraceptive recommendations. The most common etiologies include idiopathic hirsutism, polycystic ovary syndrome (PCOS), and genetic hirsutism. Other etiologies include ovarian and adrenal tumors, Cushing's syndrome, incomplete 21-hydroxylase or 11β-hydroxylase deficiency, drug-induced hirsutism, and congenital lesions such as Hurler's syndrome.

Infertility

Most androgen excess states are associated with anovulation and fertility problems. PCOS is probably the most common disorder in young adult women causing the combination of hirsutism and infertility. This disorder of the hypothalamic-pituitary-ovarian axis occurs in about 5% of the adolescent and adult populations.[142] The disorder leads to temporary or persistent anovulation and usually hyperandrogenism, with often elevated levels of testosterone, free testosterone, and dehydroepiandrosterone (DHEA) sulfate. Clinical manifestations include amenorrhea (51%) or oligomenorrhea, infertility (74%), hirsutism (69%), and obesity (41%).[143]

Pregnancy

There is no contraindication to pregnancy in women with PCOS; however, they may require clomiphene or gonadotropin therapy to correct the anovulatory state.[142] These women are at risk for developing multiple follicles with the risk of multiple pregnancies.[144] There may also be an associated high pregnancy loss, particularly in those women who are obese or have hyperandrogenism.[145] Androgen-producing adrenal and ovarian tumors should be corrected before conception.

Contraception

Idiopathic hirsutism and PCOS are two common conditions in which combination oral contraceptives may be of significant benefit.[131,143] The androgen excess in these women, being gonadotropin dependent, is decreased by the gonadotropin suppression of combined oral contraceptives and the increase in sex hormone–binding globulin.[131,146] The improvement in hirsutism in women given oral contraceptives usually takes 6 to 9 months. The best results occur from pills that are more estrogenic and less androgenic. The newer progestins are also a good alternative as they have little androgenic activity.

Some women with PCOS have an associated insulin resistance and hyperlipidemia. Because of these cardiovascular risk factors and the obesity that often is present in women with PCOS, their metabolic status should be monitored when they are treated with oral contraceptives.

Progestin-only contraceptives and the IUD are not as good a contraceptive choice for these women. Except for DMPA, none of these contraceptives would suppress luteinizing hormone and so androgen production would not be suppressed. In addition, the progestin pill, the Norplant device, and the copper IUD might exacerbate the already underlying tendency to abnormal uterine bleeding in these women. Barrier methods also do not suppress the androgen excess state and are thus not an ideal choice. Before oral contraceptives are prescribed to hirsute women, it is important to eliminate other causes of hirsutism such as adrenal or ovarian tumors.

References

1. Gregerman RI. Diabetes Mellitus. In Barker LR, Burton JR, Zieve PD, eds. Principles of Ambulatory Medicine. Baltimore, Williams and Wilkins, 1982, p 677.
2. National Diabetes Data Group. Classification and diagnosis of diabetes mellitus and other categories of glucose intolerance. Diabetes 1979;28:1039–57.
3. Francisco GE Jr. Diabetes mellitus. In DiPiro JT, Talbert RL, Hayes PE, Yee GC, Posey LM, eds. Pharmacotherapy. New York, Elsevier, 1989, pp 805–21.
4. Magee MS, Walden CE, Benedetti TJ, Knopp RH. Influence of diagnostic criteria on the incidence of gestational diabetes and perinatal morbidity. JAMA 1993;269:609–15.
5. Cahill GF Jr, Arky RA, Perlman AJ. Diabetes mellitus. In Rubenstein E, Federman DD, eds. Scientific American Medicine. New York, Scientific American, 1987.
6. Mestman JH, Schmidt-Sarosi C. Diabetes mellitus and fertility control: Contraception management issues. Am J Obstet Gynecol 1993;168:2012–20.
7. Judd SJ, Kerin J. Contraception and diabetes mellitus. Clin Reprod Fertil 1986;4:297–304
8. Guidelines on contraception and diabetes mellitus. Aust Fam Physician 1988;17:853.
9. Pedersen J, Molsted-Pedersen L. Congenital malformations: The possible role of diabetes care outside pregnancy. In Pregnancy, Metabolism, Diabetes, and the Fetus. Amsterdam, Excerpta Medica, 1979, pp 265–71.
10. Skouby SO, Jensen BM, Kuhl C, Molsted-Pedersen L, Svenstrup B, Nielsen J. Hormonal contraception in diabetic women: Acceptability and influence on diabetes control and ovarian function of a nonalkylated estrogen/progestin compound. Contraception 1985;32:23–31.
11. Burkart W, Fischer-Guntenhoener E, Standl E, Schneider HP. Menarche, menstrual cycle and fertility in diabetic patients. Geburtshilfe Frauenheilkd 1989;49:149–54.
12. Cameron DF, Rountree J, Schultz RE, Repetta D, Murray FT. Sustained hyperglycemia results in testicular dysfunction and reduced fertility potential in BBWOR diabetic rats. Am J Physiol 1990;259:E881–9.
13. Zeidler A, Shargill NS, Meehan WP, Warren DW. Reproductive defects in the male diabetic athymic nude mouse. Biochem Med Metab Biol 1987;38:240–5.
14. Barss VA. Diabetes and pregnancy. Med Clin North Am 1989;73:685–701.
15. Carstensen LL, Frost-Larsen K, Fugleberg S, Nerup J. Does pregnancy influence the prognosis of uncomplicated insulin dependent diabetes mellitus? Diabetes Care 1982;5:1–5.
16. Klein BE, Moss SE, Klein R. Effect of pregnancy on progression of diabetic retinopathy. Diabetes Care 1990;13:34–40.
17. Beecham WP. Diabetic retinopathy in pregnancy. Trans Am Ophthalmol Soc 1950;48:205–2]16.
18. Berk MA, Miodovnik M, Mimouni F. Impact of pregnancy on complications of insulin dependent diabetes mellitus. Am J Perinatol 1988;5:359–67.
19. Jovanovic R, Jovanovic L. Obstetric management when normoglycemia is maintained in diabetic women with vascular compromise. Am J Obstet Gynecol 1984;149:617–23.
20. Kitzmiller JL, Brown ER, Phillippe M, Stark AR, Acker D, Kaldany A, Singh S, Hare JW. Diabetic nephropathy and perinatal outcome. Am J Obstet Gynecol 1981;141:741–51.
21. Dicker D, Feldberg D, Peleg D, Karp M, Goldman JA. Pregnancy complicated by diabetic nephropathy. J Perinat Med 1986;14:299–307.
22. Reece EA, Coustan DR, Hayslett JP, Holford T, Coulehan J, O'Connor TZ, Hobbins JC. Diabetic nephropathy: Pregnancy performance and fetomaternal outcome. Am J Obstet Gynecol 1988;159:56–66.
23. Combs CA, Kitzmiller JL. Diabetic nephropathy and pregnancy. Clin Obstet Gynecol 1991;34:505–15.
24. Miodovnik M, Skillman C, Holroyde JC, Butler JB, Wendel JS, Siddiqi TA. Elevated maternal hemoglobin A1 in early pregnancy and spontaneous abortion among insulin-dependent diabetic women. Am J Obstet Gynecol 1985;153:439–42.
25. Miodovnik M, Mimouni F, Tsang RC, Ammar E, Kaplan L, Siddiqi TA. Glycemic control and spontaneous abortion in insulin-dependent diabetic women. Obstet Gynecol 1986;68:366–9.
26. Mills JL, Simpson JL, Driscoll SG, Jovanovic-Peterson L, VanAllen M, Aarons JH, Metzger B, Bieber FR, Knopp RH, Holmes LB. Incidence of spontaneous abortion among normal

women and insulin-dependent diabetic women whose pregnancies were identified within 21 days of conception. N Engl J Med 1988;319:1617–23.

27. Ylinen K, Aula P, Stenman UH, Kesaniemi-Kuokkanen T, Teramon K. Risk of minor and major fetal malformations in diabetics with high haemoglobin A1c values in early pregnancy. Br Med J 1984;289:345–8.

28. Miodovnik M, Mimouni F, Dignan PS, Berk MA, Ballard JL, Siddiqi TA, Khoury J, Tsang RC. Major malformations in infants of IDDM women. Diabetes Care 1988;11:713–8.

29. Lucas MJ, Leveno KJ, Williams ML, Raskin P, Whalley PJ. Early pregnancy glycosylated hemoglobin, severity of diabetes, and fetal malformations. Am J Obstet Gynecol 1989;161:426–31.

30. Rosenn B, Miodovnik M, Dignan PSJ, Siddiqui TA, Khoury J, Mimouni F. Minor congenital malformations in infants of insulin-dependent diabetic women: Association with poor glycemic control. Obstet Gynecol 1990;76:745–9.

31. Becerra JE, Khoury MJ, Cordero JF, Erickson JD. Diabetes mellitus during pregnancy and the risks for specific birth defects: A population-based case-control study. Pediatrics 1990;85:1–9.

32. Rosenn B, Miodovnik M, Combs CA, Khoury J, Siddiqi TA. Pre-conception management of insulin-dependent diabetes: Improvement of pregnancy outcome. Obstet Gynecol 1991;77:846–9.

33. Steel JM, Johnstone FD, Hepburn DA, Smith AF. Can prepregnancy care of diabetic women reduce the risk of abnormal babies? Br Med J 1990;301:1070–4.

34. Kitzmiller JL, Gavin LA, Gin GD, Jovanovic-Peterson L, Main EK, Zigrang WD. Preconception care of diabetes: Glycemic control prevents congenital anomalies. JAMA 1991;265:731–6.

35. Piacquadio K, Hollingsworth DR, Murphy H. Effects of in-utero exposure to oral hypoglycaemic drugs. Lancet 1991;138:866–9.

36. Miodovnik M, Skillman C, Hertzberg V, Harrington DJ, Clark KE. Effects of hyperketonemia on hyperglycemic pregnant ewes and their fetuses. Am J Obstet Gynecol 1986;154:394–401.

37. Hay WW. Fetal metabolic consequences of maternal diabetes. In Jopvanovic L, Peterson CM, Fuhrmann K, eds. Diabetes and Pregnancy. New York, Praeger, 1986, pp 185–227.

38. Berk M, Khoury J, Miodovnik M. Respiratory distress syndrome in infants of diabetic mothers relates to maternal hypoglycemia. Diabetes 1987;36(suppl 1):92A.

39. Stangenberg M, Persson A, Stange L, Carlstrom K. Insulin-induced hypoglycemia in pregnant diabetics. Acta Obstet Gynecol Scand 1983;62:249–52.

40. Kolodny RC. Sexual dysfunction in diabetic females. Diabetes 1971;20:557–9.

41. Fontbonne A, Basdevant A, Faguer B, Thomassin M, Buschsenschutz D. Contraceptive practice in 209 diabetic women regularly attending a specialized diabetes clinic. Diabete Metab 1987;13:411–6.

42. Adams PW, Oakley NW. Oral contraceptives and carbohydrate metabolism. Clin Enodcrinol Metab 1972;3:697.

43. Wynn V, Doar JRH. Some effects of oral contraceptives on carbohydrate metabolism. Lancet 1969;2:761–5.

44. Spellacy WN, Buhi WC, Spellacy CE, Moses LE, Goldzieher JW. Glucose, insulin and growth hormone studies in long-term users of oral contraceptives. Am J Obstet Gynecol 1970;106:173–82.

45. Spellacy WN. A review of carbohydrate metabolism and the oral contraceptive. Am J Obstet Gynecol 1979;104:448–60.

46. Aznar R. The effect of various contraceptive hormonal therapies in women with normal and diabetic oral glucose tolerance test. Contraception 1976;13:299–309.

47. Semmer JR, Diddle AW. Oral contraception medication and glucose metabolism. South Med J 1974;67:664–6.

48. Posner NA, Silverstone FA, Tobin EH, Breuer J. Changes in carbohydrate tolerance during long-term oral contraception. Am J Obstet Gynecol 1975;123:119–27.

49. Muck BR. Effect of long-term use of oral contraceptives on glucose tolerance. Arch Gynecol 1976;220:185–90.

50. Gaspard UJ, Lefebvre PJ. Clinical aspects of the relationship between oral contraceptives, abnormalities in carbohydrate metabolism, and the development of cardiovascular disease. Am J Obstet Gynecol 1990;163:334–43.

51. Hannaford PC, Kay CR. Oral contraceptives and diabetes mellitus. Br Med J 1989;299:1315–6.
52. Wingrave SJ, Kay CR, Vessey MP. Oral contraceptives and diabetes mellitus. Br Med J 1979;1:23.
53. Duffy TJ, Ray R. Oral contraceptive use: Prospective follow-up of women with suspected glucose intolerance. Contraception 1984;30:197–208.
54. Tsibris JCM, Raynor LO, Buhi WC, Buggie J, Spellacy WN. Insulin receptor in circulating erythrocytes and monocytes from women on oral contraceptives or pregnant women near term. J Clin Endocrinol Metab 1980;51:711–7.
55. Wynn V, Adams PW, Godsland I, Melrose J, Niththyananthan R, Oakley NW, Seed M. Comparison of effects of different combined oral-contraceptive formulations on carbohydrate and lipid metabolism. Lancet 1979;1:1045–9.
56. Spellacy WN, Newton RE, Buhi WC, Birk SA. Lipid and carbohydrate metabolic studies after one year of megestrol acetate treatment. Fertil Steril 1976;27:157–61.
57. Spellacy WN. Carbohydrate metabolism during treatment with estrogen, progestogen and low-dose oral contraceptives. Am J Obstet Gynecol 1982;142:732–4.
58. Godsland IF, Crook D, Simpson R, Proudler T, Felton C, Lees B, Anyaoku V, Devenport M, Wynn V. The effects of different formulations of oral contraceptive agents on lipid and carbohydrate metabolism. N Engl J Med 1990;323:1375–81.
59. Anderson FD. Selectivity and minimal androgenicity of norgestimate in monophasic and triphasic oral contraceptives. Acta Obstet Gynecol Scand Suppl 1992;156:15–21.
60. Kafrissen ME, Corson SL. Comparative review of third-generation progestins. Int J Fertil 1992;37:104–15.
61. Runnebaum B. Rabe T. New progestogens in oral contraceptives. Am J Obstet Gynecol 1987;157:1059–63.
62. Radberg T, Gustafson A, Skryten A, Karlsson K. Metabolic studies in gestational diabetic women during contraceptive treatment: Effects on glucose tolerance and fatty acid composition of serum lipids. Gynecol Obstet Invest 1982;13:17–29.
63. Kung AW, Ma JT, Wong VC, Li DF, Ng MM, Wang CC, Lam KS. Glucose and lipid metabolism with triphasic oral contraceptives in women with history of gestational diabetes. Contraception 1987;35:257–69.
64. Shoupe D, Kjos S. Effects of oral contraceptives on the borderline NIDD patient. Int J Fertil 1988;33:27–34.
65. Skouby SO, Kuehl C, Molsted-Pedersen L, Petersen K, Christensen MS. Triphasic oral contraception: Metabolic effects in normal women and those with previous gestational diabetes. Am J Obstet Gynecol 1985;153:495–500.
66. Kjos SL, Shoupe D, Douyan S, Friedman RL, Bernstein GS, Mestman JH, Mishell DR Jr. Effect of low-dose oral contraceptives on carbohydrate and lipid metabolism in women with recent gestational diabetes: Results of a controlled, randomized, prospective study. Am J Obstet Gynecol 1990;163:1822–7.
67. Skouby SO, Andersen O, Saurbrey N, Kuehl C. Oral contraception and insulin sensitivity: In vivo assessment in normal women and women with previous gestational diabetes. Clin Endocrinol Metab 1987;64:519–23.
68. Molsted-Pedersen L, Skouby SO, Damm P. Preconception counseling and contraception after gestational diabetes. Diabetes 1991;40:147–50.
69. Skouby SO. Oral contraceptives: Effects on glucose and lipid metabolism in insulin-dependent diabetic women and women with previous gestational diabetes. A clinical and biochemical assessment. Dan Med Bull 1988;35:157–67.
70. Skouby SO, Molsted-Pedersen L, Kuehl C, Bennet P. Oral contraceptives in diabetic women: Metabolic effects of four compounds with different estrogen/progestogen profiles. Fertil Steril 1986;46:858–64.
71. Steel JM, Duncan LJP. Contraception for the insulin-dependent diabetic woman: The view from one clinic. Diabetes Care 1980;3:557–60.
72. Radberg T, Gustafson A, Skryten A, Karlsson K. Oral contraception in diabetic women. Diabetes control, serum and high density lipoprotein lipids during low-dose progestogen, combined oestrogen/progestogen and non-hormonal contraception. Acta Endocrinol (Copenh) 1981;98:246–55.
73. Miller GJ, Miller NE. Plasma-high-density-lipoprotein concentration and development of ischaemic heart disese. Lancet 1975;1:16–9.

74. Miller NE, Hammett F, Saltissi S, Rao S, Van Zeller H, Coltart J, Lewis B. Relation of angiographically defined coronary artery disease of plasma lipoprotein subfractions and apolipproteins. Br Med J 1981;282:1741–4.
75. Witztum J, Schonfeld G. High density lipoproteins. Diabetes 1979;28:326–33.
76. Wynn V, Niththyananthan R. The effect of progestins in combined oral contraceptives on serum lipids with special reference to high density lipoproteins. Am J Obstet Gynecol 1982;142:766–72.
77. Knopp RH, Walden CE, Wahl PW, Hoover JJ. Effects of oral contraceptives on lipoprotein triglyceride and cholesterol: Relationships to estrogen and progestin potency. Am J Obstet Gynecol 1982;142:725–32.
78. Knopp RH. Effects of sex steroid hormones on lipoprotein levels in pre- and post menopausal women. Can J Cardiol 1990;6:31B–5B.
79. Kay CR. The RCGP oral contraceptive study. Clin Obstet Gynecol 1984;11:759–86.
80. Yeshurun D, Barak C, Blumensohn R, Rosenzweig B. A comparison of plasma cholesterol, triglycerides and high density lipoprotein cholesterol levels in women using contraceptive pills and a control group. Gynecol Obstet Invest 1984;18:169–73.
81. Godsland IF, Crook D, Wynn V. Coronary heart disease risk markers in users of low-dose oral contraceptives. J Reprod Med 1991;36:226–37.
82. Klein JBE, Moss SE, Klein R. Oral contraceptives in women with diabetes. Diabetes Care 1990;13:895–8.
83. Steel JM, Duncan LJP. Serious complications of oral contraception in insulin-dependent diabetics. Contraception 1978;17:291–5.
84. Hatcher RA, Stewart F, Trussell J, Kowal D, Guest F, Stewart GK, Cates W. Contraceptive Technology: 1990-1992. 15th rev ed. New York, Irvington Publishers, 1990.
85. Fennoy I. Contraception and the adolescent diabetic. Health Educ Wash 1989;20:21–3.
86. Dickey RP. Managing Contraceptive Pill Patients. 5th ed. Durant, OK, Creative Informatics, 1987.
87. Derman R. Oral contraceptives: A reassessment. Obstet Gynecol Surv 1989;44:662–8.
88. Breckwoldt M, Wieacker P, Geisthovel F. Oral contraception in disease states. Am J Obstet Gynecol 1990;163:2213–6.
89. Vessey MP. Contraceptive methods: Risks and benefits. Br Med J 1978;1:721–2.
90. Westrom L, Bengtsson LP, Mardh PA. The risk of pelvic inflammatory disease in women using intrauterine contraceptive devices as compared to non-users. Lancet 1976;2:221–4.
91. Gosden C, Ross A, Steel J, Springbett A. Intrauterine contraceptive devices in diabetic women. Lancet 1982;1:530–4.
92. Skouby SO, Molsted-Pedersen L, Kosonen A. Consequences of intrauterine contraception in diabetic women. Fertil Steril 1984;42:568–72.
93. Wiese J. Intrauterine contraception in diabetic women. Fertil Steril 1977;28:422–5.
94. Skouby SO, Molsted-Pedersen L, Kuehl C. Contraception in diabetic women. Acta Endocrinol (Copenh) 1986;277:125–9.
95. Craig GM, Newton JR. Contraception in diabetics. Br Med J 1981;283:1184.
96. Smith JE. Pregnancy complicated by thyroid disease. J Nurse Midwifery 1990;35:143–9.
97. Sugrue D, Drury MI. Hyperthyroidism complicating pregnancy: Results of treatment by antithyroid drugs in 77 pregnancies. Br J Obstet Gynaecol 1980;87:970–5.
98. Tunbridge WMG, Evered DC, Hall R, Appleton D, Brewis M, Clark F, Grimley Evan J, Young E, Bird T, Smith BR. The spectrum of thyroid disease in a community. Clin Endocrinol (Oxf) 1977;7:483–93.
99. Becks GP, Burrow GN. Thyroid disease and pregnancy. Med Clin North Am 1991;75:121–50.
100. Glinoer D, Soto MF, Bourdoux P, Lejeune B, Delange F, Lemone M, Kinthaert J, Robijn C, Grun J, De Nayer P. Pregnancy in patients with mild thyroid abnormalities: Maternal and neonatal repercussions. J Clin Endocrinol Metab 1991;73:421–7.
101. Parker RH, Bierwaltes WH, Elzinga KF, Spafford NR, Hassoun S. Thyroid antibodies during pregnancy and in the newborn. J Clin Endocrinol Metab 1961;21:792–8.
102. Nelson JC, Palmer FJ. A remission of goitrous hypothyroidism during pregnancy. J Clin Endocrinol Metab 1975;40:383–6.
103. Mortimer RH, Tyack SA, Galligan JP, Perry Keene DA, Tan YM. Graves' disease in pregnancy: TSH receptor binding inhibiting immunoglobulins and maternal and neonatal thyroid function. Clin Endocrinol (Oxf) 1990;32:141–52.
104. Amino N, Tanizawa O, Mori H, Iwatani Y, Yamada T, Kurachi K, Kumahara Y, Miyai K.

Aggravation of thyrotoxicosis in early pregnancy and after delivery in Graves disease. J Clin Endocrinol Metab 1982;55:108–12.

105. Hod M, Sharony R, Friedman S, Ovadia J. Pregnancy and thyroid carcinoma. A review of incidence, course, and prognosis. Obstet Gynecol Surv 1989;44:774–9.

106. Fukuda K, Hachisuga T, Sugimori H, Tsuzuku M. Papillary carcinoma of the thyroid occurring during pregnancy. Report of a case diagnosed by fine needle aspiration cytology. Acta Cytol 1991;35:725–7.

107. Burrow G. Thyroid disease. In Burrow G, Ferris T, eds. Medical Complications during Pregnancy. 3rd ed. Philadelphia, WB Saunders, 1988, pp 224–53.

108. Mestman JH: Management of thyroid diseases in pregnancy. Clin Perinatol 1980;7:371–7.

109. Momotani N, Ito K, Hamada N, Nishikawa Y, Mimura T. Maternal hyperthyroidism and congenital malformations in the offspring. Clin Endocrinol (Oxf) 1984;20:695–700.

110. Davis LE, Lucas MJ, Hankins GDV, Roark ML, Cunningham FG. Thyrotoxicosis complicating pregnancy. Am J Obstet Gynecol 1989;160:63–70

111. Montoro M, Collea J, Frasier D, Mestman J. Successful outcome of pregnancy in women with hypothyroidism. Ann Intern Med 1981;94:31–4.

112. Potter J. Hypothyroidism and reproductive failure. Surg Gynecol Obstet 1980;150:251–5.

113. Heck J, Adelson H. Amenorrhea-galactorrhea associated with hypothalamic hypothyroidism. Am J Obstet Gynecol 1981;139:736–7.

114. Davis LE, Levno KJ, Cunningham FG. Hypothyroidism complicating pregnancy. Obstet Gynecol 1988;72:108–12.

115. Cheron R, Kaplan M, Larsen P, Selenkow HA, Crigler JF Jr. Neonatal thyroid function after propylthiouracil therapy for maternal Graves' disease. N Engl J Med 1981;304:525–8.

116. Davis LE, Lucas MJ, Hankins GDV, Roark ML, Cunningham FG. Thyrotoxicosis complicating pregnancy. Am J Obstet Gynecol 1989;160:63–70.

117. Decherney AH. The use of birth control pills in women with medical disorders. Clin Obstet Gynecol 1981;24:965–75.

118. Phillips DI, Lazarus JH, Butland BK. The influence of pregnancy and reproductive span on the occurrence of autoimmune thyroiditis. Clin Endocrinol (Oxf) 1990;32:301–6.

119. Frank P, Kay CR. Incidence of thyroid disease associated with oral contraceptives. Br Med J 1978;2:1531.

120. Ramcharan S, Pellegrin FRA, Rayt RM. The Walnut Creek Contraceptive Drug Study: A prospective study of the side effects of oral contraceptives. J Reprod Med 1980;25(suppl):337–72.

121. Diaz S, Pavez M, Brandeis A, Cardenas H, Croxatto HB. A longitudinal study on cortisol, prolactin and thyroid hormones in users of Norplant subdermal implants or a copper T device. Contraception 1989;40:505–17.

122. Emans SJH, Goldstein DP. Pediatric and Adolescent Gynecology. 3rd ed. Boston, Little, Brown, 1990.

123. Olsson SE, Wide L, Odlind V. Aspects of thyroid function during use of Norplant implants. Contraception 1986;34:583–7.

124. Chaudhuri PK, Walker MJ, Briele HA, Beattie CW, Das Gupta TK. Incidence of estrogen receptor in benign nevi and human malignant melanoma. JAMA 1980;244:791–3.

125. Money SR, Muss W, Thelmo WL, Boeckl O, Pimpl W, Kaindl H, Sungler P, Kirwin J, Waclawicek H, Jaffe BM, Pertshuk DO. Immunocytochemical localization of estrogen and progesterone receptors in human thyroid. Surgery 1989;106:975–8.

126. Linn S, Schoenbaum SC, Monson RR, Rosner B, Ryan KJ. Delay in conception for former "pill users." JAMA 1982;247:629–32.

127. Kaunitz AM. Injectable contraception. Clin Obstet Gynecol 1989;32:356–67.

128. Data on file. The Upjohn Company, Kalamazoo, MI, 1993.

129. Abdel-Hamid MW, Joplin GF, Lewis PD. Incidentally found small pituitary adenomas may have no effect on fertility. Acta Endocrinol (Copenh) 1988;117:361–4.

130. Coulon G, Fellmann D, Arbez-Gindre F, Pageaut G. Latent pituitary adenoma. Autopsy study. Sem Hop Paris 1983;59:2747–50.

131. Loriaux DL, Wild RA. Contraceptive choices for women with endocrine complications. 1993;168:2021–6.

132. Fox MW, Harms RW, Davis DH. Selected neurologic complications of pregnancy. Mayo Clin Proc 1990;65:1595–618.

133. Marshall JR. Pregnancy in patients with prolactin-producing pituitary tumors. Clin Obstet Gynecol 1980;23:453–63.
134. Rowe TC, Sheaman RP, Fraser IS. Antecedent factors and outcome in amenorrhea-galactorrhea. Obstet Gynecol 1979;54:535–43.
135. Magyar DM, Marshall JR. Pituitary tumors and pregnancy. Am J Obstet Gynecol 1978;132:739–49.
136. Samaan NA, Schultz PN, Leavens TA, Leavens ME, Lee YY. Pregnancy after treatment in patients with prolactinoma: Operation versus bromocriptine. Am J Obstet Gynecol 1986;155:1300–5.
137. Badawy SZA, Rebscher F, Kohn L, Wolfe H, Oates RP, Moses A. The relationship between oral contraceptive use and subsequent development of hyperprolactinemia. Fertil Steril 1981;36:464–7.
138. Shy KK, McTiernan AM, Daling JR, Weiss NS. Oral contraceptive use and the occurrence of pituitary prolactinoma. JAMA 1983;249:2204–7.
139. Voelker W, Reitmann I, Kannengiesser U, Niesert S, Gehring WG, vonzur-Muehlen A. Oral steroid contraception in hyperprolactinemia. Geburtshilfe Frauenheilkd 1981;41:199–203.
140. Maheuz R, Jenicek M, Cleroux R, Beauregard H, De-Muylder X, Gratton NM, Van Campenhout J. Oral contraceptives and prolactinomas: A case-control study. Am J Obstet Gynecol 1982;143:134–8.
141. Hatch R, Rosenfield RL, Kim MG, Tredway D. Hirsutism: Implications, etiology, and management. Am J Obstet Gynecol 1981;140:815–30.
142. Barnes R, Rosenfield RL. The polycystic ovary syndrome: Pathogenesis and treatment. Ann Intern Med 1989;110:386–99.
143. Neinstein LS. Polycystic ovary syndrome and ovarian cysts and tumors. In Neinstein LS. Adolescent Health Care, 2nd ed. Baltimore, Urban & Schwarzenberg, 1991, pp 679–86.
144. Hamilton–Fairley D, Kiddy D, Watson H, Sagle M, Franks S. Low-dose gonadotrophin therapy for induction of ovulation in 100 women with polycystic ovary syndrome. Hum Reprod 1991;6:1095–9.
145. Homburg R, Eshel A, Armar NA, Tucker M, Mason PW, Adams J, Kilborn J, Sutherland IA, Jacobs HS. One hundred pregnancies after treatment with pulsatile luteinising hormone releasing hormone to induce ovulation. Br Med J 1989;298:809–2.
146. Givens JR, Andersen RN, Wiser WL. The effectiveness of two oral contraceptives in suppressing plasma androstanedione, testosterone, LH and FSH, and stimulating plasma testosterone-binding capacity in hirsute women. Am J Obstet Gynecol 1976;124:333.

10

Hematological Conditions

Sickle Cell Hemoglobinopathies

The most common form of sickle cell disease is the homozygous SS state, which affects 0.15 to 0.20% of African Americans in the United States or about 50,000 individuals. About 7 to 9% of the African American population has the trait.

Fertility

Fertility is not impaired in women with sickle cell disease although men are often reported to have fertility problems secondary to reduced semen volume, sperm counts, sperm mobility, and motility.[1] Another problem that males can encounter is impotence as a consequence of earlier priapism.

Effects of Pregnancy on Sickle Cell Anemia

Pregnancy in a women with homozygous sickle cell (SS) disease can have serious sequelae for both the mother and her offspring. Associated with pregnancy are changes that can accentuate sickle cell disease including a hypercoagulable state, stasis in the pelvic area, and increased metabolic demands. Complications of sickle cell disease in the pregnant woman include a higher risk of severe anemia, sickle cell crisis, pneumonia, pyelonephritis, pulmonary emboli, and cerebrovascular accidents.[2-7] Morbidity among pregnant women ranges from 4 to 100% while mortality ranges from 0 to 35%. However, the maternal mortality has dropped

116

significantly from about 4.1% in 1972 to 1.7% after the National Sickle Cell Act of 1972.[7]

Effect of Sickle Cell Anemia on Pregnancy

Sickle cell disease also has a significant impact on pregnancy and the infant. Perinatal mortality has ranged from 3 to over 50%.[4,7] Again, since the Sickle Cell Act, the infant mortality rate has decreased from over 50 to 22.7% in women with SS disease and from 33.3 to 27.3% in infants of women with sickle cell SC disease.[7] Women with sickle cell–hemoglobin C disease are at a similar risk to those with SS disease while the risk to those with sickle cell–thalassemia is increased but to a lesser degree.[2-5] In one study comparing the rates of spontaneous abortions and stillbirths with controls, the rates were 10.5% in the controls, 12.5% for SC disease, 17.5% for hemoglobin S-thalassemia, and 20% for SS sickle cell disease.[1]

Contraception and Sickle Cell Anemia

Because of the significant maternal and fetal morbidity and mortality associated with sickle cell disease, a safe and effective form of contraception is vital. In one study of women with sickle cell disease, only 33% reported use of a contraceptive method, compared with 66% in the control group.[8] Barrier methods have no contraindications but their lower effectiveness rates compared to hormonal contraceptives make them less than ideal.

Concerns have arisen about hormonal contraceptive in women with sickle cell anemia because of the possibility of a synergistic effect of these hormones on the thromboembolic problems in already susceptible women. In past years, hormonal contraceptives were often avoided in women with either sickle cell disease or trait. While research in this area is minimal and often based on anecdotal cases, available evidence does not support the notion that hormonal contraceptives are contraindicated in these women.[9]

Most of the negative reports in women with sickle cell disease are based on anecdotal cases. For example, Dunn and Haynes reported on a woman with sickle cell–thalassemia who developed a pulmonary infarction following the use of combined oral contraceptives, and reported on two women with sickle cell SC who developed venous thrombosis and a pulmonary infarction.[10,11] However, there have been reports showing no negative side effects and occasionally reports of improvement with hormonal contraceptives.[9,12-19] Lutcher found that 11 of 12 women on combined contraceptives did not experience an increased severity of their disease over 6 to 54 months.[12] In a follow-up period of up to 10 years in the Sickle Cell Clinic at the Medical College of Georgia, in unpublished data, none of their women on oral contraceptives has had a major complication.[13] Contrary to the concerns of increased thromboembolic activity with hormonal contraceptives, there have been several anecdotal reports that progesterones may decrease the risk of sickling in individuals with sickle cell anemia.[14–19] In one report, individuals with sickle cell disease using depomedroxyprogesterone acetate (DMPA) for contraception had a statistically significant reduction in the number of sickle cell attacks and improvement in hemoglobin and other laboratory test results.[17] There was also one report of a woman with sickle cell disease whose transfusion requirements were eliminated after receiving DMPA for 3 months.[19]

The findings in women with sickle cell trait are similar, with negative reports coming from isolated anecdotal cases. In one report, a 16-year-old female adolescent with sickle cell trait had a pulmonary embolus after taking oral contraceptives for 3 months,[20] while in another report, a 22-year-old woman with sickle cell trait had a stroke after taking oral contraceptives for 2 years.[21] However, Herson et al. reviewed the course of 112 women with sickle cell trait on oral contraceptives and found that none developed any serious side effects.[22]

In past years, researchers advised against the use of combined hormonal contraceptives in sickle cell disease because of the potential thromboembolic threat. However, as listed above, the evidence for problems in these women has not been well documented. In fact, in one survey among 52 women with sickle cell disease including 34 with SS Hgb, 10 with SC Hgb, and 4 with Hgb S-thalassemia, oral contraceptives were the most common form of birth control utilized.[8] Contraceptive Technology lists sickle cell disease and sickle cell SC disease as a consideration that "may suggest that pills are not the ideal contraceptive," although it no longer lists the condition as a strong relative contraindication.[23] Freie, in a review of sickle cell diseases and hormonal contraception, concluded that low-dose combination oral contraceptives are the method of choice for contraception in women with sickle cell disease.[9] Progestin-only pills, DMPA, and perhaps the Norplant implant, although not systematically studied in this population, may be beneficial. Combination oral contraceptives and DMPA have the additional benefit of reducing menstrual blood loss in women who already are anemic from their sickle cell disease. Progestin-only contraceptives probably have little, if any, effect on the coagulation system.[24,25] Thus, if the health care practitioner is concerned about combined oral contraceptives, pro-gestin-only contraceptives would be a good alternative.

The intrauterine device (IUD) could potentially be a problem in these women by worsening an already existent anemia. However, the progestin-containing IUD could be used without increasing menstrual blood loss. As in any other woman, infection is an important consideration if the individual has multiple sexual partners.

Summary

1. Fertility, while normal in women with sickle cell disease, may be reduced in males.

2. Pregnancy can have a significant impact on maternal and fetal outcome.
3. In women with sickle cell trait, combination or progestin-only contraceptives could be used with apparent safety.
4. For most women with sickle cell disease, hormonal contraceptives may be the best choice. Barrier methods are safe but not as effective. Combination oral contraceptives have not been demonstrated to increase the risk of sickling or thromboembolism in women with sickle cell anemia. If combination pills are used, low-dose estrogen/progestin combinations should be chosen.
5. Progestin-only contraceptives are another good alternative. These contraceptives, particularly DMPA, can decrease menstrual blood loss and have anecdotally been reported to improve sickle cell anemia. Further studies in the use of progestin-only contraceptive devices in these individuals would be helpful.
6. The copper IUD would not be a good alternative in women with sickle cell disease because of the tendency to increase menstrual blood loss. The progestin-containing IUD could be used in multiparous women who are in a stable, monogamous relationship.

Anemia

The most common form of anemia is iron deficiency anemia. Postpubertal females require three times the daily iron intake of men because of iron losses during menstruation.[26]

A relative anemia occurs during the midtrimester of pregnancy because of the rise in plasma volume (about 42% over nonpregnant state) that is greater than the rise in red cell mass (about 26%). During the first and third trimesters, the hemoglobin and hematocrit should be above 11 g/dL and 33%. A pregnant woman with a hematocrit less than 30% should be evaluated. The two most common causes during pregnancy are iron and folate deficiencies.

In nonpregnant women, combined oral contraception can protect against iron deficiency anemia as their use decreases the amount of menstrual flow by half or more. The incidence of iron deficiency anemia in oral contraceptives users in the Royal College of General Practitioners study was 567 per 100,000 compared to 971 per 100,000 in women never using the pill.[27] Thus, women with iron deficiency anemia needing contraception could benefit from choosing combination oral contraceptives. The reverse is true for the copper IUD because of its associated increase in menstrual flow. However, this would not be true of the progestin-containing IUD. Faundes et al. compared several IUDs and found the prevalence of an abnormal hematocrit to be 22% with the copper T compared to 2% with the progestin IUD.[28] Low ferritin levels were found in 55% of copper T users compared to 14% of the progestin IUD users.

Hypercoagulability

Inherited hypercoagulable conditions include those women with protein S deficiency, protein C deficiency, and antithrombin III deficiency. Protein S deficiency is the most common inherited hypercoagulable disorder, frequently causing superficial thrombophlebitis, deep venous thrombosis, and pulmonary emboli.[29] Women with this condition are often in the reproductive age group, with a mean age of first thrombosis of 28 years.[29] Acquired hypercoagulable states include pregnancy, myeloproliferative disorders, cancer, antiphospholipid antibody syndrome, and defects in clot lysis associated with surgery. Pregnancy is a significant risk in women with an underlying hypercoagulable state, as pregnancy increases the risk of further thromboembolic disease by both stasis and affecting coagulation factors. For example, pregnancy decreases protein S by 50%.[30]

Because of the risk of thromboembolic complications, women with acquired or inherited hypercoagulability should be excluded from using estrogen-containing contraceptives if they are not adequately anticoagulated. Estrogen/progestin oral contraceptives affect blood clotting by increasing plasma fibrinogen and the activity of coagulation factors, especially factors VII and X.[31] Antithrombin III, an inhibitor of coagulation, is usually decreased while platelet activity is often enhanced.[31] Early reports of combination oral contraceptives demonstrated an increased risk of thromboembolic disease that was dependent on dose, between 50 and 150 µg of estrogen.[30] These studies were confounded by problems with overdiagnosis of thrombophlebitis by health care providers who knew women were on oral contraceptives and by infrequent use of reliable diagnostic techniques for deep vein thrombosis and pulmonary embolism. In women taking low-dose estrogen pills, with less than 50 µg, increases in coagulation appear small and counterbalanced by increases in fibrinolytic activity.[31] In a recent study of over 230,000 women between the ages of 15 and 44 years in the Michigan Medicaid population, the relative risks of venous thrombosis between oral contraceptives with less than 50 µg of estrogen, 50 µg of estrogen, and more than 50 µg of estrogen were 1, 1.5, and 1.7.[32] However, as yet there has not been a well-controlled, randomized, blinded prospective study evaluating the risk of deep venous thrombosis and pulmonary embolism in women on newer low-dose contraceptive pills.

In women who are effectively anticoagulated, hormonal contraceptives could be considered. Even though hormonal contraceptives, particularly higher-dose estrogen-containing compounds, can increase coagulability, the benefits may outweigh the risks in these women for several reasons. First, low-dose combination pills and progestin-only contraceptives appear to have little impact on increasing coagulation.[24,25,31,33–36] Second, these women are at potential risk for negative effects of anticoagulation on a pregnancy and a fetus. Third, a pregnancy itself may place the women at significant risk for further thromboembolic disease.

Hemorrhagic Disorders

Hemorrhagic disorders include disorders involving both the coagulation system and disorders involving platelet number and function. Hereditary coagulopathies are uncommon in pregnant individuals occurring in about 1 to 2 per 10,000 individuals. The most common such disorder occurring with pregnancy is von Willebrand's disease. The defect in this condition is in the von Willebrand part of factor VIII. It is associated with an abnormal partial prothrombin time (PTT) and prolonged bleeding time. Cryoprecipitate or plasma transfusion is needed for intrapartum or postpartum hemorrhage. In hemophilia A and B, most women are protected from bleeding by rises in factors VIII and IX during gestation.

Immune thrombocytopenic purpura (ITP) may also be a cause of severe menstrual bleeding and bleeding during delivery. This disorder is caused by a production of IgG antibodies that interact with platelet surface antigens leading to platelet damage and destruction. The antibodies can cross the placenta, leading to neonatal thrombocytopenia.[37] Even mothers in remission can have infants with severe thrombocytopenia secondary to circulating antiplatelet antibodies. Steroid therapy is indicated in those mothers with platelet counts less than 75,000/mm³. Immunoglobulin therapy has also been used. With appropriate therapy, maternal mortality should not be increased. Fetal morbidity and mortality are increased, although not as high in recent studies[38,39] as in the 25% mortality found in older studies.[40,41]

Most of the reports on hormonal contraceptives in women with these coagulation and platelet problems are anecdotal, involving the use of these hormones to control abnormally heavy menstrual bleeding. Haber reported on a woman with factor X deficiency whose bleeding problems were controlled using the progestational agent norethynodrel.[42] Ozsoylu and Corbacioglu used oral contraceptives to treat nine patients with von Willebrand's disease.[43] In all of these patients, except two patients on oral contraceptives for less than 3 months, thromboplastin generation time improved. However, several other investigators did not find any improvement in controlling bleeding in individuals with hemophilia treated with oral contraceptives.[44–47] No serious side effects from contraceptives were reported in these various studies. Thus, in women with coagulopathies, hormonal contraceptives have not been reported to be a problem and may in fact help to control menorrhagia. These women may be at risk of hemoperitoneum secondary to ovulation. Combination oral contraceptives and DMPA, by suppressing ovulation, reduce this risk.

The copper IUD because of its association with heavier menstrual bleeding would be contraindicated in women with coagulopathies or platelet disorders. In women on steroid therapy for ITP, a copper IUD and the progestin IUD would be contraindicated because of reduced effectiveness.

References

1. Davies S. Obstetric implications of sickle cell disease. Midwife Health Visit Commun Nurse 1988;24:361–3.
2. Fort AT, Morrison JC, Berreras L, Diggs LW, Fish SA. Counseling the patient with sickle cell disease about reproduction: Pregnancy outcome does not justify the maternal risk. Am J Obstet Gynecol 1971;11:324–7.
3. Hendricks JP, Harrison KA, Watson-Williams EJ, Luzzatto L, Ajabor LN. Pregnancy in homozygous sickle-cell anemia. J Obstet Gynaecol Br Commonw 1972;79:396–409.
4. Morrison JC. Hemoglobinopathies and pregnancy. Clin Obstet Gynecol 1979;22:819–42.
5. Brodie JL. Sickle cell anemia—The disease of challenge. J Am Med Wom Assoc 1972;27:411–5.
6. Richardson EAW, Milne LS. Sickle cell disease and the childbearing family: An update. Am J Maternal Child Nurs 1983;8:417–22.
7. Helman NS. Sickle cell disease and pregnancy. NAACOGS Clin Issu Perinat Womens Health Nurs 1990;1:194–201.
8. Samuels-Reid JH, Scott RB, Brown WE. Contraceptive practices and reproductive patterns in sickle cell disease. J Natl Med Assoc 1984;76:879–83.
9. Freie HM. Sickle cell diseases and hormonal contraception. Acta Obstet Gynecol Scand 1983;62:211–7
10. Dunn JM, Haynes RL. Sickle cell thalassemia in pregnancy. Am J Obstet Gynecol 1967;97:574–5.
11. Haynes RL, Dunn JM. Oral contraceptives, thrombosis, and sickle cell hemoglobinopathies. JAMA 1967;200:186–8.
12. Lutcher CL. Blood coagulation studies and the effect of oral contraceptives in patients with sickle cell anemia. Clin Res 1976;24:47A.
13. Carlone JP, Keen PD. Oral contraceptive use in women with chronic medical conditions. Nurse Pract 1989;14:9–16.
14. Issacs WA, Hayhoe FG. Steroid hormones in sickle cell disease. Nature 1967;215:1139–42.
15. Issacs WA, Effiong CE, Ayeni O. Steroid treatment in the prevention of painful episodes in sickle cell disease. Lancet 1972;1:570–1.
16. Adadevoh BK, Issacs WA. The effect of megestrol acetate on sickling. Am J Med Sci 1973;265:367–70.
17. De Ceulaer K, Gruber C, Hayes R, Sergeant GR. Medroxyprogesterone acetate and homozygous sickle-cell disease. Lancet 1982;2:229–31.
18. Adedevoh BK, Dada OA. Contraception and haemoglobinopathies in Ibadan, Nigeria. Trop Geogr Med 1977;29:77–81.
19. Perkins RP. Contraception for sicklers. N Engl J Med 1971;285:296.
20. Hargus EP, Shearin R, Colon AR. Pulmonary embolism in a female with sickle cell trait and oral contraceptive use. Am J Obstet Gynecol 1977;129:697–8.
21. Greenwald JG. Stroke, sickle cell trait, and oral contraceptives. Ann Intern Med 1970;72:960.
22. Herson J, Sharma S, Crocker CL, Jones D. Physical complaints of patients with sickle cell trait. J Reprod Med 1975;14:129–32.
23. Hatcher RA, Stewart F, Trussell J, Kowal D, Guest F, Stewart GK, Cates W. Contraceptive Technology: 1990-1992. 15th rev ed. New York, Irvington Publishers, 1990.
24. Beller FK, Ebert C. Effects of oral contraceptives on blood coagulation. A review. Obstet Gynecol Surv 1985;40:425–36.
25. Jespersen J, Petersen KR, Skouby SO. Effects of newer oral contraceptives on the inhibition of coagulation and fibrinolysis in relation to dosage and type of steroid. Am J Obstet Gynecol 1990;163:396–403.
26. Oral contraceptives in the 1980s. Popul Rep [A] 1982;6.
27. Advantages or orals outweight disadvantages. Popul Rep [A] 1975;2.
28. Faundes A, Alvarez F, Brache V, Tejada AS. The role of the levonorgestrel intrauterine device in the prevention and treatment of iron deficiency anemia during fertility regulation. Int J Gynaecol Obstet 1988;26:429–33.
29. Alving BM. The hypercoagulable states. Hosp Pract 1993;29:103–21.
30. Comp PC, Zacur HA. Contraceptive choices in women with coagulation disorders. Am J Obstet Gynecol 1993;168:1990–3.

31. Bonnar J. Coagulation effects of oral contraception. Am J Obstet Gynecol 1987;157:1042–8.
32. Gerstman BB, Piper JM, Tomita DK, Ferguson WJ, Stadel BV, Lundin FE. Oral contraceptive estrogen dose and the risk of deep venous thromboembolic disease. Am J Epidemiol 1991;133:32–7.
33. Anderson FD. Selectivity and minimal androgenicity of nortgestimate in monophasic and triphasic oral contraceptives. Acta Obstet Gynecol Scand 1992;156:15–21.
34. Bonnar J, Daly L, Carroll E. Blood coagulation with a combination pill containing gestodene and ethinyl estradiol. Int J Fertil 1987;32:21–8.
35. Inauen W, Stocker G, Haeberli A, Straub PW. Effects of low and high dose oral contraceptives on blood coagulation and thrombogenesis induced by vascular subendothelium exposed to flowing human blood. Contraception 1991;43:435–46.
36. Fioretti P, Fruzzetti F, Navalesi R, Ricci C, Miccoli R, Cerri M, Melis GB. Clinical and metabolic effects of a pill containing 30 mcg ethinylestradiol plus 75 mcg gestodene. Contraception 1989;40:649–63.
37. Schlamowitz M. Membrane receptors in the specific transfer of immunoglobulins from mother to young. Immunol Commun 1976;5:481–500.
38. Jones RW, Asher MI, Rutherford CJ, Munro HM. Autoimmune (idiopathic) thrombocytopenic purpura in pregnancy and the newborn. Br J Obstet Gynaecol 1977;84:679–83.
39. Noriega-Guerra L, Aviles-Miranda A, de la Cadena OA, Espinosa LM, Chavez F, Pizzutu J. Pregnancy in patients with autoimmune thrombocytopenic purpura. Am J Obstet Gynecol 1979;133:439–48.
40. Laros RK Jr, Sweet RL. Management of idiopathic thrombocytopenic purpura during pregnancy. Am J Obstet Gynecol 1975;122:181–91.
41. Peterson OH Jr, Larson P. Thrombocytopenic purpura in pregnancy. Obstet Gynecol 1954;4:454–69.
42. Haber S. Norethynodrel in the treatment of factor X deficiency. Arch Intern Med 1964;114:89–94.
43. Ozsoylu S, Corbacioglu B. Oral contraceptives for haemophilia. Lancet 1967;1:1001.
44. Beck P, Bloom AL, Giddings JC, Sweetnam PM. A controlled trial of oral contraceptives in haemophilia. Br J Haematol 1970;19:667–73.
45. Karaca M, Kocabas A, Kabakci T, Akoguz O. Oral contraceptives in hemophilia. Lancet 1971;1:1974.
46. Bloom AL, Beck P, Giddings JC, Sweetnam PM. Coagulation studies in haemophilia patients taking oral contraceptives. J Clin Pathol 1971;24:23–6.
47. Brandt NJ, Cohn J, Hilden M. Controlled trial of oral contraceptives in haemophilia. Scand J Haematol 1973;11:225–9.

11

Rheumatological Diseases

Systemic Lupus Erythematosus

Systemic lupus erythematosus (SLE) has a predilection for women in child-bearing years so pregnancy and family planning issues become very important.

Fertility

Overall, fertility and fecundity rates do not appear to be altered by SLE.[1,2] Friedman and Rutherford found a sterility rate of 20.8% and an average of 2.3 pregnancies per fertile woman.[2] Fraga et al. found fertility rates of 3.4 and 2.1 pregnancies per woman before and after the onset of lupus, as compared to 3.6 in a control group of women.[1] These overall results have been considered to be similar to rates in women without lupus. However, it is probable that women who are seriously ill or have significant renal dysfunction have reduced fertility.[3–18]

Effect of Pregnancy on Systemic Lupus Erythematosus

There is no universal agreement about the effects of pregnancy on the course of SLE as there is a high degree of variability reported from study to study. Both exacerbations and remissions during the pregnancy and post-partum period have been reported. Several factors make comparison of these studies difficult. First, the definition of a lupus flare is not standardized. Second, the treatment of these women has changed dramatically over the past 30 to 40 years, with more steroids and immunosuppressives used during pregnancy in recent years. Early reports of the effect of pregnancy on lupus tended to report disease exacerbations during gestation or the postpartum period. Cecere and Persellin reviewed the course of 688 pregnancies occurring from the years 1950 to 1980 from 26 different reports.[3] Exacerbations occurred in about 50% of the pregnancies, 186 (27%) of 688 during pregnancy and 174 (25.2%) of 688 in the postpartum period. Nineteen percent of the women had a remission. During the last decade studied (1970–1980) only 8% of women had remissions during pregnancy. Overall, there was a 7% mortality rate, declining to 1% during the last decade of their review. They found the highest number of exacerbations occurring in the third trimester and postpartum periods. Several other studies also found evidence of lupus flares with pregnancy, particularly in the puerperium period.[4–6]

Other studies have not been able to document an increased rate of flares in pregnancy during the postpartum period as compared to nonpregnant women with lupus.[7–11] Derksen critically analyzed recent data in the literature on pregnancy in women with systemic lupus and felt that overall, pregnancy does not induce an exacerbation of the disease.[9] Donaldson and DeAlvarez examined 81 pregnancies in 54 women with active SLE.[7] During pregnancy about one-half had no change, one-third improved, and one-sixth had an exacerbation. In a prospective case-control study, Lockshin et al. compared 33 pregnancies in 28 women with matched controls and no differences were found in clinical markers of SLE activity.[8] However, this study did not include matched women with active disease at the time of conception. Earlier reports and Derksen's review indicated that the presence of disease activity at conception is associated with a higher risk for maternal morbidity during pregnancy.[9,11] For example, in one study, among 30 women with lupus in remission, 74% remained in remission while among 27 women with active disease at conception, disease activity remained the same or worse in 70%.[11]

Another concern with pregnancy in women with SLE has focused on renal disease and function. Fine et al. reported on 52 pregnancies in 39 women seen between 1963 and 1978.[12] They did not find an increased prevalence of major systemic nonrenal manifestations of SLE in these women and found that exacerbations in the immediate postpartum period were less (9.5% versus 31%) in those women who received steroids in the intrapartum and postpartum period. Renal disease was evaluated by stratifying the women into those with prior minimal, mild, or moderate renal disease. None of their patients with moderate renal disease became pregnant. Of the study women, no measurable change in renal function occurred in 40, while 7 women had transient and reversible deterioration. In 5 (9.6%) of the women, renal function deteriorated during the pregnancy and remained worse during a 3- to 12-month follow-up period. One women died 2 months postpartum. None of the 15 women who had first-trimester abortions had a worsening in renal function. Samuels and Pfeifer reviewed six studies involving 242 pregnancies in 156 women.[13] Of these women, 30.2% had transient renal dysfunction during pregnancy while 7.1% had a permanent decline in renal function. However, there was no comparison with nonpregnant women with renal disease.

One problem in evaluating these studies is that it may be difficult to differentiate a renal lupus flare from preeclampsia. Both can lead to hypertension, proteinuria, and edema. The distinction is important, not only for evaluating past studies but also for treatment as therapy is markedly different for the two. A lupus flare requires increasing medications while preeclampsia often necessitates an early delivery. The presence of other lupus characteristics such as arthralgias, skin rash, and pleuritis suggests a lupus flare while the presence of thrombocytopenia, elevated serum transaminases, and hyperuricemia without other lupus symptoms suggests preeclampsia. Complement (C3 and C4) levels may be valuable in differentiating the two conditions, as complement values fall with a lupus flare but rise with preeclampsia.[14] It is important to consider that complement levels rise in the normal pregnancy so that following levels may be helpful. Antibodies to double-stranded DNA (dsDNA) may also increase prior to a SLE flare.

In summary, there is no universal agreement about the effects of pregnancy on SLE but it appears that women with more inactive disease fare better than those with active disease. More recent studies that have a comparison group of nonpregnant women with lupus are more reassuring regarding pregnancy not exacerbating the disease. While some women may have an exacerbation during pregnancy, overall there is no long-term effect on the course of lupus with pregnancy. While there does not appear to be a strong contraindication to pregnancy during active disease, most authors recommend a period of about 6 months of inactive disease before conception.[13,15] In one study, a successful pregnancy outcome was demonstrated in 92% of women who had been in remission for at least 6 months.[15]

Effects of Systemic Lupus Erythematosus on Pregnancy

While there is some controversy about the effect of pregnancy on lupus activity, there is less question about the potential negative impact of lupus on the outcome of a pregnancy. SLE can affect fetal outcome both early and late in pregnancy, leading to spontaneous abortions, prematurity, stillbirths, and neonatal lupus, with most reports demonstrating an increase in fetal morbidity and mortality rates. Dombroski reviewed eight studies evaluating the outcome of pregnancies in women with lupus.[16] These showed spontaneous abortion rates of 5 to 30%, intrauterine fetal death rates of 1 to 44%, and term delivery rates of only 31 to 62%.[16] In general, most studies seem to indicate that those women with milder disease are at less risk for fetal complications and that outcomes since 1980 appear better.[16–18] Ramsey-Goldman reviewed seven studies of fetal outcome involving 742 pregnancies and found an adverse outcome in 34 to 72% (mean, 42%), with miscarriages in 16% (10–29%), prematurity in 20% (6–50%), and stillbirths in 6% (1–16%).[17] Out et al. reviewed 21 studies between 1962 and 1987 that demonstrated fetal loss rates from either spontaneous abortions or stillbirths of between 11 and 46% (median rate, 29%) as compared to 15% in the general population.[19] The median rate of premature births was 15%, compared to 8 to 9% in the general population. In the review by Fine et al. of 58 pregnancies in 44 patients over a 20-year period, there were 10 stillbirths (17.2%) and three spontaneous abortions (5.1%), for a fetal loss rate of 22.4%. Of these women, 14 (24%) delivered prematurely.[12] Mintz et al. found a 49% prevalence of prematurity in women with SLE, increasing to 59% in mothers with active SLE. Rates of small-for-gestational-age newborns were 23% in the total group of women with SLE and 65% in mothers with active SLE.[20]

One factor involved in the adverse outcome of these newborns may relate to changes in placental size. Hanly et al. demonstrated an overall reduction in placental size in women with SLE compared to either women without a chronic illness or women with diabetes.[21] They also found several pathological changes in the placenta including placental infarction, intraplacental hematoma, deposition of immunoglobulin and complement, and thickening of the trophoblast basement membrane.

Lupus nephritis also appears to be associated with increased risk of fetal loss.[12] In Fine's study, renal dysfunction correlated with fetal loss.[12] Women with proteinuria of over 300 mg/24 hours had a fetal loss rate of 38.5%, while a creatinine clearance rate of less than 100 mL/min was associated with fetal losses in 45.5% of pregnancies, and with both criteria present, the fetal loss rate was over 80%. Burkett also compared fetal losses in those women with and those without renal disease and found that the fetal loss rate was 36% in women with active renal disease and 15% if renal disease was inactive.[22]

Not all studies have reported high fetal loss rates. Wong et al., in a study of 29 pregnancies in 22 patients, reported a spontaneous fetal loss rate of 6.9%.[23] McHugh et al. compared pregnancy loss among a group of women with SLE, systemic sclerosis, or rheumatoid arthritis and healthy controls.[24] The women with SLE had similar fetal loss rates to the control group and those with rheumatoid arthritis.

The risk of fetal morbidity and mortality is correlated with activity of the disease and the degree of renal dysfunction. However, in recent years, several serological markers have also been strongly correlated with fetal losses. Antibodies to negatively charged phospholipids have been reported to be associated with early fetal losses while the development of neonatal lupus syndrome has been correlated to the presence of Ro antibody-positive mothers. While both of these entities occur in mothers with clinical lupus, they also occur in women without clinical evidence of disease. It remains to be seen whether these women without disease have a precursor to a collagen vascular disease or whether SLE needs redefining to include women with these conditions.

Antiphospholipid Antibody Syndrome

The antiphospholipid antibody syndrome is the association of antibodies to negatively charged phospholipids measured as either a biological false-positive test result for syphilis (VDRL), the lupus anticoagulant (LA), or anticardiolipin (ACL) antibodies, with several clinical complaints including recurrent fetal loss, arterial and venous thrombosis, and thrombocytopenia as well as several other clinical diseases. The syndrome may occur either in women with known collagen vascular diseases or in individuals who do not have other evidence of a collagen vascular disease. Despite extensive research in the past 5 to 10 years, the pathophysiology of this syndrome remains unclear. Antiphospholipid antibodies have also been associated with fetal growth restriction.[25]

Phospholipid antibodies include both the LA and ACL. Cardiolipin is a phospholipid located in the inner mitochondrial membranes of eukaryocytes.[16] ACL antibodies are present in 25 to 30% of SLE patients.[17] Cardiolipins are also the substrate for the VDRL. The LA is an IgG or IgM antibody that can cause prolonged clotting times in coagulation tests dependent on phospholipids.[19] The antibody prolongs coagulation times by binding to the phospholipid portion of the prothrombin activator complex.[16,19,26] LA is found in about 10% of SLE patients while about 50% of individuals with LA have SLE.[16] The antibody is usually detected by a prolonged PTT by a 1:1 mixture of the patient's and control plasma, and proved if the abnormality is due to an inhibitor whose activity is directed against phospholipid and not any specific coagulation proteins.[19,26]

The first antiphospholipid antibody explored was that associated with syphilis. Women with only a false-positive VDRL result are not at increased risk of fetal losses without the presence of other antiphospholipid antibodies. This was demonstrated in a study by Koskela et al., in which 134 women with false-positive VDRL test results were examined and the fetal loss rate (7%) was found to be similar to the RPR-negative controls.[27] Women with a false-positive VDRL result often have an autoimmune disorder and LA or ACL antibody.[26] The relative implications and meaning of a false-positive result for the VDRL, LA, or ACL antibody are not entirely clear at present.

Women with LA do not have bleeding problems unless there is another problem such as thrombocytopenia; however, they have been reported to be at increased risk for venous and arterial thrombosis,[8,26,28] thrombocytopenia,[29] pulmonary hypertension,[28,30] central nervous system disease,[31] lupus retinopathy,[32] livedo reticularis,[33] hemolytic anemia,[34] and excess fetal losses.[8,26,28,35,36]

Just as with LA, ACL antibody has been associated with recurrent pregnancy losses and recurrent thrombosis.[17,37–40] Pregnancy losses seem to be associated with ACL IgG antibodies and occasionally IgM antibodies. The pathophysiology is thought to be secondary to thrombosis of the utero-placental unit and vasoconstriction resulting from the binding of the immunoglobulins to platelet and endothelial membrane phospholipids.[39] Deleze et al. compared women with lupus with and without fetal loss to women without lupus with and without fetal loss.[41] The results demonstrated that women with SLE and a high titer of IgG antiphospholipid had a 10.5-fold risk of fetal loss. However, even women with high titers of antibodies can have normal pregnancies. Ishii and coworkers were able to divide individuals with lupus into two groups based on IgG ACL antibodies.[42] One group had persistently positive antibodies and while having milder lupus, had a high prevalence of thromboses, spontaneous abortions, and LA. Another group only had the antibodies in the active phase of lupus. This group had a higher prevalence of renal disease and anti-dsDNA. The rate of spontaneous abortions was 34% in the first group versus 6% in the second group. Some studies did not find an association between ACL antibodies and fetal loss.[24,43] Infante-Rivard et al. conducted a hospital-based case-control study of 331 women with spontaneous abortion or fetal death and 993 controls.[44] Only those women who had no previous spontaneous fetal loss were included. Both LA and IgG ACL antibodies were identified. There was no higher risk of these antibodies in women with fetal loss compared to controls in this study.[44]

It is not clear whether measuring LA or direct measurement for ACL antibody is a more sensitive predictor for fetal losses. In one study of 55 women with a history of recurrent fetal losses, 27% had ACL antibodies while only 7% had evidence of LA by a prolonged PTT.[39] In general, the prevalence of LA in women with recurrent fetal loss varies from 5.2 to 48.2% while the prevalence of antiphospholipid antibodies ranges from 7.7 to 42.4%.[26] The LA assay is often poorly controlled and performed differently at various institutions.

The efficacy of treatment for women with recurrent fetal losses and the presence of these antibodies is controversial. Treatment approaches have included both immunosuppression with steroids and antithrombogenic medications such as aspirin or heparin.[18] Gatenby et al. studied 15 women with SLE who previously had a 88% rate of fetal death or abortions and 22 women with definite SLE who had a prior fetal loss rate of 79%.[18] The women were treated with either prednisone alone or prednisone plus low-dose aspirin, 75 to 100 mg/day. Following treatment, the fetal loss rate was 55% in the women with SLE and 25% in the women without SLE. The largest success seemed to be in the women without definite SLE. Other studies have used steroids with some success but they were small and uncontrolled.[44–46] Heparin has not been well studied in this regard. Rosove et al. performed a small uncontrolled study of 14 women with a history of abnormal pregnancy outcomes.[47] In these high-risk women, with either LA or ACL antibodies, 14 of 15 pregnancies resulted in live births. Both high-dose gamma-globulin and plasmapheresis have also been reported to be successful in case reports but not in controlled studies.[48]

Another risk to pregnant women with lupus is the presence of maternal antibodies to ribonuclear proteins Ro(SSA) and La(SSB). These have been associated with congenital heart block and neonatal lupus syndrome.[16,29,49] About 50% of these infants will have heart disease and the other 50% will have hematological and dermatological abnormalities.[50] Most infants born with isolated congenital heart block have anti-SSA, passively acquired from their mothers.[18] These infants may also develop myocarditis and fibroelastosis. The prognosis for these infants is related to the degree of heart involvement.[50] Those without cardiac involvement generally have a good course. Neonates with isolated heart block may require cardiac pacing. Those with involvement of heart muscle and structural lesions may have a poor prognosis. The risk of any clinical manifestation in infants whose mothers have these antibodies appears to be about 25% but less than 3% for complete heart block.[45] The neonatal lupus syndrome also appears in infants of mothers with these antibodies who clinically do not appear to have lupus.

Thus, some antibodies are associated with fetal complications (SSA and SSB with neonatal lupus syndrome and heart block) and some antibodies with pregnancy outcome (antiphospholipid antibodies). The question of which of these antibody tests should be ordered as well as possible treatments is still open to debate. Those women with a history of recurrent fetal loss should have more aggressive diagnostic and therapeutic management.

Effect of Systemic Lupus Erythematosus Medications on Pregnancy

Aside from the effects of lupus on the pregnancy and fetus, the physician and family are also often concerned about medications' effects on the fetus.

ASPIRIN

While aspirin crosses the placenta and can produce congenital anomalies in animals, there is no evidence, in prospective studies, of fetal malformations in humans.[51,52] However, since the medication can result in lengthening of labor and hemorrhagic problems, it should be discontinued several weeks before anticipated delivery.

NONSTEROIDAL ANTIINFLAMMATORY DRUGS

These medications may lead to pulmonary hypertension in the fetus but long-term risks are not known. No evidence exists that these medications act as teratogens. Their use needs to be balanced against need. These drugs should also be discontinued several weeks before delivery to avoid hemorrhagic complications.

ANTIMALARIAL DRUGS

These drugs should be avoided because of their potential teratogenic effects on the eyes and ears of the fetus. Chloroquine and hydroxychloroquine both cross the placenta and can accumulate in the uveal tract of the fetus. It is best to discontinue these drugs at least 2 months before conception or to discontinue immediately after discovery of an unplanned pregnancy.

CORTICOSTEROIDS

These can be used if needed and appear to be relatively safe for use during pregnancy. Animal studies have demonstrated an increased risk of cleft lip and palate, which does not seem to be a significant problem in humans.[53] High doses of steroids during pregnancy have been associated with intrauterine growth retardation.

AZATHIOPRINE

While teratogenicity is possible and has been reported in animals, the potential in humans seems to be low and normal pregnancies have been reported.[11,54–61] Azathioprine does cross the placenta and has been associated with immunosuppression and serious infections in the newborn.[11] Long-term effects on the fetus are unknown.

CYCLOPHOSPHAMIDE

This is a known teratogen and should be avoided during pregnancy.[62–66] It is reported to cause multiple congenital anomalies including absent toes, palatal grooves, and hernias.

Contraception

With the increased risk of fetal complications in these women and the multisystem disease that many of these individuals have, the choice of a contraceptive becomes an integral part of their care. Contraception needs to be effective, reversible, and safe without exacerbating their lupus. Concerns have arisen over the use of combination hormonal contraceptives because of the risk that these hormones might exacerbate the disease. This concern arose out of the observation that the disease has a female-male ratio of 9:1 and that some women during pregnancy have a flare of their disease.

While several reports exist about possible problems of women on combination oral contraceptives, no controlled studies have been carried out in this population. Most of the reports are either case reports or small uncontrolled studies. Chapel and Burns reported on two women with lupus who had a lupus flare after starting combination oral contraceptives.[67] In another case report, four women with SLE were reported to have developed excessive fluid retention and one developed thrombophlebitis after starting combination oral contraceptives.[68] Iskander and Khan commented on three women who developed chorea as a presenting symptom of SLE after starting combination oral contraceptives.[69] All three had ACL antibodies, indicating the possibility that oral contraceptives could unmask SLE in individuals with ACL antibodies. Jungers et al. examined the effects of combination oral contraceptives and progestin-only contraception on the disease activity in 26 women with SLE.[70] A lupus flare occurred in 9 (43%) of the 20 women on combination pills within 3 months of starting. Five of the women were on a pill containing 30 μg of ethinyl estradiol. No exacerbations occurred in the 11 women who were on progestin-only oral contraceptives for up to 30 months (included 5 women previously on combination pills). Several other reports of a lupus flare associated with the start of combination oral contraceptives have been published.[71–74] However, none of these studies involved a large group of women or a control group. Mintz et al. evaluated progestin-only contraceptives in women with systemic lupus.[75] Ten women with systemic lupus received 200 mg of norethisterone enanthate intramuscularly, 15 women received 0.03 mg/day of oral levonorgestrel, and 18 women with systemic lupus on no hormonal contraceptives served as controls. There were no significant differences in the numbers of episodes of active SLE between the three groups. There are no studies examining the use of medroxyprogesterone or the Norplant implant in this population.

Many authorities would advise against the use of combination estrogen/progestin pills in these women. If hormonal contraceptives are utilized, it is probably wise to use progestin-only contraceptives. Before prescribing hormonal contraceptives, the physician should consider the extent and degree of organ damage. Estrogen-containing pills should probably only be considered for those women with very mild lupus and with no hypertension or vascular involvement. If combination pills are used, a very low dose of estrogen should be used. In those women with liver involvement, hormonal contraception is probably best avoided.

The intrauterine device (IUD) is not a good alternative in these individuals. As these women may already be at increased risk of infection, the addition of another source of infection is not desirable. In addition, if the woman is on steroids, the efficacy of the IUD may be reduced. There are no contraindications to barrier methods in individuals with SLE. While barrier devices have the least number of side effects, these devices are associated with a greater risk of pregnancy.

Summary

1. Fertility rates do not seem affected by SLE except in women who are seriously ill or have significant renal disease.
2. The effect of pregnancy on SLE is variable. Some women will experience an exacerbation during or after pregnancy, with the first trimester and

the puerperium being the most common periods. It is recommended that women wait 6 months with their disease in an inactive state before a pregnancy is contemplated. While maternal deaths do occur during pregnancy, the rate is very small.

3. Fetal complications including spontaneous abortions, prematurity, and stillbirths are more common in women with SLE. Women with milder disease are at lower risk while those with renal dysfunction are at a higher risk. Women with antiphospholipid antibodies (either LA or ACL antibody) are also at greater risk of recurrent fetal losses. Women with anti-SSA and anti-SSB are at greater risk for having an infant with neonatal lupus syndrome.

4. Barrier methods have the least number of associated side effects in women with SLE; however, they are associated with a higher rate of pregnancy.

5. Progestin-only contraceptives appear safe in most women with lupus. Combination hormonal contraceptives could be considered in women with SLE without hypertension and vascular complications.

6. The IUD is probably not desirable because of concerns about infections in an already immunocompromised individual.

Rheumatoid Arthritis

Fertility

Fertility rates do not appear to be lower in individuals with rheumatoid arthritis. However, sexuality and sexual libido could be affected if there is either joint pain or a significant limitation of joint motion. This in turn could affect the number of pregnancies. In addition, medications such as steroids may affect libido.

Traditionally, advice to women on motherhood is often based on perceptions of the medical profession without significant regard to the response of women to their pregnancies and motherhood. Ostensen examined these issues in a study of women with rheumatic disease.[76] Among women with either juvenile rheumatoid arthritis (JRA) or rheumatoid arthritis, 10% received no information about gestation and their disease and 27% were advised against pregnancy by either health professionals, family, or other patients. These women often remarked about receiving notes of caution but rarely positive advice or competent information. They found that answers were often global and did not focus on their particular form of illness. Only 8% had received complete answers to their questions and felt comfortable about going through with a pregnancy. Most of the women wished for two children. Ostensen recommended that competent and extensive information be provided to these women before a pregnancy.[76] This information should include not only medical facts but also practical aids including how to solve problems after delivery. More important than the effects of the disease may be the individual coping skills and access to help with child caring. Spacing of pregnancies may be important to discuss. In addition, the spouse should be included in the decision-making process at all times as he will be important in parental responsibilities.

Effect of Pregnancy on Rheumatoid Arthritis

Pregnancy can alter the disease activity in women with various collagen vascular diseases. Pregnancy in women with rheumatoid arthritis probably has the most consistent effect among the various collagen vascular diseases. First noted over 50 years ago by Hench and by many others since, rheumatoid arthritis is associated with a remission during the pregnancy and often with a postpartum flare.[77–80] In Persellin's review of 308 pregnancies, a remission occurred in 73%, with no change or a worse course in 27%.[78] In those with a remission, 75% occurred during the first trimester, 20% in the second trimester, and 5% in the third trimester. If there is a remission, it usually will persist throughout pregnancy, often reaching maximal improvement in the third trimester.[78,81] Of note is that these remissions occur in many individuals despite a large reduction or even elimination of antirheumatic medications.[78,82,83] The severity or duration of disease does not seem to be predictive of which women will have a remission during pregnancy. However, if improvement occurs with one pregnancy, improvement tends to occur with other pregnancies.[78,82]

Contrary to the course during pregnancy, over 90% of women experience a relapse after delivery. In Persellin's review, 9% of the relapses occurred within the first 2 weeks postpartum, 17% between 2 and 4 weeks, 27% between 4 and 6 weeks, 12% between 6 and 8 weeks, and 35% after 8 weeks.[78] Most women require the restart of their medications postpartum. The severity of disease postpartum usually returns to the level of disease activity before the pregnancy.

While the exact cause of the pregnancy-related remission is unknown, the most common hypothesis is related to pregnancy-induced immunosuppression secondary to either fetal suppression of the maternal immune system, depression of cell-mediated immunity, or suppression of inflammatory reactions.[80] Numerous circulating factors have been hypothesized as possible causes of this immunosuppression. These include estrogen, progesterone, alpha-fetoproteins, corticosteroids, and several proteins produced in the placenta such as pregnancy-associated plasma protein A (PAPP-A), pregnancy-associated alpha$_2$-globulin (PAG), pregnancy-specific beta$_1$-glycoprotein (SPa), and placental protein 14 (PP-14).[80]

Effect of Rheumatoid Arthritis on Pregnancy

There has been no strong evidence for any increase in risk to a pregnancy or to the fetus as a consequence of rheumatoid arthritis. Several reports demonstrated a good maternal and fetal outcome associated with rheumatoid arthritis, with no evidence of obstetric complications, prematurity, or fetal loss.[79,82,84–86] However, studies examining only women with severe systemic disease have not been reported.

Effect of Rheumatoid Arthritis Medications on Pregnancy

Another consideration in these women either when planning a pregnancy or after a pregnancy is the effect of their medication on the fetus. These women have the possibility of being on many different medications including salicylates, nonsteroidal antiinflammatory drugs, corticosteroids, gold, antimalarials, D-penicillamine, methotrexate, and azathioprine. Many of these women will be able to cut down or eliminate their medication during pregnancy. If needed, salicylates appear to be a safe medication for use during pregnancy. However, because of the risk of antepartum or postpartum hemorrhage in infants, it is recommended to discontinue the medication for several weeks before delivery. In prospective studies, no significant congenital malformations were found in humans using salicylates.[51,52] Significant reports of teratogenicity have also not been reported with the nonsteroidal antiinflammatory drugs, although the clinical experience during pregnancy is less than that with salicylates. Because of their unknown effects, many authors have recommended switching to aspirin during pregnancy. Nonsteroidals, when used, should also be discontinued several weeks before delivery. When needed, corticosteroids appear to be relatively safe for use during pregnancy. Although gold has not been reported to be teratogenic in humans, because of reports of teratogenicity in animals and because it is a second-line drug, it should probably be discontinued during pregnancy. However, gold has been used during pregnancy without fetal problems.[86,87] Antimalarials including chloroquine and hydroxychloroquine have been associated with both retinal damage and nerve deafness and should be discontinued before pregnancy is contemplated. Most women on D-penicillamine have no complications with their offspring.[88,89] However, there are two reports of fetal connective tissue disease when mothers took D-penicillamine during pregnancy.[90,91] Thus, the drug is not advisable for use during pregnancy if the disease can be controlled without it. The effect of methotrexate during pregnancy in women with rheumatoid arthritis was examined in one study of eight women with 10 pregnancies.[92] The mean number of weeks of gestation while taking the methotrexate was 7.5. The 10 pregnancies ended with three spontaneous abortions, two therapeutic abortions, and five full-term uncomplicated deliveries. All five children were normal and had normal growth and development at a mean age of 11.5. In this study, there was no proof of teratogenicity, but there was a suggestion of a higher rate of spontaneous abortion. However, congenital malformations have been reported.[93,94] Since, the potential for tetratogenicity exists, a therapeutic abortion, while not mandatory, is a consideration and certainly once a pregnancy is diagnosed, the drug should be stopped. In addition, if a pregnancy is planned, the medication should be stopped several months before conception. Recommendations for the use of azathioprine are similar. Normal infants have resulted from pregnancies when the mother was on azathioprine.[80] However, congenital malformations have been reported to occur in women on azathioprine with prednisone so that it would be advised to discontinue azathioprine before a pregnancy is planned or after one is diagnosed.[95,96] In addition, reports of lymphopenia and decreased immunoglobulin levels in the infants of mothers taking azathioprine have been reported.[95,96]

Other considerations in these women are the difficulties they may have with maternity clothes and positioning during pelvic examinations and during delivery. Women with significant joint limitation of movement or pain may have trouble placing their feet in the stirrups of the examination and delivery table and abducting their legs for the examination and delivery. It might be useful to have a family member available to help support the woman's legs or for the examiner to conduct the examination in the side-lying position. Maternity dresses may also need to be altered with Velcro openings to allow the women to open and close the dresses with greater ease.

Contraception

In early studies, combination oral contraceptives were actually used as a therapy for rheumatoid arthritis because of the positive effect of pregnancy in these women. However, there has been no benefit in active arthritis from the use of oral contraceptives. Most of the research in relation to oral contraceptives and rheumatoid arthritis has been in evaluating the relative prevalence of rheumatoid arthritis in users and nonusers of oral contraceptives. Several studies showed a protective effect.[97–100] For example, in one case-control study, nulliparous women never having used oral contraceptives had four times the risk of developing rheumatoid arthritis as multiparous women who had used oral contraceptives.[97] The initial results from the Royal College of General Practitioners (RCGP) also demonstrated a decreased prevalence among oral contraceptives users; however, a more recent analysis of the RCGP data failed to show a protective effect in oral contraceptive users.[101,102] Other studies also failed to show a protective effect.[103–106] Two meta-analyses of this question have been conducted. One of these suggested that oral contraceptives may have a positive effect, not by preventing the disease but by decreasing the number of individuals who progress from mild to severe disease.[107] The other meta-analysis involving 12 prior studies demonstrated a small but statistically insignificant protective effect.[108]

While it has been presumed that hormonal contraceptives do not negatively affect the course of the disease in rheumatoid arthritis, there are few studies that actually demonstrate this. Hazes et al. conducted a study of 10 women with active rheumatoid arthritis and placed them on a high-dose oral contraceptive to try and improve their disease.[109] There was no improvement in the clinical or laboratory course of the disease. However, there was no increase in severity while the women were taking oral contraceptives. Overall, there is no evidence that hormonal contraceptives have any negative impact on rheumatoid arthritis. There is the possible problem of oral contraceptive packages being too difficult to handle by women with severe deformities of their hands. The intrauterine device (IUD) does not have any special contraindications except in those women on steroids or other immunosuppressives where there have been reports of IUD failure. Barrier methods might present a problem if the individual is severely disabled and may not have adequate dexterity for insertion or removal of these barrier devices. Partners may need to take an active role in these situations.

Summary

1. Fertility rates are normal in women with rheumatoid arthritis.
2. Most women experience a remission during pregnancy that usually starts in the first trimester. Most women also experience a flare of their disease postpartum.
3. The course of the pregnancy and fetal outcome is not altered by rheumatoid arthritis but the potential exists for fetal problems in women taking certain medications such as methotrexate. Because most women will have an improvement or remission during pregnancy, medications should be tapered down when possible.
4. Hormonal contraceptives are fully acceptable in women with rheumatoid arthritis. However, while they provide effective contraception, there is little to suggest they will reduce the severity of the disease.
5. Barrier devices are acceptable but may be a problem for those women with severe disabilities of their hands or hips.
6. The IUD has no specific contraindications, with the exception of women on steroids or immunosuppressives where a decrease in efficacy could occur.

Juvenile Rheumatoid Arthritis

Ostensen evaluated the relationship between pregnancy and those women with JRA.[110] She collected data from 76 pregnancies in 51 women with JRA in a retrospective study. In those women with quiescent JRA, disease activity did not change during gestation. In those women with minor symptoms at conception and in those with active inflammation, most showed improvement or remission in the second half of pregnancy. Of the 76 pregnancies, 74 resulted in a normal healthy-weight infant, with one infant of low birthweight and one stillborn. A flare occurred 3 to 6 months postpartum in 45 pregnancies. A higher frequency of cesarean sections was performed, with bilateral hip prosthesis being the main reason. In those women with cervical spine, temporomandibular joint, and cricoarytenoid joint involvement, warnings about possible complications of general anesthesia should be given. These data suggest a good outcome for mother and infant in those women with JRA. However, the long-term effects of prior drug treatment were not evaluated in this study. Contraceptive recommendations for these women would be similar to those for women with rheumatoid arthritis.

Ankylosing Spondylitis

Much less is known about pregnancy in women with ankylosing spondylitis than with rheumatoid arthritis. There is little to suggest that there is the type of improvement seen with rheumatoid arthritis. Reports indicate that about one-third of women get better and one-third get worse.[111] Many will experience a temporary exacerbation within the first 6 months postpartum that usually lasts about 2 to 4 months.[11] After this, the majority will return to their prepregnancy state. There have been no reports of an increase in fetal complications or losses. There does not appear to be any specific contraindications or considerations with contraceptive devices in individuals with ankylosing spondylitis.

Systemic Sclerosis

Fertility problems have been reported in individuals with systemic sclerosis.[112,113] However, in one series of 86 women with systemic sclerosis there was no difference in fertility rates compared to those in matched controls.[114]

The combination of pregnancy and systemic sclerosis is uncommon, as this disease has only a prevalence in the United State of about 3 to 12 per 100,000. In one large review study, 39% of women had a worsening of their condition while in 22% there was an improvement and 39% had no change.[115] There was no control group of nonpregnant women with systemic sclerosis in this study. In another study, those women with early rapidly progressive diffuse skin thickening were at higher risk of developing a renal crisis with accelerated hypertension.[116] In this study 48 pregnant women with systemic sclerosis were compared to 48 pregnant women with rheumatoid arthritis and a control group of 48 pregnant women. There was no change in the disease symptoms in 88% of pregnancies while there was an exacerbation in 7% and an improvement in 5%. The investigators also found no difference in survival rates between the pregnant and nonpregnant women with systemic sclerosis. There were also no differences in rates of miscarriages or perinatal death in the women with systemic sclerosis compared to women with rheumatoid arthritis or the control group. However, preterm births occurred slightly more frequently in the women with systemic sclerosis and rheumatoid arthritis. Overall, the investigators reported a 5% perinatal mortality rate and a 3% fetal mortality rate in women with systemic sclerosis, as well as a 10% incidence of intrauterine growth retardation and an 8% incidence of preterm delivery. Two other studies suggested a higher rate of abortions in women with systemic sclerosis.[113,114]

No information or studies that examined the effects of hormonal contraceptives and other contraceptive devices in these women have been found. Use of hormonal contraceptives would have to be on an individual basis, using caution and either progestin-only contraceptives or combination contraceptives with low doses of hormones.

References

1. Fraga A, Mintz G, Orozco J, Orozco JH. Sterility and fertility rates, fetal wastage and maternal morbidity in systemic lupus erythematosus. J Rheumatol 1974;1:293–8.
2. Friedman EA, Rutherford JW. Pregnancy and lupus erythematosus. Obstet Gynecol 1956;8:601–9.
3. Cecere FA, Persellin RH. The interaction of pregnancy and the rheumatic diseases. Clin Rheum Dis 1981;7:747–68.
4. Garsenstein M, Pollak VE, Karik RM. Systemic lupus erythematosus and pregnancy. N Engl J Med 1962;276:165–9.
5. Zurier RG, Argyros T, Urman J, Warren J, Rothfield NF. Systemic lupus erythematosus: Management during pregnancy. Obstet Gynecol 1978;51:178–80.
6. Nossent HC, Swaak TJ. Systemic lupus erythematosus VI. Analysis of the interrelationship with pregnancy. J Rheumatol 1990;17:771–6.
7. Donaldson LB, DeAlvarez RR. Further observations on LE associated with pregnancy. Am J Obstet Gynecol 1961;83:1461–73.
8. Lockshin MD, Reinitz E, Druzin ML, Murrman M, Estes D. Lupus pregnancy. Case-control prospective study demonstrating absence of lupus exacerbation during or after pregnancy. Am J Med 1984;77:893–98.
9. Derksen RH. Systemic lupus erythematosus and pregnancy. Rheumatol Int 1991;11:121–5.
10. Estes D, Larson DL. Systemic lupus erythematosus and pregnancy. Clin Obstet Gynecol 1965;8:307–21.
11. Meehan RT, Dorsey JK. Pregnancy among patients with systemic lupus erythematosus receiving immunosuppressive therapy. J Rheumatol 1987;14:252–8.
12. Fine LG, Barnett EV, Danovitch G, Nissenson AR, Conolly ME, Lieb SM, Barrett CT. SLE in pregnancy. Ann Intern Med 1981;94:667–77.
13. Samuels P, Pfeifer SM. Autoimmune disease in pregnancy. The obstetricians' view. Rheum Dis Clin North Am 1989;15:307–22.
14. Buyon JP, Cronstein BN, Morris M, Tanner M, Weissmann G. Serum complement values (C3 and C4) to differentiate between systemic lupus activity and pre-eclampsia. Am J Med 1986;81:194–200.
15. Hayslett JP, Lynn RI. Effect of pregnancy in patients with lupus nephropathy. Kidney Int 1980;18:207.
16. Dombroski RA. Autoimmune disease in pregnancy. Med Clin North Am 1989;73:605–21.
17. Ramsey-Goldman R. Pregnancy in sytemic lupus erythematosus. Rheum Dis Clin North Am 1988;14:169–85.
18. Gatenby PA. Systemic lupus erythematosus and pregnancy. Aust N Z J Med 1989;19:261–78.

19. Out HJ, Derksen RH, Christiaens GC. Systemic lupus erythematosus and pregnancy. Obstet Gynecol Surv 1989;44:585–91.
20. Mintz G, Niz J, Guttierez G, Gardia Alonso A, Karchmer S. Prospective study of pregnancy in systemic lupus erythematosus. Results of a multidisciplinary approach. J Rheumatol 1986;13:732–9.
21. Hanly JG, Gladman DD, Rose TH, Laskin CA, Urowitz MB. Lupus pregnancy. A prospective study of placental changes. Arthritis Rheum 1988;31:358–66.
22. Burkett G. Lupus nephropathy and pregnancy. Clin Obstet Gynecol 1985;28:310–23.
23. Wong KL, Chan FY, Lee CP. Outcome of pregnancy in patients with systemic lupus erythematosus: A prospective study. Arch Intern Med 1991;151:269–73.
24. McHugh NJ, Reilly PA, McHugh LA. Pregnancy outcome and autoantibodies in connective tissue disease. J Rheumatol 1989;16:42–6.
25. Polzin WJ, Kopelman JN, Robinson RD, Read JA, Brady K. The association of antiphospholipid antibodies with pregnancies complicated by fetal growth restriction. Obstet Gynecol 1991;78:1108–11.
26. Triplett DA. Antiphospholipid antibodies and recurrent pregnancy loss. Am J Reprod Immunol 1989;20:52–67.
27. Koskela P, Vaarala O, Makitalo R, Palosuo T, Aho K. Significance of false positive syphilis reactions and anticardiolipin antibodies in a nationwide series of pregnant women. J Rheumatol 1988;15:70–3.
28. Harvey CJ, Verklan T. Systemic lupus erythematosus: Obstetric and neonatal implications. NAACOGS Clin Issu Perinat Womens Health Nurs 1990;1:177–85.
29. Parke AL. Antiphospholipid antibody syndromes. Rheum Dis Clin North Am 1989;15:275–86.
30. Asherson RA, Mackworth-Young CG, Boey ML, Hull RG, Saunders A, Gharawi AE, Hughes GRV. Pulmonary hypertension in systemic lupus erythematosus. Br Med J 1983;287:1024–5.
31. Levine SR, Welch KMA. Cerebrovascular ischemia associated with lupus anticoagulant. Stroke 1987;18:257–63.
32. Levine SR, Crofts JW, Lesser R, Floberg J, Welch MA. Visual symptoms associated with the presence of a lupus anticoagulant. Ophthalmology 1988;95:686–91.
33. Weinstein C, Miller MH, Axtens R, Buchanan R, Littlejohn GO. Livedo reticularis associated with increased titers of anticardiolipin antibodies in systemic lupus erythematosus. Arch Dermatol 1987;123:596–600.
34. Deleze M, Alarcon-Segovia D, Oria CV. Occurrence of both hemolytic anemia and thrombocytopenic purpura (Evans'syndrome) in systemic lupus erythematosus. Relationship to antiphospholipid antibodies. J Rheumatol 1988;15:611–5.
35. Scott JR, Rote NS, Branch DW. Immunologic aspects of recurrent abortion and fetal death. Obstet Gynecol 1987;70:645.
36. Lubbe WF, Butler WS, Palmer SJ, Liggins GC. Lupus anticoagulant and pregnancy. Br J Obstet Gynaecol 1984;91:357–63.
37. Lockshin MD, Druzin ML, Goei S, Qamar T, Magid MS, Jovanovic L, Ferenc M. Antibody to cardiolipin as a predictor of fetal distress or death in pregnant patients with systemic lupus erythematosus. N Engl J Med 1985;313:152–6.
38. Harris EN, Chan JKH, Sherson RA, Asherson RA, Aber UR, Gharari AE, Hughes GRV. Thrombosis, recurrent fetal loss and thrombocytopenia, Predictive value of the anticardiolipin antibody test. Arch Intern Med 1986;146:2153–6.
39. Lockwood CJ, Reece EA, Romero R, Hobbins JC. Antiphospholipid antibody and pregnancy wastage. Lancet 1986;2:742–3.
40. Lockshin MD, Qamar T, Levy RA, Druzin ML. Pregnancy in systemic lupus erythematosus. Clin Exp Rheumatol 1989;7:S195–7.
41. Deleze M, Alarcon-Segovia D, Valdes-Machon E, Oria CV, Poncede-Leon S. Relationship between antiphospholipid antibodies and recurrent fetal loss in patients with systemic lupus erythematosus and apparently healthy women. J Rheumatol 1989;16:768–72.
42. Ishii Y, Nagasawa K, Mayumi T, Niho Y. Clinical importance of persistence of anticardiolipin antibodies in systemic lupus erythematosus. Ann Rheum Dis 1990;49:387–90.
43. Hanly JG, Dafna DG, Rose TH, Laskin CA, Urowitz MB. Lupus pregnancy. A prospective study of placental changes. Arthritis Rheum 1988;31:358–66.
44. Infante-Rivard C, David M, Gauthier R, Rivard GE. Lupus anticogulants, anticardiolipin antibodies and fetal loss. N Engl J Med 1991;325:1063–6.

45. Lubbe WF, Butler WS, Palmer SJ, Ligins GC. Fetal survival after prednisone suppression of maternal lupus anticoagulant. Lancet 1983;1:1361–3.
46. Branch WB, Scott JR, Kochenour NK, Hershgold E. Obstetric complications associated with the lupus anticoagulant. New Engl J Med 1985;313:1322–6.
47. Rosove MH, Tabsh K, Wasserstrum N, Howard P, Hahn BH, Kalunian KC. Heparin therapy for pregnant women with lupus anticoagulant or anticardiolipin antibodies. Obstet Gynecol 1990;75:630–4.
48. Lockshin MD. Pregnancy associated with systemic lupus erythematosus. Semin Perinatol 1990;14:130–8.
49. Scott JS, Maddison PJ, Taylor PV, Esscher E, Scott O, Skinner RP. Connective tissue disease, antibodies to ribonucleoprotein and congenital heart block. N Engl J Med 1983;309:209–12.
50. Watson RM, Lane AT, Barnett NK, Bias WB, Arnett FC, Provost TT. Neonatal lupus erythematosus: A clinical, serological and immunogenetic study with review of the literature. Medicine 1984;63:362–78.
51. Lee P. Anti-inflammatory therapy during pregnancy and lactation. Clin Invest Med 1985;8:328–32.
52. Sloan D, Heinonem OP, Siskind V, Kaufman DW, Monson RR, Shapiros S. Aspirin and congenital malformations. Lancet 1976;1:1373–75.
53. Gabbe SG. Drug therapy in autoimmune disease. Clin Obstet Gynecol 1983;26:635–41.
54. Tuchmann-Duplessis H, Mercier-Parot L. Production in rabbits of malformations of the limbs by azathioprine and 6-mercaptopurine. C R Soc Biol 1966;166:501–6.
55. Rosenkrantz JG, Githens JH, Cos SM, Kellum DL. Azathioprine (Imuran) in pregnancy. Am J Obstet Gynecol 1967;97:387.
56. Erkman J, Blyth JG. Azathioprine therapy complicated by pregnancy. Obstet Gynecol 1972;40:708–10.
57. Farber M, Kennison RD, Jackson HT. Successful pregnancy after renal transplantation. Obstet Gynecol 1976;48(suppl 1):25–45.
58. Registration Committee of the European Dialysis and Transplant Association. Successful pregnancies in women treated by dialysis and kidney transplantation. Br J Obstet Gynaecol 1980;87:839–45.
59. Davidson AM, Guillon PJ. Successful pregnancies reported to the registry up to the end of 1982. Proc Eur Dialysis Transplant Assoc London 1984;21:54–5.
60. Gaudier FL, Santiago-Delphin E, Rivera J, Gonzales Z. Pregnancy after renal transplantation. Surg Gynecol Obstet 1988;167:533–43.
61. Hou S. Pregnancy in organ transplant recipients. Med Clin North Am 1989;734:667–83.
62. Greenberg LH, Palos V, Tanaka KR. Congenital anomalies probably induced by cyclophosphamide. JAMA 1964;188:423–6.
63. Toledo TM, Harper RC, Moser RH. Fetal effects during cyclophosphamide and irradiation therapy. Ann Intern Med 1971;74:87–91.
64. Coates A. Cyclophosphamide in pregnancy. Aust N Z J Obstet Gynaecol 1970;10:33–4.
65. Murray CL, Reichert JA, Anderson J, Twiggs LB. Multimodal cancer therapy for breast cancer in the first trimester of pregnancy. JAMA 1984:252:2607–8.
66. Sweet DL, Kinzie J. Consequences of radiotherapy and antineoplastic therapy for the fetus. J Reprod Med 1976;17:241–6.
67. Chapel TA, Burns RE. Oral contraceptives and exacerbation of lupus erythematosus. Am J Obstet Gynecol 1971;110:366–9.
68. Rothfield N. General consideration in the treatment of systemic lupus erythematosus. Mayo Clin Proc 1969;44:691–6.
69. Iskander MK, Khan M. Chorea as the initial presentation of oral contraceptive related systemic lupus erythematosus. J Rheumatol 1989;16:850–1.
70. Jungers P, Dougados M, Pelissier C, Kuttenn F, Tron F, Lesaure P, Back JF. Influence of oral contraceptive therapy on the activity of systemic lupus erythematosus. Arthritis Rheum 1982;25:618–23.
71. Travers RL, Hughes GR. Oral contraceptive therapy and systemic lupus erythematosus. J Rheumatol 1978;5:448–51.
72. Pimstone BL. Systemic lupus erythematosus exacerbated by oral contraceptives. S Afr J Obstet Gynecol 1966;4:62–3.
73. Hadida M, Sayag J. Lupus erythemateux subaign apparu apres une cure de norluten chez une malade atteinte de lupus erythemateux chronique. Bull Soc Fr Dermatol Syphil 1968;75:616–7.

74. Garovich M, Agudelo C, Pisko E. Oral contraceptives and systemic lupus erythematosus. Arthritis Rheum 1980;23:1396–8.
75. Mintz G, Gutierrez G, Deleze M, Rodriguez E. Contraception with progestagens in systemic lupus erythematosus. Contraception 1984;30:29–38.
76. Ostensen M. Counselling women with rheumatic disease—How many children are desirable? Scand J Rheumatol 1991;20:121–6.
77. Hench PS. The ameliorating effect of pregnancy on chronic atrophic (infectious rheumatoid) arthritis, fibrosis, and intermittent hydrarthrosis. Proc Mayo Clin 1938;13:161.
78. Persellin RH. The effect of pregnancy on rheumatoid arthritis. Bull Rheum Dis 1977;27:922–7.
79. Nicholas NS. Rheumatic diseases in pregnancy. Br J Hosp Med 1988;39:50–3.
80. Klipple GL, Cecere FA. Rheumatoid arthritis and pregnancy. Rheum Dis Clin North Am 1989;15:213–39.
81. Bulmash JM. Rheumatoid arthritis and pregnancy. Obstet Gynecol 1985;8:223–76.
82. Ostensen M, Husby G. A prospective clinical study of the effect of pregnancy on rheumatoid arthritis and ankylosing spondylitis. Arthritis Rheum 1983;26:1155–9.
83. Unger A, Kay A, Griffin AJ, Panayi GS. Disease activity and pregnancy associated alpha-2 glycoprotein in rheumatoid arthritis during pregnancy. Br Med J 1983;286:750–2.
84. Morris WIC. Pregnancy in rheumatoid arthritis and systemic lupus erythematosus. Aust N Z J Obstet Gynaecol 1969;9:136–44.
85. Ostensen M, Aune B, Husby G. Effect of pregnancy and hormonal changes on the activity of rheumatoid arthritis. Scand J Rheumatol 1983;12:315–8.
86. Huskisson EC, Berry H. Some immunologic changes in rheumatoid arthritis among patients receiving penicillamine and gold. Postgrad Med J 1974;505:59–61.
87. Thurnau GR. Rheumatoid arthritis. Clin Obstet Gynecol 1983;26:558–78.
88. Lyle WH. Penicillamine in pregnancy. Lancet 1978;1:606–7.
89. Scheinberg IH, Sternlieb I. Pregnancy in penicillamine treated patients with Wilson's disease. N Engl J Med 1975;293:1300–2.
90. Solomon L, Abram G, Dinner M, Berman L. Neonatal abnormalities associated with D-penicillamine treatment during pregnancy. N Engl J Med 1977;296:54–5.
91. Mjolnerod IK, Rasmussen K, Dommerud SA, Gjeroldsen ST. Congenital connective tissue defect probably due to penicillamine treatment during pregnancy. Lancet. 1971;1:673–5.
92. Kozlowski RD, Steinbrunner JV, MacKenzie AH, Clough JD, Wilek WS, Segal AM. Outcome of first trimester exposure to low dose methotrexate in eight patients with rheumatic disease. Am J Med 1990;88:589–92.
93. Decker JL. Toxicity of immunosuppressive drugs in man. Arthritis Rheum 1973;16:58–74.
94. Milunsky A, Graef JW, Gaynor MF Jr. Methotrexate-induced congenital malformations. J Pediatr 1968;72:790–5.
95. Penn I, Makowski EL. Parenthood in kidney and liver transplant recipients. Transplant Proc 1981;13:36–9.
96. O'Connell PJ, Caterson RJ, Steart JH, Mahony JF. Problems associated with pregnancy in renal allograft recipients. Int J Artif Organs 1989;12:147–52.
97. Hazes JM, Silman AJ, Brand R, Spector TD, Waler DJ, Vandenbroucke JP. A case control study of oral contraceptive use in women with rheumatoid arthritis and their unaffected sisters. Br J Rheumatol 1989;28(suppl I):35–45.
98. Hazes JM, Kijkmans BC, Vandenbroucke JP, deVries RR, Cats A. Reduction of the risk of rheumatoid arthritis among women who take oral contraceptives. Arthritis Rhuem 1990;33:173–9.
99. Hazes JM, Silman AJ, Brand R, Spector TD, Walker DJ, Vandenbroucke JP. Influence of oral contraception on the occurrence of rheumatoid arthritis in female sibs. Scand J Rheumatol 1990;19:306–10.
100. Spector TD, Roman E, Silman AJ. The pill, parity, and rheumatoid arthritis. Arthritis Rheum 1990;33:782–9.
101. Wingrave S, Kay CR. Reduction in incidence of rheumatoid arthritis associated with oral contraceptives. Lancet 1978;1:569–71.
102. Hannaford PC, Kay CR. Oral contraceptives and rheumatoid arthritis: New data from the Royal College of General `Practitioners' Oral Contraception Study. Br J Rheumatol 1989;28(suppl I):36.
103. Linos A, Worthington JW, O'Fallon WM, Kurland LT. Case-control study of rheumatoid arthritis and prior use of oral contraceptives. Lancet 1983;1:1299–300.

104. Del Junco DJ, Annegers JF, Luthra HS, Coulam CB, Kurland LT. Do oral contraceptives prevent rheumatoid arthritis? JAMA 1985;254:1938–41.
105. Vessey MP, Villard-Mackintosh L, Yeates D. Oral contraceptives, cigarette smoking and other factors in relation to arthritis. Contraception 1987;35:457–64.
106. Hernandez-Avila M, Liang MH, Willett WC, Stampfer MJ, Colditz GA, Rosner B, Chang RW, Hennekens CH, Speizer FE. Exogenous sex hormones and the risk of rheumatoid arthritis. Arthritis Rheum 1990;33:947–53.
107. Spector TD, Hochberg MC. The protective effect of the oral contraceptive pill on rheumatoid arthritis: An overview of the analytical. Br J Rheumatol 1989;28:18–23.
108. Romieu I, Hernandez-Avila M, Liang MH. Oral contraceptives and the risk of rheumatoid arthritis: A meta-analysis of a conflicting literature. Br J Rheumatol 1989;28:13–7.
109. Hazes JM, Dijkmans BA, Vandenbroucke JP, Cats A. Oral contraceptive treatment for rheumatoid arthritis: An open study in 10 female patients. Br J Rheumatol 1989;28:28–30.
110. Ostensen M. Pregnancy in patients with a history of juvenile rheumatoid arthritis. Arthritis Rheum 1991;34:881–7.
111. Ostensen M, Husby G. Ankylosing spondylitis and pregnancy. Rheum Dis Clin North Am 1989;15:241-54.
112. Leinwant I, Duryee AW, Richter MN. Scleroderma (based on a study of over 150 cases). Ann Intern Med 1954;41:1003–41.
113. Silman AJ, Black C. Increased incidence of spontaneous abortion and infertility in women with scleroderma before disease onset: A controlled study. Ann Rheum Dis 1988;47:441–4.
114. Giordano M, Valentini G, Lupoli S, Giordano A. Pregnancy and systemic sclerosis. Arthritis Rheum 1985;28:237–8.
115. Johnson TR, Bannes EA, Winkelman RK. Scleroderma and pregnancy. Obstet Gynecol 1964;23:467–9.
116. Steen VD, Conte C, Day N, Ramsey-Goldman R, Medsger TA Jr. Pregnancy in women with systemic sclerosis. Arthritis Rheum 1989;32:151–7.

12

Cardiovascular Diseases

Cardiovascular diseases cover a wide range of conditions. This chapter focuses on valvular disease, atherosclerotic heart disease, hyperlipidemia, and hypertension.

Physiological Cardiovascular Changes of Pregnancy

Pregnancy is associated with many changes that help meet the demands of the growing fetus.[1,2] Many of these involve the cardiovascular system. This is no problem for the healthy woman but the woman with cardiac diseases may not be able to meet these demands. These changes include

- A blood volume that increases by about 50%
- An extravascular fluid increase associated with edema particularly in the lower extremities
- A lowered systemic vascular resistance secondary to the placental bed acting as a large arteriovenous shunt
- A cardiac output that increases about 30 to 40% from about 4.5 to 6.0 L/min

Maternal cardiac output increases after about 12 weeks of gestation and continues to increase thereafter until about the 32nd week. Cardiac output plateaus at that time until about the 38th week when there is a slight decrease until term. Another increase in cardiac output occurs during labor secondary to the effects of pain and the increase in blood released from uterine contractions.

The increase in cardiac output associated with pregnancy is a result of an increase in both stroke volume and rate.[1] Stroke volume increases mainly in the first half of pregnancy and then declines to normal levels in the third trimester. Heart rate, after rising by about 10 beats/min by the end of the second trimester, falls slightly.

Aside from cardiac output changes, the enlarged uterus can compress the inferior vena cava, leading to a large fall in venous return as well as causing changes in the cardiac location by pushing the diaphragm upward and the heart laterally. In pregnant women, there is also an increase in coagulability that is of particular concern to some women with cardiac problems.

Some of the normal cardiovascular changes of pregnancy can cause alterations in physical examination signs that can be mistaken for cardiac abnormalities. The increase in cardiac volume can cause neck vein distension, a cervical venous hum, and a bounding pulse. In addition, the increased volume can increase the first heart sound and cause a systolic ejection murmur at the left sternal border. Also an S_3 and S_4 might be heard. The enlarged uterus can push the heart into a more horizontal position and thus appear enlarged on x-ray films.

Infertility and Cardiovascular Disease

In most cardiovascular diseases, fertility is preserved. However, if the congenital heart disease is associated with a significant chromosomal derangement, it is likely the individual will have a reduced life span or reduced fertility.[3] Fertility was examined in women with coarctation of the aorta and found not to be adversely affected.[4] Fertility in women who have undergone cardiac surgery for either valvular disease or coronary artery disease has also been examined.[5,6] Nunley et al. examined 208 women retrospectively who had undergone cardiac surgery and required cardiopulmonary bypass.[5] The largest categories of surgery were septal defect repairs (921), commissurotomies (60), and valve replacements (46). Fertility appeared to be similar as compared to the general population. Singh et al. followed 27 women after surgical correction for tetralogy of Fallot and found that infertility was uncommon.[6] In men, hyperlipidemia has been suggested to adversely affect testicular function, leading to poor semen quality.[7]

Effects of Pregnancy on Valvular Heart Disease

A woman with normal cardiac function can handle the physiological changes of pregnancy without difficulty, although she may have signs and symptoms usually associated with a cardiac problem such as tachycardia, murmurs, edema, and dyspnea. However, with an underlying cardiac condition, the additional stresses can lead to cardiac decompensation. If the woman has a condition where she cannot increase her cardiac stroke volume, such as with aortic regurgitation or constrictive pericarditis, she will often be able to compensate through an increase in heart rate. However, those women who have a slowed left ventricular filling, as with severe mitral stenosis or severe cardiomyopathies, may experience severe difficulties. Those with fixed right ventricular outflow obstruction, such as pulmonary stenosis or pulmonary hypertension with a septal defect, may have an increase in right-to-left shunting with a consequent fall in maternal oxygen tension and possible intrauterine growth retardation.

The most common cardiac problems that would put women at risk as a consequence of pregnancy are predominantly valvular in origin. Congenital defects now make up a large percentage of high-risk cardiac pregnancies. This is a result of the decline in the prevalence of rheumatic heart disease and the rise in the number of women living into childbearing age as a result of better management of congenital defects.[1] Estimates are that 71% of individuals with congenital heart disease currently survive to at least the age of 20.[8] Currently about three to four times as many high-risk cardiac pregnancies are related to congenital conditions as compared to rheumatic heart disease. While the prognosis for pregnant women with acquired and congenital heart defects has improved, pregnancy in these women is still associated with dangers to both mother and infant and remains the most important nonobstetric reason for maternal death.[9] This is particularly true for those women with either pulmonary hypertension or pulmonary edema. Women with pulmonary hypertension are at particular risk for permanent worsening of their disease by the pregnancy.[9] The additional demands placed on the heart in women with congenital heart disease can worsen already existing cardiac failure. However, most pregnancies associated with maternal heart disease have a favorable outcome for both mother and fetus.[10] In fact, one British study demonstrated that the perinatal mortality rate in these women was 19 per 1000, or slightly lower than that in the overall obstetric population.

Those conditions associated with the highest degree of maternal and fetal risks are outlined in Tables 12–1 and 12–2. The most common congenital defects associated with survival into adulthood include atrial septal defect, patent ductus arteriosus, pulmonic valve stenosis, ventricular septal defects, coarctation of the aorta, aortic valve disease, and tetralogy of Fallot. The effects of pregnancy on these conditions and others are briefly listed below.

Atrial Septal Defect (Secundum)

Atrial septal defects are the most common congenital lesions seen in pregnant women, with a secundum defect being the most common congenital defect not recognized until adult age.[9] Most pregnant women with this

Table 12–1   Cardiac Conditions Associated with Maternal Mortality
Low risk of maternal mortality (less than 1%)
Uncomplicated septal defects
Patent ductus arteriosus, uncomplicated
Pulmonic/tricuspid disease
Corrected tetralogy of Fallot
Bioprosthetic valve
Mitral stenosis, New York Heart Association classes I and II
Moderate risk of maternal mortality (5–15%)
NYHA classes III and IV mitral stenosis
Aortic stenosis
Marfan's syndrome with normal aorta
Uncomplicated coarctation of the aorta
Past history of myocardial infarction
Mitral stenosis with atrial fibrillation
Artificial valve
Uncorrected tetralogy of Fallot
High risk of maternal mortality (25–50%)
Eisenmenger's syndrome
Pulmonary hypertension
Marfan's syndrome with abnormal aortic root
Periportal cardiomyopathy

Adapted from Gianopoulos JG, Medical Clinics of North America 73:641, 1989 and Clark SL, Critical Care Obstetrics. Oradell, NJ, Medical Economics Books, 1987.

defect will not have significant cardiac complications and tolerate pregnancy well. Some of these women, particularly those over the age of 40, will develop either atrial fibrillation, atrial flutter, or a supraventricular tachycardia. Such arrhythmias during pregnancy can lead to cardiac decompensation and right-side heart failure. There is an increase in the left-to-right shunt through the atrial septal defect secondary to the hypervolemia of pregnancy. Although this increases right ventricular work, most patients tolerate this well. Pulmonary hypertension is rare in these individuals and if it occurs, is usually in the fourth or fifth decade of life.[9]

Patent Ductus Arteriosus

Most individuals have surgical closure done in childhood, so that this lesion is less common during adulthood and with pregnancy. Women with uncomplicated patent ductus arteriosus tolerate pregnancy well. The women at risk for fetal problems include those with a nonrestrictive patent ductus arteriosus and a right-to-left shunt as a result of very high pulmonary vascular resistance. In these individuals, the fall in systemic vascular resistance with pregnancy could lead to a worsening of the right-to-left shunt and further desaturation of blood to the fetus.

Table 12–2   Cardiac Conditions Associated with Fetal Risk

1. Pulmonary hypertension
2. Cyanotic congenital heart disease
3. Need for oral anticoagulants

Adapted from Oakley.[9]

Pulmonic Valve Stenosis

Most women with mild to moderate pulmonic valve stenosis tolerate pregnancy well. Even with severe pulmonic stenosis the pregnancy may be tolerated without significant problems.

Ventricular Septal Defects

Uncorrected ventricular septal defects are uncommon by the age of pregnancy. In those women with uncorrected small and moderate-sized defects, pregnancy is usually well tolerated although the risk for endocarditis is increased. Those women with large defects may be at significant risk if development of pulmonary hypertension occurs with the development of a right-to-left shunt (Eisenmenger's syndrome).

Pulmonary Hypertension

Pulmonary hypertension can be isolated or a consequence of congenital or rheumatic heart disease. Women with pulmonary hypertension and a left-to-right shunt may tolerate pregnancy, although their pulmonary hypertension may worsen and temporary heart failure may develop. However, the risk to the mother and the fetus with advancing pulmonary vascular disease and the development of a right-to-left shunt is very high. The risk in those women with Eisenmenger's complex during pregnancy, labor, delivery, and the puerperium is between 30 and 70%.[1] In these women, small hemodynamic changes, such as vasovagal faints or straining during labor, can provoke a sudden fall in cardiac output, with the risk of maternal and fetal death.[1,9,11] Many authors advocate termination of pregnancy in all those women with Eisenmenger's syndrome.[9]

Primary pulmonary hypertension is often diagnosed during or after pregnancy in a previously healthy woman. As the condition often becomes worse following pregnancy, pregnancy would not be recommended for these women.[12]

Coarctation of the Aorta

While coarctation of the aorta is ideally corrected before pregnancy, it may not be discovered until pregnancy has occurred. The risk to women with a coarctation during pregnancy ranges from 0 to 17%, with 50% of the mortality associated with the first pregnancy.[13] The risk to the mother appears to be less in a more recent study, especially in women with New York Heart Association (NYHA) class I or II (Table 12–3) prior to pregnancy.[14] In this study of 83 pregnancies in 23 women, there were no maternal deaths or permanent cardiac complications. The major risk appears to be in women with an aortic or intervertebral aneurysm, or aneurysm of the circle of Willis, where mortality may be as high as 15%.[13] There is an additional risk that with pregnancy, aortic rupture or dissection could result.[1]

Aortic Valvular Disease

Congenital aortic valve stenosis is usually the result of a congenitally bicuspid aortic valve but is five times more likely in men than women.[9] Two potential serious problems with this condition during pregnancy include an increased risk of bacterial endocarditis and the risk of syncope and sudden death. This latter problem can occur as a result of the vasodilatation of pregnancy and the inability of the individual to compensate by increasing stroke volume because of severe outflow obstruction. Labor and delivery comprise a particularly hazardous time for those women with severe outflow obstruction. In contrast, congenital aortic regurgitation usually does not cause significant problems to either the mother or the fetus during pregnancy. With the increase in cardiac rate and stroke volume and decrease in peripheral vascular resistance, the regurgitant flow usually decreases.

**Table 12–3   New York Heart Association:
Functional Classification of Cardiac Disease**

Class I
  No functional limitation of activity
  No symptoms of cardiac decompensation with activity

Class II
  Mild amount of functional limitation
  Patients are asymptomatic at rest
  Ordinary physical activity results in symptoms

Class III
  Limitation of most physical activity
  Asymptomatic at rest
  Minimal physical activity results in symptoms

Class IV
  Severe limitation of physical activity
  Patients may be symptomatic at rest
  Any physical activity results in cardiac symptoms

Adapted from the Criteria Committee of the New York Association. Nomenclature and Criteria for Diagnosis of Diseases of the Heart and Great Vessels. 8th ed. New York, New York Heart Association, 1970.

Tetralogy of Fallot

Tetralogy of Fallot is the most common cyanotic congenital heart problem allowing survival into the childbearing ages. These individuals are at risk for an increase in a right-to-left shunt secondary to the gestational fall in systemic vascular resistance, an augmented cardiac output, and an obstructed right ventricle. This leads to a fall in oxygenation and a rise in the hematocrit. While this is often well tolerated, it can put the mother at risk, particularly at the time of labor and delivery, and can also be a cause of intrauterine growth retardation, spontaneous abortions, and prematurity. Women with a corrected tetralogy of Fallot appear to tolerate pregnancy well, whereas with uncorrected lesions mortality ranges from 4 to 15%, with a 30% fetal mortality rate.[13]

Ebstein's Anomaly of the Tricuspid Valve

These women may cope poorly with the increase in cardiac output that occurs during pregnancy. In addition, the condition may be associated with arrhythmias including paroxysmal atrial tachycardia, atrial flutter, and most serious, ventricular tachycardia leading to possible sudden death.

Corrected Heart Lesions

Most women who have had their congenital heart lesions corrected as children, including those women with corrected atrial and ventricular septal defects, will tolerate pregnancy well. Women with cyanotic heart disease with right-to-left shunts may tolerate the pregnancy but their offspring are at increased risk of intrauterine growth retardation depending on the degree of deoxygenation. The risks for those women with a bioprosthetic porcine or homograft valve who are in functional class I or II are lower than those in women with a mechanical valve or who are in functional class III or IV.[15] Patients who are class III or IV should be warned about the significant risk of pregnancy. Pregnancy should be discouraged in these patients until their classification can be improved to I or II via medical or surgical therapy.

There has been considerable discussion over which type of heart valve is preferred for women in their childbearing years. Mechanical heart valves require the use of anticoagulation with inherent risks to the mother and infant. Badduke et al. reviewed a series of women who went through pregnancy with biological valvular prostheses.[16] In this group of 17 patients with 37 pregnancies, the pregnancies were well tolerated and the spontaneous abortion rate was 16.2%, a rate similar to that seen in the general population. However, there was a marked increase in the need for early reoperation because of prosthetic obstruction from calcification.

Rheumatic Heart Disease and Mitral Stenosis

Rheumatic heart disease still exists, resulting primarily in mitral stenosis. Mitral stenosis can be a serious problem in pregnancy and is the number one cause of cardiac mortality in pregnant women. To compensate for the incomplete emptying of the left atrium, the normal tachycardia of pregnancy becomes even more pronounced. This in turn only further enhances the incomplete emptying of the obstructed atrium, leading to further reductions in stroke volume of the ventricle and further tachycardia. Ultimately, there can be significant elevations in left atrial pressure and pulmonary edema. The tachycardia associated with labor and delivery may also exacerbate this problem, leading to a significant decrease in cardiac output and blood pressure. This may require a beta-blocker during labor or delivery. There is probably little risk to the mother whose cardiac function is class I before pregnancy. However, a pregnant women in class III or IV can have a mortality as high as 5% and up to 15% if atrial fibrillation is also present.[17]

Other Valvular Lesions

AORTIC STENOSIS AND INSUFFICIENCY

Aortic stenosis is also usually rheumatic in origin. If mild to moderate, aortic stenosis is well tolerated during pregnancy. However, women with gradients over 100 mm Hg are at significant risk with a reported mortality of 17%.[18] With any decrease in preload, cardiac output can fall significantly, leading to myocardial ischemia and sudden death. These women are at special risk during delivery or termination of pregnancy. Aortic insufficiency, also most common secondary to rheumatic fever, is well tolerated during pregnancy. Both aortic stenosis and insufficiency secondary to rheumatic fever are often associated with mitral valve disease as well. In both aortic stenosis and insufficiency, bacterial endocarditis prophylaxis is indicated and should be used during labor and delivery.

MITRAL INSUFFICIENCY

Women with mitral insufficiency usually tolerate pregnancy well. However, these women are at risk for atrial enlargement and fibrillation with an increased risk during pregnancy. Bacterial endocarditis prophylaxis is indicated.

MITRAL VALVE PROLAPSE

Mitral valve prolapse, caused by enlargement of one or both of the mitral leaflets, is the most frequent congenital heart condition, present in up to 12 to 17% of women of childbearing age.[19] This lesion is also associated with redundant chordae and disrupted collagen bundles in the fibrosal layer that are replaced with myxomatous tissue.[2] Mitral valve prolapse in most individuals is transmitted genetically, with 30 to 50% of first-degree relatives of individuals with mitral valve prolapse also having mitral valve prolapse.[20] Mitral valve prolapse usually has an uneventful course.[21,22] Although there is a concern that pregnancy can lead to an increase in cerebrovascular events, this has not been well documented. In one review of 42 pregnancies in 25 women with mitral valve prolapse, there were no remarkable cardiac complications other than one episode of congestive heart failure associated with the use of a beta$_2$-sympathomimetic drug.[23] Similar findings were found in a study by Tang et al.[24] Occasional cases of serious complications of mitral valve prolapse during pregnancy such as a cerebrovascular event or endocarditis have been reported, but these seem to be highly unusual.[2] The main risk in women with mitral valve prolapse is the development of bacterial endocarditis, particularly in those women with a structural abnormality of the mitral valve. This can result in chordal rupture, mitral insufficiency, and congestive heart failure.

As with the murmur of mitral and aortic regurgitation, the murmur of mitral valve prolapse may decrease with pregnancy.[2,25] During pregnancy, the increase in blood volume increases left ventricular end-diastolic volume, which can favorably realign the mitral valve and decrease the click.

There is still quite a bit of discussion as to which individual with mitral valve prolapse should receive antibiotic prophylaxis. The American Heart Association suggests antibiotic prophylaxis for only those individuals with mitral valve prolapse complicated by mitral insufficiency while acknowledging that complete information to guide therapy in this area is limited.[26] Uncomplicated vaginal delivery and cesarean section rarely, if ever, precipitate endocarditis. It is recommended to provide prophylaxis to those with mitral valve prolapse who have mitral insufficiency at the time of delivery and to those without mitral insufficiency if the delivery is complicated.

Effects of Valvular Heart Disease on Pregnancy

Valvular heart disease can threaten the growth and health of the developing fetus by either reducing uterine blood flow in the case of heart failure or by desaturation of oxygen in the case of cyanotic conditions.[1] The fetus is also at risk for congenital cardiac malformations in hereditary valvular conditions and for the side effects of cardiac medications ingested by the mother. The risk to the fetus is dependent on the severity of the heart disease, the amount of right-to-left shunting, and the success of surgical corrections of valvular and congenital abnormalities prior to pregnancy. The overall outcome, however, can be quite good. McFaul et al. reported on the outcome of 519 pregnant women with previous heart disease.[10] Of these women, 60% had rheumatic heart disease; 31%, congenital heart diseases; and the remaining had conditions such as arrhythmias, ischemic heart disease, and cardiomyopathies. As a group, 87% of the infants were born at term. The perinatal mortality rate was 19 per 1000, which was lower than the 25 per 1000 of the overall obstetric population during this time period. The frequency of congenital malformation was 5.9%, which was also similar to that in the overall obstetric population. In a study of the outcome of pregnancies comparing 37 women with mitral valve prolapse and 282 pregnant women without mitral valve prolapse, there were no differences in length of labor, birthweight, prematurity rate, and mortality rate.[24]

Effects of Pregnancy in Other Cardiac Conditions

Several other cardiac conditions may be complicated by pregnancy. Women with constrictive pericarditis usually tolerate pregnancy well, as they can compensate for the lack of an increase in stroke volume with a rise in heart rate. On the other hand, women with Marfan's syndrome do not do as well during pregnancy. The risk of aortic dissection, an increase in mitral regurgitation, or rupture of a dilated aortic root increases. Those women who have a strong family history of these problems do particularly poorly. As the condition is transmitted as a dominant trait, genetic counseling is warranted.

Another cardiac condition not infrequently discovered during pregnancy is hypertrophic obstructive cardiomyopathy. This condition involves hypertrophy of the septum of the left and often the right ventricle. The severity and manifestations of the condition vary greatly but of major concern is the small prevalence of sudden death in asymptomatic individuals. The condition may be discovered during pregnancy from either symptoms, a murmur, or an abnormal electrocardiogram (EKG) or chest x-ray film. Pregnancy is usually tolerated by these individuals and treatment is given if the individual has either symptoms or an arrhythmia. Infants born to mothers with this condition are usually normal although they may also have hypertrophic obstructive cardiomyopathy.

A dilated cardiomyopathy, often following a viral infection, can be found in some young women. Women with a large dilated left ventricle and poor exercise tolerance usually do quite poorly during pregnancy and in these individuals, pregnancy would not be advisable.

Bacterial endocarditis is unusual during pregnancy, but is a serious problem when encountered. The mortality in women with bacterial endocarditis appears similar in pregnant and nonpregnant women.[27] However, bacterial endocarditis is associated with a higher maternal mortality rate than heart disease in general.[27] While the diagnosis and management are similar to those in nonpregnant women, antibiotics should be chosen with regard to their effects on the fetus.

Uncommon during childbearing ages, the incidence of myocardial infarction during pregnancy is estimated at 1 in 10,000 deliveries.[28] Hankins et al. reviewed 68 cases and found a 45% mortality rate with third-trimester infarctions compared to 23% if the infarction occurred in the first or second trimester.[29] If delivery occurs within 2 weeks of the myocardial infarction, the mortality rate rises dramatically.[20] While often these women have associated risk factors such as smoking, hypertension, hyperlipidemia, and a family history, in Hankin's study only 13% were diagnosed with coronary artery disease prior to pregnancy. More women with myocardial infarctions during pregnancy have normal coronary arteries than do other individuals with a myocardial infarction.[9] Smaller myocardial infarctions are tolerated in pregnancy and do not exclude a normal pregnancy and delivery. However, the closer the event is to labor, the more risk there is for maternal mortality associated with the stress of labor. The fetal mortality rate for mothers who have had a myocardial infarction is about 34%.[20]

Another group of individuals who may experience cardiac problems under the stresses of pregnancy are those women with severe kyphoscoliosis. During pregnancy these women may have heart failure and cor pulmonale exacerbated by chronic hypoxemia and hypercapnia. In addition, respiratory distress may worsen during pregnancy because of pressure from the enlarging uterus on the diaphragm in those individuals with shortened spinal columns. Delivery will often require a cesarean section.

Hypertension is another cardiovascular condition that may impact on pregnancy. Hypertension is associated with a 20 to 30% increase in the risk of preeclampsia during pregnancy.[20] In addition, pregnancies in women with uncontrolled hypertension are at risk for abruptio placentae, disseminated intravascular coagulation, acute tubular necrosis, and renal cortical necrosis.[20] Despite the potential for these problems, the overall mortality to pregnant women with hypertension is low. The prognosis is worse in the presence of underlying renal disease. Sibai and Anderson evaluated the maternal and perinatal outcome associated with continuing pregnancy in 44 women with severe chronic hypertension in the first trimester.[30] There were no maternal deaths but there was significant morbidity, including 19 women with transient and 1 with permanent renal deterioration. Twenty-three of the women developed superimposed preeclampsia, 1 woman developed pleural effusion, and 1 woman had postpartum hypertensive encephalopathy. There was a perinatal mortality rate of 25%, including 10 stillbirths and one neonatal death. Seventy percent of the infants were delivered before 37 weeks' gestation, and 19 infants (43%) were small for gestational age.

Moderate to severe hypertension during pregnancy should be treated. Many drugs including methyldopa, hydralazine, beta-blockers, and calcium channel blockers have been used with success in pregnancy.[20] Methyldopa has the longest record of safety for the neonate and infant.[31] Beta-blockers appear safe for use in the third trimester but can cause intrauterine growth retardation when used for longer periods.[31] Calcium channel blockers appear to have a lot of potential although long-term experience during pregnancy is more limited. Because of the possibility of adverse fetal effects of angiotensin-converting enzyme (ACE) inhibitors in animal and human studies, these medications should probably be avoided during pregnancy.[31–34] These studies suggested that ACE inhibitors could be associated with a decrease in fetal renal blood flow, renal tubular dysgenesis, and underdeveloped skull bones.

Effect of Cardiac Medications on Pregnancy

Another concern for women with cardiac problems during pregnancy is the effect of their cardiac medications on the developing fetus. Unfortunately, there is little information about the teratogenic risks of many cardiac drugs and recommendations are usually the result of uncontrolled studies, animal studies, and case reports. Most cardiac medications should be continued throughout pregnancy to keep the mother in a cardiac compensated state.[35,36]

One group of medications with significant risks to the developing fetus are the anticoagulants.[37–40] However, fetal outcome is usually good even with anticoagulation. The most common problems include early spontaneous abortions and congenital defects.[41] Warfarin crosses the placenta, unlike heparin, and may be associated with both warfarin embryopathy and central nervous system abnormalities.[42] Warfarin embryopathy includes punctate calcifications, saddle-nose deformities, and stippled epiphyses. In one study, warfarin was associated with a 26.1% prevalence of adverse outcomes, compared to 3.6% for heparin.[43]

Heparin appears to be the safest of the anticoagulants to use during pregnancy. However, it is associated with a decrease in fertility. Some authors advise switching to heparin before conception and if conception is a problem, to use the warfarin drugs and then switch back to heparin as soon as pregnancy is diagnosed. Warfarin drugs are associated with a specific syndrome, warfarin embryopathy,[44] that appears to have its greatest effects between the sixth and ninth weeks of gestation. At that time, it can result in damage to the epiphyseal ends of long bones and developing cartilaginous bones, leading to chondrodysplasia punctata.[9] It has also been associated with fetal losses, neurological damage, and bleeding events, when given later in gestation.[1] In one series of 418 pregnancies in women using warfarin derivatives, 16.6% resulted in an abnormal live-born infants, 16.6% in abortion or stillbirth, and 66% in normal infants.[15] Most physicians feel that heparin is the anticoagulant of choice during pregnancy, but there is concern that heparin is less effective in preventing thromboembolism from artificial valves and may itself lead to retroplacental hemorrhage, stillbirths, and prematurity.[9,36] Heparin has also been reported to cause reversible bone demineralization, thrombocytopenia, and hyperkalemia.[45] Some physicians recommend not switching from warfarin derivatives until 2 weeks before term, and then switching to avoid delivering a baby with a prolongation of the prothrombin time. Heparin is not excreted into breast milk and clotting times have been normal in nursing mothers during warfarin treatment.[36]

Diuretics have been discouraged during pregnancy as they may interfere with the physiological volume expansion of pregnancy.[46] Thiazides have also been reported to cause maternal and fetal thrombocytopenia.[36] Methyldopa and hydralazine have not been reported to be associated with adverse fetal effects.[1] Propranolol has been reported to be associated with intrauterine growth retardation, neonatal hypoglycemia, and an abnormal heart rate response to movement.[47] As mentioned above, ACE inhibitors should be avoided during pregnancy.

Many antiarrhythmic drugs such as digoxin, lidocaine, and quinidine have been used for years without reports of significant adverse fetal effects.[35,36] Experience with verapamil is more limited, but this drug also seems to be unassociated with teratogenic effects.[1]

Some women with cardiovascular problems are on lipid-lowering drugs. Lovastatin and niacin are contraindicated during pregnancy and lactation. Lovastatin has caused skeletal abnormalities in animal studies.[48]

The other risk to the fetus that women with cardiac problems face is exposure to radiation secondary to diagnostic x-ray studies. Radiological studies should be performed if needed, but a lead abdominal shield should be used and the studies delayed, if possible, until after the first trimester. Radioisotope scans should be avoided, as the isotope may concentrate in the fetus, with unknown side effects.

Overall, most women with cardiac problems can tolerate pregnancy with a good maternal and fetal prognosis. However, for many of these women, pregnancy will be better tolerated at a younger age when their cardiac condition is better. There are several indications for a therapeutic abortion during pregnancy because of the severe danger to maternal life. Oakley reviewed these indications (Table 12–4).[49] In addition to these, Pitkin et al. also considered complicated aortic coarctation, complicated atrial septal defect, and complicated patent ductus arteriosus to be contraindications to pregnancy.[1] Management of these pregnant women should be done by an obstetrician trained in high-risk cardiac pregnancies in combination with a cardiologist with a knowledge of obstetric manifestations of cardiac disease.

Contraception and Cardiac Diseases

It is important to provide women with cardiac conditions appropriate guidance on both the need and choice of contraceptive methods. Concerns regarding contraceptive choices include the cardiovascular sequelae of pregnancy should the contraceptive fail and the potential adverse circulatory effects of various contraceptive methods. The best choice of contraception will vary based on the individual's cardiac condition and preferences.

Table 12–4   Cardiac Indications for Therapeutic Abortion
1. Pulmonary hypertension, either primary or Eisenmenger's syndrome with central right-to-left shunt 2. Dilated cardiomyopathy 3. Marfan's syndrome with cardiovascular involvement 4. Pulmonary arteriovenous fistulas 5. Complicated aortic coarctation 6. Complicated atrial septal defect 7. Complicated patent ductus arteriosus 8. Any uncorrectable cardiac condition with class III symptoms before conception

Adapted from Pitkin et al.[1] and Oakley CM. Cardiovascular disease in pregnancy. Can J Cardiol 1990;6:3B–9B.

However, specific considerations for different cardiac conditions are discussed in this section.

It is important to begin a discussion of sexuality and contraception early as these individuals are similar to their peers in sexual activity but may not be using appropriate contraception. In a study of adolescents with congenital heart disease, only 21% were found to have knowledge of appropriate birth control methods.[50] At the same time, their sexual interest and activity were found to parallel those of their adolescent peers without a chronic illness.

Hormonal Contraceptives and Cardiac Disease

The contraceptive method that usually is associated with the greatest degree of concern among physicians and women with cardiac diseases is hormonal contraception. Certain effects of hormonal contraceptives may have a negative impact on cardiac diseases. On the other hand, many women with cardiac conditions can take hormonal contraceptives safely. Potential concerns of hormonal contraceptives include worsening of embolic disease, hypertension, fluid and water retention, and hyperlipidemia.

Estrogens increase hepatic production of serum globulins, of which some are involved in the coagulation process, such as factor VII and fibrinogen.[51] Combination oral contraceptives may cause a hypercoagulable state and increase the risk for the development of thrombosis in certain individuals. The Royal College of General Practitioners (RCGP) study demonstrated a 5.7 times relative risk of deep thrombosis of the legs.[52] The risk appears related to the dose of estrogen, and recent evidence suggests that in users of pills with less than 50 μg of estrogen, the rate of thromboembolic disease is substantially lower.[53]

In certain groups of individuals, such as those women with pulmonary hypertension or with coarctation of the aorta complicated by vascular accidents, oral contraceptives would be contraindicated. Women with cardiac conditions associated with heart failure, cyanosis, left ventricular outflow obstruction, and significant cardiac arrhythmias would also be poor candidates for oral contraceptives as they would be at greater risk for thrombotic complications. Hormonal contraceptives also have the possibility of exacerbating existing heart failure or other symptoms through fluid retention or hypertension. Both combination oral contraceptives and progestins alone have been implicated in fluid retention related to both the estrogen and progestin components.[54–56]

Intrauterine Devices

There are two important considerations in using the intrauterine device (IUD) in women with cardiac problems. These include the risk of infection and the occurrence of the vagal syndrome during insertion. There is no evidence that the IUD alters hemodynamics, blood pressure, blood coagulation, or metabolic status.

Infection with an IUD could be devastating to the woman with a congenital heart problem or acquired valvular disease. The IUD may be associated with an increased risk of endometritis, particularly in women with multiple sexual partners or a history of pelvic inflammatory disease.[57,58] Cobbs reported on a case of a 22-year-old woman with mitral valve disease who developed endometritis and endocarditis 1 month after the insertion of an IUD. This patient required a mitral valve prosthesis.[59] Because of the potential risk of endometritis and bacterial endocarditis, if bacteremia resulted during insertion or with an infection, IUDs would not be recommended in women with valvular problems or other cardiac problems that would predispose them to endocarditis. Some clinicians would still consider the use of an IUD in women with valvular disease if prophylactic antibiotics are given during insertion. This would include ampicillin, 2 g intramuscularly or intravenously, plus gentamicin, 1.5 mg/kg intramuscularly or intravenously given ½ to 1 hour before the procedure. A follow-up dose could be given 8 hours later. For penicillin allergic patients, vancomycin, 1.0 g intravenously slowly over 1 hour, plus gentamicin, 1.5 mg/kg intramuscularly or intravenously given 1 hour before the procedure, should be given. This could be repeated once 8 to 12 hours later.

During IUD insertion, vagal reflexes can cause cardiac rate and rhythm changes including bradycardia, tachycardia, syncope, diaphoresis, and seizures.[60,61] In one study of 87 IUD insertions, 18 were associated with tachyarrhythmias and 11 with bradycardia or other arrhythmias.[62] The incidence is less than 1% with smaller copper devices.[63] Thus, while the IUD could function as a good choice in select women with a cardiac problem, the physician must be aware of the risks of infection and the possibility of a vagal response.

There are no contraindications to barrier methods in women with cardiac disease although they are less effective than hormonal contraceptives or the IUD. However, in motivated couples, particularly if the woman is at low risk if she becomes pregnant, barrier methods would be a good alternative. The combination of a spermicidal agent and a condom would provide both effective and safe contraception.

Contraceptives and Mitral Valve Prolapse

There has been a degree of controversy over the use of combination oral contraceptives in women with mitral valve prolapse. Concern has been expressed that the abnormal hemodynamics of the mitral valve might promote thrombus formation with associated cerebrovascular accidents.[64] In one report, there was a 13.3 times increased risk of thromboembolic cerebrovascular insufficiency in oral contraceptive users with mitral valve prolapse compared to nonuser controls.[65] The study also documented a hypercoagulable state in these individuals by showing decreased plasma antithrombin II activity, increased platelet coagulant activity, and elevated plasma beta-thromboglobulin levels. However, all but one of the eight women with mitral valve prolapse on oral contraceptives who had a cerebrovascular accident either was a smoker or had a documented history of migraine headaches. Both of these are also associated with an elevated risk of cardiovascular complications when used in conjunction with hormonal contraceptives. Some of the studies suggest that there is a subgroup of mitral valve prolapse patients who have coagulation problems.[20] It may be that the combination of oral contraceptives, mitral valve prolapse, and abnormal coagulation patterns is dangerous. At present, the factors in defining which women are susceptible are not clear.

Combination oral contraceptives could be prescribed to women with mitral valve prolapse with several precautions. The individual should not have a history of other risk factors such as smoking, hypertension, migraine headaches, or prior thrombotic complications. They should not have mitral valve prolapse–associated symptoms such as tachycardia, chest pain, and shortness of breath. They also should not have overt mitral regurgitation. There have been no studies examining the use of progesterone-only contraceptives in these conditions, but the presumed negligible risk of altering coagulation parameters and causing embolic disease would make them a worthwhile alternative. IUD insertion in women with mitral valve prolapse is probably safe if there is no mitral regurgitation and antibiotic prophylaxis is used.

Contraceptives and Atherosclerotic Heart Disease

Hormonal contraceptives may have an impact on atherosclerotic heart disease. Extensive literature exists that evaluates the risks of myocardial infarction related to hormonal contraceptives.[66–68] Early studies demonstrated an elevated risk in oral contraceptive users. However, most of these studies (the Oxford Family Planning Association Study, the RCGP study, and the Walnut Creek Cohort Study) linking oral contraceptive use with myocardial infarction were based on women ingesting combination formulations with 50 μg of estrogen or more.[68-70] Also contraindications to oral contraceptive use were different than currently advised, so that oral contraceptives were prescribed to older women with risk factors such as hypertension, diabetes, and hypercholesterolemia. Even in these older studies, an elevated risk was found primarily in older users who had additional risk factors such as smoking and hypertension.[71,72] Newer data on lower doses of hormones do not seem to support an elevated risk in appropriately chosen women. An analysis of data from a large cohort study with formulations containing less than 50 μg of estrogen and using only healthy pill users and controls (65,000 women) demonstrated no myocardial infarctions in any contraceptive user and a relative risk of strokes of 0.9 compared to that in nonusers.[73,74] In a meta-analysis of 13 studies, there were no differences between past users and never users in the rate of cardiovascular disease.[75] The final report of the Walnut Creek study showed no differences in myocardial infarction in current or past oral contraceptive users.

Cardiovascular disease and cerebrovascular disease that occur in women on the pill seem to be related more to thrombosis than atherosclerosis.[76] Hormonal contraceptives, particularly those with an estrogen component, are probably protective against atherosclerosis.[20] This conclusion is based on studies that demonstrate no elevated risk of myocardial infarction in former hormonal contraceptive users,[75,77] that the incidence of cardiovascular disease does not correlate with the duration of use,[71] and that even though oral contraceptives lower high-density-lipoprotein (HDL) cholesterol levels, they may have a protective effect against atherosclerosis in cynomolgus macaque monkeys.[78] One study of women who had a history of myocardial infarction and who were 50 years or less found the prevalence of coronary atherosclerosis confirmed by angiographically to be double in nonoral contraceptive users as compared to oral contraceptive users.[20] Overall, while hormonal contraceptives do not seem to be associated with an increased risk of cardiac disease in healthy women, they could not be recommended to women with a history of myocardial infarction or to women with preexisting atherosclerotic heart disease, particularly with a history of other cardiac risk factors. Smoking in particular is a significant risk factor for women over 35 years old who are also on oral contraceptives.[48] Progestin-only contraceptives including the progestin-only oral contraceptive, depomedroxyprogesterone acetate (DMPA), and the Norplant implant would also appear to have similar indications and contraindications in women with atherosclerotic disease. The progestin-only contraceptives do not appear to affect coagulation, which would appear to be a plus in these women. However, because of their lack of estrogen, they may have less of a protective effect against atherosclerosis.

The IUD is an alternative in women with atherosclerotic heart disease. If there is associated arrhythmias, the possible effects of a vasovagal reaction and stress during insertion would have to be kept in mind. In those women on anticoagulation, the progestin-containing IUD would probably be preferred to avoid increased blood loss.

Contraceptives and Hyperlipidemia

Hormonal contraceptives have a potential impact on lipids. This would be of particular concern to those women with already underlying hyperlipidemia or atherosclerotic heart disease. Both the estrogen and progesterone components have been studied in this regards. Estrogen seems to have a beneficial effect on lipid metabolism by lowering low-density-lipoprotein (LDL) levels and increasing HDL cholesterol levels.[76] However, alkylated estrogens (ethinyl estradiol and mestranol) and equine estrogens (equilin) as opposed to natural estrogens elevate triglycerides and very-low-density lipoproteins (VLDL).[79] The complete mechanism of estrogen-associated LDL cholesterol reduction is not entirely understood. However, estrogens appear to increase the binding and uptake of LDL particles in the liver.[79] Estrogens also reduce the activity of hepatic lipase on the luminal surface of liver endothelial cells, resulting in reduced catabolism of HDL (primarily HDL_2, not HDL_3).

The progestins in combination oral contraceptives and progestin-only pills are related to 19-nortestosterone and may be subclassified as gonanes or estranes.[80] The gonanes include desogestrel, norgestimate, levonorgestrel, and gestodene while the estranes include norethindrone, norethindrone acetate, ethynodiol diacetate, lynestrenol, and norethynodrel. The gonanes have an ethyl substitution at the 13 carbon of the steroid nucleus and the estranes have a methyl substitution. The gonane progestins have greater androgenic and progestational potency. However, the newer gonanes, including gestodene, desogestrel, and norgestimate, seem to have a very favorable pharmacological profile. These steroids appear to have potent progestational activity and low androgenic activity with no detrimental effects on lipid or carbohydrate metabolism.[81]

The most commonly used gonane progestin is norgestrel. Norgestrel is made up of two isomers, levonorgestrel and dextronorgestrel. Levonorgestrel is the active component, so that a pill with norgestrel is 50% as active as one with only levonorgestrel. Among the estranes, only norethindrone is an active steroid, with all other estranes being metabolized by the liver to norethindrone. The 17-hydroxyprogesterones include megestrol acetate, medroxyprogesterone acetate, and cyproterone acetate.

In general, progestins tend to have an opposite effect as estrogens on lipids in that they decrease triglycerides, increase LDL, and decrease HDL and HDL_2.[82] HDL_2 levels appear more predictive for cardiovascular disease than total HDL or HDL_3 levels. However, while some progestins decrease levels of HDL and raise LDL levels, this is often counterbalanced by the estrogen component, leading to no overall significant effect on lipoproteins.[83,84] The mechanism of progestin's effects on lipoprotein metabolism is not fully understood, but they seem to increase hepatic lipase and thus increase the catabolism of HDL cholesterol.

The effect of progestins on lipoprotein metabolism seems dependent on the type of progestin, the dose, and the balance of estrogen and progestin in an oral contraceptive pill.[79] In general, in doses used in oral contraceptives, the 19-nortestosterone derivatives (norethindrone, levonorgestrel) affect lipoprotein metabolism to a greater extent than the 17-hydroxyprogesterones (e.g., megestrol acetate, medroxyprogesterone acetate).[79]

Several studies have examined the relationship between dose and type of oral contraceptive and lipid levels. Godsland et al. studied 1060 women on nine different types of oral contraceptives used for at least three cycles, compared to 418 women off hormonal contraceptives.[85] The contraceptives included pills with levonorgestrel in low (150 µg), high (250 µg), and triphasic (50–125 µg) doses; norethindrone in low (500 µg), high (1000 µg), and triphasic (500–1000 µg) doses; and a new desogestrel pill in one dose, 150 µg. All of the pills contained 30 to 40 µg of ethinyl estradiol. Two additional pills contained progestin only. Women taking combination pills, as compared to controls, did not have an increased total cholesterol level but did have increases of 13 to 75% in fasting triglyceride levels. LDL cholesterol levels were reduced by 14% in women taking the combination pill containing desogestrel and by 12% in those taking low-dose norethindrone. Levels of HDL cholesterol were lowered by 5 and 16% by the combination pills containing low-dose and high-dose levonorgestrel. These were due to reductions of 29 and 43% in HDL_2. High-dose norethindrone pills had no effect on HDL whereas low-dose norethindrone pills increased HDL by 10%. Desogestrel combination pills increased HDL by 12%. The progestin-only formulations had only minor metabolic effects. Overall, the pills with the best metabolic effects on lipoprotein metabolism were combination pills with either low-dose norethindrone or desogestrel or progestin-only formulations. LaRosa studied women on 50 µg of ethinyl estradiol combined with either 1 mg of ethynodiol diacetate, 0.5 mg of levonorgestrel, or 1 mg of norethindrone.[86] Trigylceride and total cholesterol levels increased with all three; however, norgestrel significantly elevated LDL, with HDL and HDL_2 levels falling. The LDL/HDL ratio significantly increased with the pill containing norgestrel compared with the other two contraceptives. Krauss and coworkers examined lipid levels in women receiving 35 µg of ethinyl estradiol combined with either 0.3 mg of *dl*-norgestrel or 0.4 mg of norethindrone. HDL cholesterol levels increased in women using norethindrone while they were unchanged in the norgestrel group.[87] In a similar study, but comparing triphasic and biphasic oral contraceptives containing levonorgestrel and norethindrone, Percival-Smith et al. demonstrated that the contraceptive containing levonorgestrel was associated with a decrease in HDL and an increase in LDL, while the norethindrone oral contraceptive was associated with a slight increase in

HDL and an unchanged LDL level.[88] Results of several other studies demonstrated similar differences between the progestins.[89,90]

Another consideration with hormonal contraceptives and lipids is their relative effect on HDL_2 and HDL_3 levels. HDL_2 is associated with a protective effect against cardiovascular disease while HDL_3 has no such effect.[91] Thus, some contraceptives may alter the lipid profile without actually altering the total level of HDL. For example, in studies using combination oral contraceptives containing norgestrel, lowered HDL_2 levels and increased HDL_3 levels were found, with the total HDL unchanged.[92,93] Conversely, in several studies examining combination pills containing norethindrone, HDL_2 levels remained unchanged.[87,94]

Overall, most of the newer, low-dose oral contraceptives seem to have only minimal, if any, impact on the lipid profile. However, because of their potential impact, women with atherosclerotic heart disease, multiple cardiac risk factors, or a history of moderate to severe hyperlipidemia would not be good candidates for these pills. In women with borderline to mild hyperlipidemia or a family history of hyperlipidemia, a low-dose combination pill with a low dose of norethindrone could be tried. Alternatively, a combination pill with one of the newer progestins, norgestimate or desogestrel, could be tried. These progestins appear to have less androgenic effects and also maintain a more favorable LDL/HDL ratio and levels of HDL cholesterol than either norgestrel or norethindrone.[95] In one study of 31 healthy women, a pill containing 30 µg of ethinyl estradiol plus 75 µg of gestodene had no significant modifications in total cholesterol, triglycerides, HDL cholesterol, LDL cholesterol, or HDL_2 cholesterol.[95] HDL_3 cholesterol levels were significantly increased.

Dash et al. conducted a study on the lipid changes associated with the Norplant implant.[96] In this study, 35 women were evaluated from the third month to the end of the second year after insertion. There were significant decreases in all lipid values up to the sixth month followed by a gradual rise of all lipid parameters except HDL, which remained significantly below the control level. However, more studies evaluating lipid levels in women with the Norplant implant are still underway. If these devices are used in women with lipid problems, close monitoring of lipid values would be recommended.

Several studies have examined DMPA in relation to lipid profile. Fajumi, in a study of 63 women followed for 3 to 30 months, found a slight decrease in total cholesterol levels.[97] Liew et al., in a small study comparing combination oral contraceptives and DMPA, found lipid levels unchanged in women on both drugs.[98] In another study, Liew et al. found cholesterol levels higher at 24, 36, and 60 months in 157 women treated with DMPA for an average of 43 months.[99]

IUDs have no effects on lipids and thus their appropriateness would have to be judged on grounds other than lipid considerations. The IUD may be an ideal contraceptive for a woman in a stable monogamous relationship who has significant hyperlipidemia or multiple cardiovascular risk factors. Studies are not available on the progestin-containing IUD although because the plasma progestin levels are low, metabolic side effects should be minimal.

Contraceptives and Hypertension

Another consideration in women with cardiac problems using contraceptives would be their impact on blood pressure. Oral contraceptives can lead to a small increase in the incidence of hypertension.[100] Hormonal contraceptives can increase angiotensinogen, leading to an increase in angiotensin II and an increase in blood pressure in some individuals.[101] In one study, 704 women using an oral contraceptive were compared with 703 using an IUD.[102] The women on oral contraceptives developed systolic blood pressures that were 3.6 to 5.0 mm Hg higher than those using the IUD, while the diastolic blood pressure was 1.9 to 2.7 mm Hg higher.[102] Other studies also demonstrated an increased incidence of hypertension in women on oral contraceptives. As in studies of myocardial infarctions and lipids, earlier studies using higher doses of hormones tended to show more impact on blood pressure.[68,103] The use of a combined oral contraceptive in women with blood pressure over 140/90 mm Hg would not be recommended. For those women with cardiac disease and borderline hypertension, contraceptives would have to be selected even more cautiously. Smoking, combined with oral contraceptives and hypertension, can increase cardiovascular risks significantly, so that either smoking or oral contraceptives would have to be discontinued. In younger women who are nonsmokers with well-controlled hypertension, combination low-dose oral contraceptives could be used, with careful monitoring of blood pressure.

Progestin-only contraceptives could be tried in those women with borderline or mild hypertension, and continued depending on the blood pressure response. Women with only a history of preeclampsia could take oral contraceptives as there is no indication that preeclampsia would predispose them to hypertension while on oral contraceptives.

Summary

1. In most cardiovascular diseases, fertility is preserved.
2. Most women with cardiac disease will tolerate pregnancy without significant problems. However, women with the following conditions are at significantly higher risk: pulmonary hypertension, functional class III or IV, severe mitral stenosis, and severe cardiomyopathies. Those women with a right-to-left shunt may have their shunt increased with a resultant fall in oxygen saturation and risk of intrauterine growth retardation. Mitral valve prolapse is not a significant problem during

pregnancy, although prophylaxis may be indicated in selected patients.

3. The overall fetal outcome in women with cardiac disease is good. With certain maternal problems such as myocardial infarction or severe hypertension during pregnancy, fetal mortality can rise significantly.

4. Most cardiac medications appear relatively safe during pregnancy and should be used, if needed, to maintain a good cardiac status. Warfarin drugs have been associated with a specific warfarin embryopathy and heparin with infertility. Diuretics should be avoided during pregnancy. Propranolol has been associated with intrauterine growth retardation and ACE inhibitors should be avoided because of possible fetal abnormalities. Lovastatin and niacin are also contraindicated during pregnancy.

5. The best choice of contraception in women with cardiac problems will vary depending on the individual cardiac problem and with their own preferences.

6. Combination oral contraceptives are contraindicated in women with pulmonary hypertension, cyanotic heart disease, heart failure, preexisting uncontrolled hypertension, thromboembolic disorders, moderate to severe hyperlipidemia, or atherosclerotic heart disease. More than one cardiac risk factor (smoking, diabetes, hypertension, hyperlipidemia, or obesity) would also contraindicate combination oral contraceptive use.

7. When combination oral contraceptives are used in women with cardiovascular conditions, they should be started with a dose of 35 μg of ethinyl estradiol or less and the equivalent of 1 mg or less of norethindrone. The newer progestins such as desogestrel should also be considered.

8. Progestin-only contraceptives may be a good alternative in some of these women, as progestins do not result in significant alterations of the coagulation system.

9. Conventional methods of contraception such as condoms, foam, and the diaphragm may be offered to the motivated couple. However, because of lower overall effectiveness and the potential high risk of pregnancy in some cardiac conditions, their use must be considered carefully.

10. While an IUD can be considered, it is not recommended in the woman with a prior history of pelvic inflammatory disease, a history of multiple sexual partners, or with valvular disease. Because of the IUD's lack of metabolic or thrombotic side effects, the IUD could be an excellent contraceptive choice in some women with cardiac problems who are in a stable monogamous relationship.

11. Specific conditions:
    Mitral valve prolapse: Combination oral contraceptives could be used in women without a history of other cardiovascular risk factors, prior thrombotic complications, migraine headaches, symptomatic mitral valve prolapse, or overt mitral regurgitation. The risk with progestin-only

contraceptives should be even less. IUD insertion should be preceded with antibiotic prophylaxis and should be avoided in women with overt mitral regurgitation.

Atherosclerotic heart disease: Hormonal contraceptives should be avoided in those women with a history of myocardial infarction or in women with preexisting atherosclerotic heart disease and other cardiac risk factors (particularly smoking). The IUD may be a good alternative in these women. The progestin-containing IUD would be preferred in those women on anticoagulation.

Hyperlipidemia: Most of the low-dose combination oral contraceptives have minimal impact on lipid profile but should be avoided in those women with moderate to severe hyperlipidemia or those with women with hyperlipidemia and either atherosclerotic heart disease or multiple cardiac risk factors. A combination oral contraceptive with one of the newer progestins may also be a good alternative. Progestin-only contraceptives may be associated with mild rises in LDL cholesterol and small decreases in HDL cholesterol. If these devices are used in women with hyperlipidemia, cholesterol levels should be monitored. IUDs have no effect on cholesterol and could be used depending on other risk-benefit considerations.

Hypertension: The use of combined oral contraceptives should be avoided in women with uncontrolled blood pressure over 140/90 mm Hg. Combination oral contraceptives used in women who smoke and with hypertension would also be contraindicated. Progestin-only contraceptives are another alternative to combination pills. IUDs should have no effect on hypertension other than at the time of insertion.

References

1. Pitkin RM, Perloff JK, Koos BJ, Beall MH. Pregnancy and congenital heart disease. Ann Intern Med 1990;112:445–54.
2. Cowles T, Gotnik B. Mitral valve prolapse in pregnancy. Semin Perinatol 1990;14:34–41.
3. Hoffman JI. Congenital heart diease: incidence and inheritance. Pediatr Clin North Am 1990;37:25–43.
4. Garcia-Machado R, Del-Castillo W. Aortic coarctation and pregnancy. Arch Inst Cardiol Mex 1988;58:203–7.
5. Nunley WC Jr, Kolp LA, Dabinett LN, Kitchin JD, Bateman BG, Craddock GB Jr. Subsequent fertility in women who undergo cardiac surgery. Am J Obstet Gynecol 1989;161:573–6.
6. Singh H, Bolton PJ, Oakley CM. Pregnancy after surgical correction of tetralogy of Fallot. Br Med J 1982;285:168–70.
7. Padron RS, Mas J, Zamora R, Riverol F, Licea M, Mallea L, Rodriguez J. Lipids and testicular function. Int Urol Nephrol 1989;21:515–9.
8. Moller J, Anderson R. 1000 Consecutive children with a cardiac malformation 26-37 year follow-up. Am J Cardiol 1992;70:661–7.
9. Oakley CM. Pregnancy in heart disease: Pre-existing heart disease. Cardiovasc Clin 1989;19:57–80.

10. McFaul PB, Dornan JC, Lamki H, Boyle D. Pregnancy complicated by maternal heart disease. A review of 519 women. Br J Obstet Gynaecol 1988;95:861–7.
11. Spinnato JA, Karaynack BJ, Cooper MW. Eisenmenger's syndrome in pregnancy: Epidural anesthesia for elective cesarean section. N Engl J Med 1981;304:1215–7.
12. Oakley CM, Somerville J. Oral contraceptives and progressive pulmonary vascular disease. Lancet 1968;1:890–3.
13. Clark SL. Cardiac disease in pregnancy. Obstet Gynecol Clin North Am 1991;18:237–56.
14. Deal K, Wooley CF. Coarctation of the aorta and pregnancy. Ann Intern Med 1973;78:706–10.
15. McColgin SW, Martin JN Jr, Morrison JC. Pregnant women with prosthetic heart valves. Clin Obstet Gynecol 1989;32:76–88.
16. Badduke BR, Jamieson WRE, Miyagishima RT, Munro AI, Gerein AN, MacNab J, Tyers GFO. Pregnancy and childbearing in a population with biologic valvular prostheses. J Thorac Cardiovasc Surg 1991;102:179–86.
17. Szekely P, Snaith L. Atrial fibrillation and pregnancy. Br Med J 1961;1407–10.
18. Arias F, Pineda J. Aortic stenosis and pregnancy. J Reprod Med 1978;20:229–32.
19. Savage DD, Garrison RJ, Devereux RD, Castelli WP, Anderson SJ, Levy D, McNamara PM, Stokes J III, Kannel WB, Feinleib M. Mitral valve prolapse in the general population. I. Epidemiologic features: The Framingham study. Am Heart J 1983;106:571–76.
20. Sullivan JM, Lobo RA. Considerations for contraception in women with cardiovascular disorders. Am J Obstet Gynecol 1993;168:2006–11.
21. Bergh PA, Hollander D, Gregori CA, Breen JL. Mitral valve prolapse and thromboembolic disease in pregnancy: A case report. Int J Gynaecol Obstet 1988;27:133–7.
22. Degani S, Abinader EG, Scharf M. Mitral valve prolapse and pregnancy: A review. Obstet Gynecol Surv 1989;44:642–9.
23. Rayburn WF, Fontana ME. Mitral valve prolapse and pregnancy. Am J Obstet Gynecol 1981;141:9–11.
24. Tang LC, Chan SY, Wong VCW, Ma HK. Pregnancy in patients with mitral valve prolapse. Br J Gynaecol Obstet 1985:23:217–21.
25. Haas JM. The effect of pregnancy on the midsystolic click and murmur of the prolapsing posterior leaflet of the mitral valve. Am Heart J 1976;92:407–8.
26. Shulman ST, Amren DP, Bisno AL, Dajani AS, Durack DT, Ferber MA, Kaplan EL, Millard D, Sanders WE, Scwartz RH, Watanakvnakorn C. Prevention of bacterial endocarditis: A statement for health professionals by the Committee on Rheumatic Fever and Infective Endocarditis of the Council on Cardiovascular Disease in the Young. Circulation 1984;70:1123A–27A.
27. Cox SM, Leveno KJ. Pregnancy complicated by bacterial endocarditis. Clin Obstet Gynecol 1989;32:48–53.
28. Ginz B. Myocardial infarction in pregnancy. J Obstet Gynaecol Br Commonw 1970;77:610–5.
29. Hankins GDV, Wendel GD, Leveno KJ, Stoneham J. Myocardial infarction during pregnancy: A review. Obstet Gynecol 1985;65:139–46.
30. Sibai BM, Anderson GD. Pregnancy outcome of intensive therapy in severe hypertension in the first trimester. Obstet Gynecol 1986;67:517–22.
31. Kyle PM, Redman CW. Comparative risk-benefit assessment of drugs used in the management of hypertension in pregnancy. Drug Safety 1992;7:223–34.
32. The 1988 report of the Joint National Committee on detection, evaluation, and treatment of high blood pressure. Arch Intern Med 1988;148:1023–38.
33. Martin RA, Jones KL, Mendoze A, Barr M Jr, Benirschke K. Effect of ACE inhibition on the fetal kidney: Decreased renal blood flow. Teratology 1992;46:317–21.
34. Barr M Jr, Cohen MM Jr. ACE inhibitor fetopathy and hypocalvaria: the kidney-skull connection. Teratology 1992;44:485–95.
35. Sheapard TH. Catalog of Teratogenic Agents. 5th ed. Baltimore, Johns Hopkins University Press, 1986, pp 342, 344-5, 489–95.
36. Briggs GG, Freeman RK, Yaffe SJ. Drugs in Pregnancy and Lactation. 2nd ed. Baltimore, Williams & Wilkins, 1986, pp 26–31, 80–3, 106–9, 142–4, 457.
37. Fillmore SJ, McDevitt E. Effects of coumarin compounds on the fetus. Ann Intern Med, 1970;73:731–51.
38. Hirsch J, Cade JF, Gallus AS. Anticoagulants in pregnancy. A review of indications and complications. Am Heart J 1972;82:301–6.

39. Hall JG, Paul RM, Wilson KM. Maternal and fetal sequelae of anticoagulation during pregnancy. Am J Med 1980;68:122–40.
40. Stevenson RE, Burton OM, Ferlauto GS, et al. Hazards of oral anticoagulants during pregnancy. JAMA 1980;24:1549.
41. Oakley CM. Valve prostheses and pregnancy. Br Heart J 1987;58:303–5.
42. Harrington R, Ansell J. Risk-benefit assessment of anticoagulant therapy. Drug Safety 1991;6:54–69.
43. Ginsberg JS, Hirsh J. Anticoagulants during pregnancy. Annu Rev Med 1989;40:79–86.
44. Jones K. Smith's Reconizable Patterns of Human Malformation. 4th ed. Philadelphia, WB Saunders, 1988, pp 224–5, 172, 276, 470–1, 491–9, 502–5, 508–11, 545.
45. Gianopoulos JG. Cardiac disease in pregnancy. Med Clin North Am 1989;73:639–51.
46. Sibai BM, Grossman RA, Grossman HG. Effects of diuretics on plasma volume in pregnancies with long-term hypertension. Am J Obstet Gynecol 1984;150:831–5.
47. Rubin PC. Current concepts: Beta blockers in pregnancy. N Engl J Med 1981;305:1323–6.
48. Knopp RH, LaRosa JC, Burkman RT. Contraception and dyslipidemia. Am J Obstet Gynecol 1993;168:1994–2005.
49. Oakley CM. Cardiovascular disease in pregnancy. Can J Cardiol 1990;6:3B–9B.
50. Uzark K, VonBargen Mazza P, Messiter E. Health education needs of adolescents with congenital heart disease. J Pediatr Health Care 1989;3:137–43.
51. Meade TW. Risks and mechanisms of cardiovascular events in users of oral contraceptives. Am J Obstet Gynecol 1988;158:1646–52.
52. Royal College of General Practitioners Oral Contraceptive Study. Oral contraceptives, venous thrombosis, and varicose veins. J R Coll Gen Pract 1978;28:393–9.
53. American College of Obstetrics and Gynecology. Oral contraceptives. ACOG Technical Bulletin, no. 106, July 1987.
54. Spellacy WN, Birk SA. Effect of intrauterine devices, oral contraceptives, estrogens and progestogens on blood pressure. Am J Obstet Gynecol 1972;112:912–3.
55. Dalen JE, Hickler RB. Oral contraceptives and cardiovascular disease. Am Heart J 1981;101:912–3.
56. Leiman G. Depo-medroxyprogesterone acetate as a contraceptive agent. Its effect on weight and blood pressure. Am J Obstet Gynecol 1972;114:97–102.
57. Shafer MA, Irwin CE, Sweet RL. Medical progress: Acute salpingitis in the adolescent female. J Pediatr 1982;100:339–50.
58. Flesh F, Weiner JM, Corlett RC, Boice C, Mishell D, Wolf RM. The intrauterine device and acute salpingitis. Am J Obstet Gynecol 1979;135:402–8.
59. Cobbs GC. Intrauterine device and endocarditis. Ann Intern Med 1973;78:451.
60. Conrad CC, Ghazi M, Kitay DZ. Acute neurovascular sequelae of intrauterine device insertion or removal. J Reprod Med 1973;11:211–2.
61. Johnson FL, Doerffer FR, Tyson JEA. Clinical experience with the Marguiles intrauterine contraception device. Can Med Assoc J 1966;95:14–20.
62. Acker D, Boehm FH, Askew DE, Rothman H. EKG changes with intrauterine contraceptive device insertion. Am J Obstet Gynecol 1973;115:458–61.
63. Newton J, Elias J, McEwan J. Intrauterine contraception using the copper seven device. Lancet 1972;2:951–4.
64. Carlone JP. Oral contraceptive use in women with chronic medical conditions. Nurse Pract 1989;14:9–16.
65. Elam MB, Viar MJ, Ratts TE, Chesney CM. Mitral valve prolapse in women with oral contraceptive related cerebrovascular insufficiency—Associated persistent hypercoagulable state. Arch Intern Med 1986;146:73–7.
66. Ory HW, Forrest JP, Lincoln R. Making Choices. Evaluating the Health Risks and Benefits of Birth Control Methods. New York, Alan Guttmacher Institute, 1983.
67. Oliver MF. Oral contraceptives and myocardial infarction. Br J Med 1970;2:210–3.
68. Royal College of General Practitioners. Oral Contraceptives and Health. New York, Pitman, 1974.
69. Ramcharan S, Pellegrin FA, Ray R, Hsu JP. The Walnut Creek Contraceptive Drug Study. A prospective study of the side effects of oral contraceptives. 1981. DHEW publication no. 74-562. Washington, DC.
70. Vessey MP, Doll R, Peto R, Johnson B, Wiggins P. A long-term follow-up study of women using different methods of contraception. An interim report. J Biosoc Sci 1976;8:375.

71. Royal College of General Practitioners' Oral Contraceptive Study. Further analysis of mortality in oral contraceptive users. Lancet 1981;1:541–6.
72. Mann JI, Doll R, Thorogood M, Vessey MP, Waters WE. Risk factors for myocardial infarction in young women. Br J Prev Soc Med 1976;30:94–100.
73. Porter JB, Hunter J, Danielson DA, Jick H, Stergachis A. Oral contraceptives and nonfatal vascular disease—A recent experience. Obstet Gynecol 1982;59:299–302.
74. Porter JB, Hunter J, Jick H, Stergachis A. Oral contraceptives and nonfatal vascular disease. Obstet Gynecol 1985;66:1–4.
75. Stampfer MJ, Willett WC, Colditz GA, Speizer FE, Hennekens CH. Past use of oral contraceptives and cardiovascular disease: A meta-analysis in the context of the Nurses' Health Study. Am J Obstet Gynecol 1990;163:285–91.
76. Mishell DR Jr. The pharmacologic and metabolic effects of oral contraceptives. Int J Fertil 1989;34:21–6.
77. Layde PM, Ory HW, Schlesselman JJ. The risk of myocardial infarction in former users of oral contraceptives. Fam Plann Perspect 1982;14:78–80.
78. Adams MR, Clarkson TB, Koritnik DR, Nash HA. Contraceptive steroids and coronary artery atherosclerosis in cynomolgus macaques. Fertil Steril 1987;47:1010–8.
79. Burkman RT. Lipid and lipoprotein changes in relation to oral contraception and hormonal replacement therapy. Fertil Steril 1988;49:39S–50S.
80. Crook D, Godsland IF, Wynn V. Oral contraceptives and coronary heart disease: Modulation of glucose tolerance and plasma lipid risk factors by progestins. Am J Obstet Gynecol 1988;158:1612–20.
81. Belaiesch J. Progress in combined oral contraception: Gestodene, a third generation progestogen. Rev Fr Gynecol Obstet 1989;84:455–9.
82. Kafrissen ME. Prevention of cardiovascular risk in women. A new concern for the obstetrician/gynecologist. Acta Obstet Gynecol Scand Suppl 1990;152:13–20.
83. Wahl P, Walden C, Knopp R, Hoover J, Wallace R, Heiss G, Rifkind B. Effect of estrogen/progestin potency on lipid/lipoprotein cholesterol. N Engl J Med 1983;308:862–7.
84. Knopp RH, Walden CE, Wahl PW, Hoover JJ. Effect of oral contraceptives on lipoprotein triglyceride and cholesterol: Relationships to estrogen and progestin potency. Am J Obstet Gynecol 1982;142:725–31.
85. Godsland IF, Crook D, Simpson R, Proudler T, Felton C, Lees B, Anyaoku V, Devenport M, Wynn V. The effects of different formulations of oral contraceptive agents on lipid and carbohydrate metabolism. New Engl J Med 1990;323:1375–81.
86. LaRosa JC. The varying effects of progestins on lipid levels and cardiovascular disease. Am J Obstet Gynecol 1988;158:1621–9.
87. Krauss RM, Roy S, Mishell DR Jr, Casagrande J, Pike MC. Effects of two low dose oral contraceptives on serum lipids and lipoproteins: Differential changes in high-density lipoprotein subclasses. Am J Obstet Gynecol 1983;145:446–52.
88. Percival-Smith RLL, Morrison BJ, Sizto R, Abercrombie B. The effect of triphasic and biphasic oral contraceptive preparations on HDL cholesterol and LDL cholesterol in young women. Contraception 1987;35:179–87.
89. Knopp RH. Effects of sex steroid hormones on lipoprotein levels in pre- and post menopausal women. Can J Cardiol 1990;6:31B–5B.
90. Lipson A, Stoy DB, LaRosa JC, Muesing RA, Cleary PA, Miller VT, Gilbert PR, Stadel B. Progestins and oral contraceptive induced lipoprotein changes: A prospective study. Contraception 1986;34:121–34.
91. Miller DR, Hammett F, Saltissi S, Rao S, Van Zeller H, Coltart J, Lewis B. Relation of angiographically defined coronary artery disease to plasma lipoprotein subfractions and apolipoproteins. Br Med J 1982;282:1741–4.
92. Briggs MH. Implications and assessments of metabolic effects of oral contraceptives. In New Considerations in Oral Contraception. New York, BMI Publications, 1982, pp 131–51.
93. Marz W. Effect of oral contraceptives on serum lipoprotein patterns in healthy women. In Rolland R (ed.). Advances in fertility control and treatment of sterility. Proceedings of Symposium at the 11th World Congress, Dublin, Boston, MTP Press, 1984, pp 99–109.
94. Wynn V, Niththyananthan R. The effect of progestins in combined oral contraceptives on serum lipids with special reference to high-density lipoproteins. Am J Obstet Gynecol 1982;142:766–72.

95. Fioretti P, Fruzzetti F, Navalesi R, Ricci C, Miccoli R, Cerri M, Melis GB. Clinical and metabolic effects of a pill containing 30 μg ethinylestradiol plus 75 mcg gestodene. Contraception 1989;40:649–63.
96. Dash DS, Das S, Nanda U, Tripathy BB, Samal K. Serum lipid profile in women using levonorgestrel contraceptive implant, Norplant-2. Contraception 1988;37:371–81.
97. Fajumi JO. Alterations in blood lipids and side effects induced by Depo-Provera in Nigerian women. Contraception 1983;27:161–75.
98. Liew DF, Ng CS, Heng SH, Ratnam SS. A comparative study of the metabolic effects of injectable and oral contraceptives. Contraception 1986;33:385–94.
99. Liew DF, Ng CS, Yong YM, Ratnam SS. Long-term effects of Depo-Provera on carbohydrate and lipid metabolism. Contraception 1985;31:51–64.
100. Beller FK, Ebert C. Effects of oral contraceptives on blood coagulation. A review. Obstet Gynecol Surv 1985;40:425–36.
101. Wilson ESB, Cruickshank J, McMaster M, Weir RJ. A prospective controlled study of the effect on blood pressure of contraceptive preparations containing different types and dosages of progestogen. Br J Obstet Gynaecol 1984;91:1254–60.
102. The WHO multicentre trial of the vasopressor effects of combined oral contraceptives: 1. Comparisons with IUD. Task Force on Oral Contraceptives. WHO Special Programme of Research, Development and Research Training in Human Reproduction. Contraception 1989;40:129–45.
103. Greenblatt DJ, Koch-Weser J. Oral contraceptives and hypertension: A report from the Boston Collaborative Drug Surveillance Program. Obstet Gynecol 1974;44:412–7.

13

Oncological Conditions

About 45,000 persons in the United States are survivors of childhood cancer that was diagnosed between 1955 and 1982.[1] Over 65,000 persons under 45 are estimated to develop cancer each year, with over 90% surviving long term. This leaves a large number of adults in the reproductive age group who have concerns about the effects of their treatment on fertility, pregnancy, and the health of their children. They may also have concerns about possible side effects of pregnancy and contraception on the course of their disease.

Fertility

Cancer and treatment for cancer have the potential to decrease fertility by several mechanisms. These include direct damage by the cancer to the reproductive tract or neuroendocrine pathways, psychosexual sequelae of any disfigurement or uncertain prognosis, direct teratogenic effect on offspring, and mutation of the germ cells through interruption of cellular metabolism and cell division and interference with DNA.[2–7] There are also the surgical effects of removal of gonads, neurogenic dysfunction, and direct damage to genitals. However, much of the existing data are from experiments in animals, which may not extrapolate accurately to humans. It is also not clear how often mutations lead to a clinical problem. Data from survivors of the atomic bomb in Japan suggest that human germ cells are five times more resistant to radiation than a mouse.[2]

Radiation therapy has been associated with a decrease in fertility and an increase in fetal wastage.[8] Stillman et al. reported on 208 patients, aged 0 to 17, with various tumors including Wilms', lymphoma, sarcoma, neuroblastoma, leukemia, osteogenic sarcoma, and others.[8] Of these individuals, 52%

received radiation and 47% chemotherapy. Following radiation therapy, 12% developed ovarian failure and all of these had received radiation. None of the women developed ovarian failure if at least one ovary was outside the treatment field, while 14% developed ovarian failure if the ovaries were on the edge of the field and 68% if both ovaries were inside the treatment field. The results were similar regardless of the chemotherapy used or the type of cancer. Since 1968, women with Hodgkin's disease at Stanford University Medical Center have had their ovaries moved to the midline during the staging laparotomy and a pelvic shield has been used during therapy.[9] With this technique, the authors reported a 59% ovarian function rate and successful pregnancies. This technique decreases the dose of radiation to the ovary by 80 to 90%.[8] Jaffe et al. studied 27 long-term male survivors of childhood cancers treated with radiation during the prepubertal and pubertal period.[10] Infertility was observed in males who received testicular radiation alone or in combination with chemotherapy.[10] Clinical examination or gonadotropin and testosterone values were not predictive of infertility. The dose of radiation to the testes has been implicated to be related to the prevalence of infertility.[11–14] In Jaffe's study, scatter radiation of about 140 rads was associated with azoospermia or oligospermia. In several other studies, radiation in doses of less than 250 rads did not result in permanent sterility while doses in excess of 250 were usually associated with azoospermia.[12,13] However, spermatogenesis may return even after treatment with 600 to 900 rads. Several other studies found that as little as 15 rads can cause transient oligospermia, with transient aspermia seen with doses above 50 rads. With 200 to 300 rads, sperm production can take about 3 years to recover and almost 45 years with 400 to 600 rads. Above 600 rads, aspermia is usually permanent.[13,14]

Fertility may be underestimated by sperm counting. In the study by Asbjornsen et al., two males who were able to conceive an offspring were oligo/azoospermic on examination just months from conception.[12] In a study of males treated for Hodgkin's disease, 17 males treated with radiation were followed by luteinizing hormone (LH), follicle-stimulating hormone (FSH), and testosterone and sperm counts.[15] While there was a transient decrease in sperm counts and a rise in FSH, full recovery occurred within 18 months. There were no changes in LH and testosterone levels.

In women, ovarian dysfunction is most common with doses over 150 rads. With doses over 500 to 600 rads, most women will become permanently amenorrheic.[16] However, gonadal exposure in women is compounded by the fact that the ovaries are located in the pelvis, are more difficult to shield, and lie more directly in the field of radiation.

Chemotherapy also has the potential of destroying testicular germinal cells and ovarian primordial follicles, leading to amenorrhea and infertility. This has been reported in individuals with rheumatological, renal, and oncological problems receiving certain drugs.[17] The most damaging drugs appear to be procarbazine and the alkylating agents including cyclophosphamide (Cytoxan), chlorambucil, and melphalan, particularly in combination regimens.[18,19] For example, the combination of mechlorethamine, vincristine, procarbazine, and prednisone (MOPP) has been implicated to produce permanent infertility in at least 90% of patients who receive more than three cycles.[20] In a study of MOPP combination chemotherapy, 8 of 14 women became amenorrheic with elevated LH and FSH levels.[19] In another study, Gershenson reported that only 3 of 39 women had serious menstrual difficulties following combination chemotherapy for malignant ovarian germ cell tumors.[21] Similar findings were found in a study of 17 women undergoing cisplatin chemotherapy for ovarian germ cell tumors, of which none developed menstrual problems afterward.[22]

Several studies have examined the question of infertility in males who have received chemotherapy.[23-32] Males treated with antimetabolites alone usually have normal spermatogenesis.[23] In a study by Jaffe et al. of 27 long-term male survivors of childhood cancers treated during the prepubertal and pubertal period, sterility was associated with large doses of single alkylating agents or reduced doses administered with other agents in combination regimens.[10] The doses of alkylating agents associated with permanent infertility average about 20 g/m² of cyclophosphamide or 1.4 g/m² of chlorambucil.[12] Patients receiving cumulative doses in excess of 400 mg of chlorambucil were uniformly azoospermic.[23] In another study, 42 of 49 patients with Hodgkin's developed azoospermia after treatment with mustine, vinblastine, procarbazine, and prednisolone (MVPP).[24] A comparison between MOPP with doxorubicin (Adriamycin), bleomycin, vinblastine, and dacarbazine (ABVD) demonstrated a 100% prevalence of azoospermia in MOPP-treated patients versus only 35% with ABVD, and recovery was seen in some of the ABVD patients.[23] In another study, boys treated for acute lymphocytic leukemia were compared to age-matched controls.[25] In treated boys, the fertility rate was shown to be significantly less than control rates, but to improve as time went on.

Nijman et al. studied gonadal function in 54 males with disseminated nonseminomatous testicular tumors who had combination chemotherapy including cisplatin, vinblastine, and bleomycin and surgery with either hemiorchiectomy and retroperitoneal lymph node dissection or hemiorchiectomy only (N = 17).[25] Significantly, even before treatment, 72% showed azoospermia or oligospermia, while 2 years after discontinuation of chemotherapy, 48% had azoospermia or oligospermia while 28% had more than 60 x 10⁶ spermatozoa/mL. Eight pregnancies occurred, with seven normal offspring and one spontaneous abortion. In those treated with surgery alone, testosterone remained lower and FSH higher than normal. Recovery continued even 1 to 2 years after treatment. Nearly 50% had a normal sperm count 2 years after completion of therapy.

Sperm banking is a consideration in males treated with combination chemotherapy, particularly with alkylating agents. However, in some conditions such as Hodgkin's disease and testicular cancer, as many as 50% of male patients are severely oligospermic or azoospermic before receiving any therapy. Some recent studies indicated that fewer than 20% of lymphoma patients have sperm that have characteristics suggesting a good chance of fertility (sperm concentration of at least 20 x 10^{-5}/mL, post-thaw motility > 40%, and postthaw progression > 2+).[27] In the study by Redman et al., 11 couples attempting artificial insemination using cryopreserved semen resulted in three pregnancies.[27] In another study of 99 males who had banked sperm, only 1 of 99 males had a useful outcome.[28] Of the 99 patients, 44 had adequate posttreatment sperm count. Of the other patients, only 4 actually used the deep-frozen sperm, with only 1 resulting in a pregnancy. Cryopreservation and artificial insemination are thus only a partial solution to this problem, with alternative methods needed to decrease gonadal toxicity. Experiments are in progress in using testosterone or gonadotropins to try and protect the testis from damage during chemotherapy.

There seems to be an association between the development of gonadal failure and the age of the individual when receiving chemotherapy, as less damage occurs to prepubertal gonads due to their quiescent state.[8,18] In a study of 35 women on chemotherapy for leukemia, ovarian failure or hypothalamic-pituitary dysfunction developed in 1 of 17 prepubertal females and 6 of 18 pubertal or postpubertal female adolescents.[29] In another study, Rivkees and Crawford found that pubertal individuals were more susceptible than midpubertal ones, who were in turn more susceptible than those prepubertal individuals.[30] However, even prepubertal males sustained damage when treated with high doses of the alkylating agent cyclophosphamide. Overall, the sequelae were dose related and worse in males. The gonadal problems appear related to a primary gonadal problem and not pituitary or hypothalamic damage.[31]

Contrary evidence suggests that damage is worse to prepubertal gonads. Clayton et al. examined the degree of testicular damage after chemotherapy for childhood tumors and grouped the individuals by maturation level.[32] Fifty boys received carmustine (BCNU) or lomustine (CCNU) after radiotherapy. Their median age was 16.2 years (10.5–25.2 years). Twenty-nine were alive to get samples and 22 had sequential data available. Of 21 males receiving chemotherapy before the age of 16 who were now adults, 20 showed evidence of primary testicular damage. Both of the two adult males who had chemotherapy after age 16 had normal study results. Germinal epithelium appears more susceptible than Leydig cells. This study demonstrated no signs of a decline in Leydig cell function but neither did it demonstrate any signs of germinal cell recovery. A similar study explored the effect of chemotherapy and radiation in relation to pubertal development in 21 females.[33] The girls were treated with neuroaxis irradiation followed by adjuvant chemotherapy with carmustine or lomustine and procarbazine. Thirteen of the girls received chemotherapy before the age of 11 and of these, 10 remained prepubertal, with 9 of the 10 having biochemical evidence of primary ovarian failure. The other 3 who received chemotherapy before age 11 were pubertal or adult with normal FSH and LH levels. These 3 females did have abnormalities of gonadotropin secretion. Eight of the girls received chemotherapy after the age of 11. All of this group entered or progressed through puberty spontaneously, with only three having either an elevated FSH or exaggerated FSH response to gonadotropin-releasing hormone (GnRH).

The long-term effects of combination chemotherapy and radiation have been studied in a longitudinal study by the National Cancer Institute.[34] The National Cancer Institute studied long-term childhood cancer survivors, which included results from the cancer registries of the Connecticut Tumor Registry, the California Tumor Registry in the San Francisco Bay area, and University Hospital registries in Iowa, Kansas, and Texas. This retrospective study examined 2283 survivors from 1945 to 1975 who had a diagnosis made before age 20, who survived for at least 5 years, and who had reached age 21. Three thousand two hundred seventy controls were also selected from the patients' siblings. Married cancer survivors were less likely than their sibling controls to have ever begun a pregnancy (relative risk, 0.85; confidence interval, 0.78–0.92). Fertility was decreased by about 25% in both sexes who had radiation therapy directed below the diaphragm. In males, fertility was decreased by about 60% when chemotherapy was used with alkylating agents with or without radiation to sites below the diaphragm. In contrast, among women, there was no apparent decrease in fertility when alkylating agents were administered alone and only a moderate decrease in fertility when alkylating agents were combined with radiation below the diaphragm (relative risk, 0.81). The study also demonstrated that fertility rates varied considerably related to sex, site of cancer, and type of treatment. Fertility rates of less than one were only observed among survivors of Hodgkin's disease and tumors of the male genital system. Nonalkylating agents did not seem to affect fertility. The worst combination affecting fertility was alkylating agents and radiation below the diaphragm in males, then alkylating alone, followed by radiation alone and then surgery. Overall, fertility in women was much less affected than in men.

In another study, Byrne et al. examined the prevalence of early menopause in long-term survivors of cancer during adolescence.[35] Women survivors of a cancer diagnosed between the ages of 13 and 19 had a risk of menopause four times greater than that in controls during the ages of 21 to 25. The greatest relative risk occurred after treatment with either radiotherapy along (3.7) or alkylating agents alone (9.2). The risk of menopause between the ages of 21 and 25 was 27-fold for women treated with both radiation below the diaphragm and alkylating agent chemotherapy. While 5% of controls had reached menopause at age 31, 42% of these treated women had reached menopause.

Hinterberger-Fischer et al. examined the effects of bone marrow transplantation on fertility.[36] They studied 9 patients with severe aplastic anemia and 14 patients with a hematological malignancy. Among the individuals with aplastic anemia, 7 who were less than 26 years old had normal gonadal function while 2 women over the age of 26 developed premature ovarian failure. All 8 of the females with hematological malignancies developed premature ovarian failure. Among the males, 4 of 6 had elevated FSH, with normal LH and testosterone levels, while 1 had normal LH, FSH and testosterone levels and 1 had elevated LH and FSH and decreased testosterone. Two women and one man with aplastic anemia parented four healthy children while none of the individuals with hematological malignancies had children.

Cancer can also alter reproductive rates through psychosocial factors. The emotional scars of cancer were evaluated in a study on the long-term effects of testicular cancer on sexual functioning in married couples.[37] Thirty-four couples were followed for 4 years after treatment. About one-fourth of the patients felt less attractive as a result of treatment, even though none of the spouses shared this feeling. All couples reported a decrease in the frequency of intercourse as compared to the frequency of intercourse before the cancer was diagnosed.

Effect of Pregnancy on Cancer

A significant question in a woman with cancer who becomes pregnant is the effect of the pregnancy on the course of the tumor. In general, there seems little evidence to suggest that pregnancy has adverse effects on non–hormonal-dependent tumors common in young adults such as Hodgkin's disease, lymphoma, and leukemia.[38–40]

Several tumors including breast cancer have been looked at specifically. While in the past, it was thought that pregnancy worsened the prognosis for breast cancer, more recent studies do not necessarily confirm this. In a study of women who became pregnant after treatment for breast cancer, there was no difference in prognosis compared to a group of nonpregnant women with breast cancer.[41] Sutton et al. examined a group of women with breast cancer treated with doxorubicin adjuvant chemotherapy and also examined the medical literature on the effect of pregnancy on breast cancer prognosis.[42] Pregnancy did not have an adverse effect on the clinical course of the disease. The evidence that does exist, suggesting that breast cancer is more aggressive during pregnancy, may relate to the delay in diagnosis and treatment in these women compared to nonpregnant women.[43] In most instances of small breast lesions, the lesion should be treated similarly to that in nonpregnant women and the pregnancy allowed to continue. If the tumor is advanced, requiring chemotherapy, then termination should be considered. If the women needs chemotherapy and the pregnancy is continued, then if possible, chemotherapy should be withheld during the first 12 weeks of gestation to lower the teratogenic potential of the chemotherapy.

In another review of the literature examining Hodgkin's disease, there were no adverse effects on the mean survival of women who had Hodgkin's disease and became pregnant.[44] However, because of the limited number of cases of non-Hodgkin's lymphoma in pregnant women, it is difficult to assess the full impact of pregnancy on this condition.

Effects of Cancer on Pregnancy

Of additional concern to the parents of cancer victims is the effect of the cancer or cancer treatment on offspring. Most of the information about outcomes of pregnancies in cancer survivors is from either case reports or retrospective case studies.[31] Most of the reports include primarily women who had cancer as a child or young adult and usually had finished their cancer treatment before a pregnancy. When reviewed, there were a total of 1573 pregnancies with a prevalence of a major birth defect of 4% (46) among the 1240 live-born infants, which was comparable to that in the general population. In a separate recent retrospective survey, 306 men and women treated for pediatric cancer were questioned.[44] Of this group, 100 reported 202 pregnancies, with a frequency of congenital anomalies of 8.1% (5/62) among the live-born children of the women and 7.9% (3/38) among the live-born children of the men. This was no greater than the 13% rate in the general population. However, structural congenital cardiac defects were identified in 2 (10%) of the 20 children of women who had been treated with dactinomycin compared with 144 (0.6%) among 24,153 children in a multicenter survey of fetal anomalies. This suggests the possibility of an adverse effect of dactinomycin on children of such patients. Van der Kolk et al. examined the effect of platinum-based combination chemotherapy for disseminated testicular carcinoma.[45] In this study, of 146 patients available for follow-up, 15 patients fathered 20 children and none had evidence of congenital malformations. Those who were fertile seemed to have normal children. Other prior studies also identified no increase in the frequency of congenital anomalies in the offspring of treated cancer victims.[46–48] Thus, if a pregnancy occurs after therapy is finished, there is no indication of an excess risk of congenital or genetic problems.

Mulvihill et al. examined the question of cancer risk in the offspring of treated cancer survivors.[49] They found a slight excess of cancer in the offspring of case survivors during the first 5 years, but after the age of 5 years there was no statistical difference between case survivors and control offspring, with prevalence rates of 0.3% in case survivors and 0.23% in controls.

Oncology Medications and Pregnancy

Other studies have examined the effect of chemotherapy given during pregnancy. In a study of 16 pregnant women with non-Hodgkin's lymphoma, all of whom had received chemotherapy during some part of the pregnancy, there was no evidence of congenital malformation in any offspring.[50] Fifteen of the babies were reported to be alive, healthy, and normal for their age, 3 to 11 years after birth. Sieber and Adamson reviewed the medical literature on the effects of chemotherapy on the fetus.[17] Overall, the offspring were normal. Reports of pregnancies in women on chemotherapy after the first trimester indicate normal babies with a tendency toward low birthweight.[9,51,52]

Other reports indicate that the risk of spontaneous abortion or fetal abnormalities is higher if alkylating agents or antimetabolites are used during the first trimester of pregnancy.[17,52–54] Kozlowski and coworkers reviewed the effects of high-dose aminopterin/methotrexate used in pregnancy.[55] They found evidence of high doses leading to an increased prevalence of spontaneous abortions and teratogenicity including bony and cerebral abnormalities. The adverse effects seemed dose related, with the higher doses used in cancer treatment (75–150 mg/week) more toxic than doses needed for rheumatoid arthritis (7.5–10.0 mg/week). Cyclophosphamide use in a mother with Hodgkin's disease has been reported to cause congenital anomalies including absent toes, palatal grooves, and hernias.[56] Subsequently seven malformed infants were also reported to have congenital anomalies after first-trimester exposure to cyclophosphamide, although all of these other cases received other cytotoxic agents or radiation besides cyclophosphamide.[57–60] Sutton et al. examined the effects of doxorubicin adjuvant chemotherapy on pregnancy in women with breast cancer.[42] Of these pregnancies 10 were terminated; 2 women had a spontaneous abortion and 19 gave birth to full-term offspring without fetal malformations. Nicholson stressed that the effect of cytotoxic therapy was critically dependent on the time of exposure.[53] Most authors recommend avoidance of chemotherapy during the first trimester of pregnancy.[38,40,61] It is also recommended to avoid pregnancy, if possible, until 1 year after successful chemotherapy.[62]

Radiation therapy may also have adverse effects on the fetus, leading to fetal loss and malformations.[38] Most of these effects occur with radiation delivered during the first trimester and with greater than 10 rads to the fetus. The effects of radiation on the fetus later as a child or adult are unknown.

Hinterberger-Fischer et al. studied the effects of bone marrow transplantation on pregnancies and offspring complications.[36] Those patients with severe aplastic anemia had four healthy children among three of nine patients receiving transplanted marrow. However, there was a high incidence of complications in the offspring including persistence of fetal circulation syndrome, erythroblastosis fetalis, and prolonged newborn icterus.

Contraception and Cancer

With timing of pregnancy an important consideration in women with a malignancy, particularly if chemotherapy or radiation is required, family planning becomes crucial in the overall care of these individuals. While there do not appear to be any adverse effects of hormonal contraceptives on non–estrogen-dependent tumors, there is very little reported in the literature on the effect of any contraceptive device, including hormonal contraceptives, on malignancies. Most prior studies are on the effects of hormonal contraceptives in women in the general population, on the prevalence of gynecological tumors.

The most closely examined malignancy in relation to hormonal contraception has been breast cancer. Overall, in reviewing data from multiple studies, there appears to be no increased risk of breast cancer in women using oral contraceptives followed to the age of 55 or 60.[63–65] In most studies, the relative risk of breast cancer is less than or equal to 1.0. Romieu et al. conducted a meta-analysis of the epidemiological literature on oral contraceptives and breast cancer and found no increase in the risk for women who had ever used oral contraceptives, even after a long duration of use.[66] In some studies, certain subgroups appear to be at increased risk, but the risk factors vary from study to study.[67] Some of these studies suggested that there could be an increased risk to long-term oral contraceptive users who begin use at an early age.[64,66] Some researchers have suggested that oral contraceptives may have a similar effect on the rate of breast cancer as pregnancy.[68] That is that both oral contraceptives and pregnancy may decrease the lifetime risk of breast cancer but increase the risk in women under 45. However, if this risk exists, it is more than likely offset by the protective effect with age and the protective effect against ovarian and endometrial cancer. In the largest case-control study examining the relationship between oral contraceptives and breast cancer, there was no elevated risk related to use at a younger age, before a first pregnancy, in women with a family history of breast cancer, or in women with benign breast disease.[68] These results were also similar for progestin-only oral contraceptives.

Studies examining this relationship are confounded by the fact that breast cancer risk is elevated by lower parity and delaying childbearing, both factors that are increased by use of oral contraceptives.[68] In addition, women receiving oral contraceptives often receive more regular medical screening during prescription renewal and so detection of tumors could occur more readily in these women.

Overall, current evidence supports the conclusions that use of oral contraceptives during an early age, the type of oral contraceptive formulation, and a family history of breast cancer do not increase the risk of breast cancer in pill users. However, because of the possibility of estrogen dependency in women with a history of breast cancer, hormonal therapy would not be advised in these individuals or in individuals with a known estrogen-dependent tumor.

Staffa et al. reviewed the literature on the relationship between progestin-only contraceptives and the risk of breast cancer.[69] The studies failed to show consistent evidence of an association between progestins and breast cancer. However, it was felt that further research was needed on potentially high-risk groups such as those with extended hormone exposure before the age of 25 and/or the first full-term pregnancy or those with exposure in the postmenopausal period.

Studies examining the relationship between hormonal contraceptives and cervical cancer have been inconclusive.[70] Recent studies showed mixed results and confounding factors that make interpretation difficult.[71–73] These factors include the observations that oral contraceptive users have been found to have an earlier onset of sexual activity and a higher number of sexual partners, a higher frequency of Papanicolaou smears, and a higher history of smoking or sexually transmitted diseases. Monsonego et al. demonstrated a high level of progesterone receptors in condyloma of the cervix and high-grade cervical intraepithelial neoplastic lesions, which suggests the possibility of hormonal effects on human papillomavirus lesions.[74]

Another question is the advisability of the use of hormonal contraceptives in women with existing cervical dysplasia. Firm data are lacking on the use or nonuse of hormonal contraceptives in these women. While there is no strong evidence to support avoiding use in women with cervical dysplasia, further studies are needed. There is no strong evidence to support withholding hormonal contraceptives in those women with a family history of cervical cancer. Lassise et al. examined the role of intrauterine devices (IUDs) in cervical cancer and found a nonsignificant reduced risk with the use of the copper IUD and no effect with an inert IUD.[75]

Oral contraceptives have been found to be protective against ovarian cancer and endometrial cancer. The protective effect for endometrial cancer in women who have ever used combined oral contraceptives is about 50%.[76,77] The protection against endometrial cancer persists for at least 15 years after discontinuation of oral contraceptives.[77,78] Protection is greatest for nulliparous women and occurs for all three main histological types of endometrial cancer.

Four years of oral contraception confers a 50% reduction in ovarian cancer risk and 7 years or more confers a 60 to 80% reduction.[76] Reductions in the prevalence of ovarian cancer can occur with as little as 6 months of use and can persist for at least 15 years after oral contraceptives are stopped.[79,80] Reductions in the risk for ovarian cancer are more marked in those who were younger (< 25 years) at first use.[68]

One tumor that may contraindicate the use of hormonal contraceptives is meningioma. These tumors are twice as common in women as men and have been noted to be altered by pregnancy. In addition, these tumors have steroid hormone receptors, particularly progesterone receptors.[81] In the study by Grunberg et al., mifepristone, an antiprogesterone agent, was noted to have antitumor effects in patients with meningiomas. Thus, it would seem prudent to avoid steroid contraceptives in women with these tumors.

Summary

1. Radiation therapy has been associated with a decrease in fertility and an increase in fetal wastage. The infertility rate is reduced in women by moving the ovaries outside the field of radiation.
2. Chemotherapy can also affect fertility, particularly with regimens that include procarbazine or alkylating agents.
3. The worse treatment in relation to fertility appears to be the combination of alkylating agents and radiation below the diaphragm in males.
4. Sperm banking is a consideration for males treated with radiation therapy and/or chemotherapy with alkylating agents. However, infertility may be problem in some individuals with gonadal cancer and other malignancies even before therapy is given. Information should be provided about the prospects of infertility, the option of sperm banking, and the possibility of healthy children if fertility is preserved.
5. There is no evidence of a significant adverse effect of pregnancy on non–hormone-dependent tumors. There is also no strong evidence of an adverse effect of pregnancy on the prognosis of breast cancer.
6. Patients with a history of treated cancer have no higher rate of congenital malformations in their offspring than does the general population. However, the pregnancy should probably be monitored with ultrasound, with the usual indications for amniocentesis observed.
7. Overall, chemotherapy during pregnancy is tolerated but alkylating agents or antimetabolites used in the first trimester are associated with spontaneous abortion and fetal abnormalities. It is recommended to wait at least 1 year after finishing chemotherapy before planning a pregnancy.
8. Timing of pregnancies should be based on the severity of disease, the therapy schedule, the prognosis, and the wishes of the family.
9. Effective contraception during chemotherapy should be given. Hormonal contraceptives appear safe in women with non-estrogen-dependent tumors but would be contraindicated in those with estrogen-dependent tumors. Barrier methods are safe but may not be as effective as other methods. The IUD would be effective with the exception of a decrease in effectiveness if used in combination with steroids or other immunosuppressive drugs.

10. Consideration of a therapeutic abortion is appropriate if radiation or chemotherapy is received during the first trimester of pregnancy.
11. Oral contraceptives do not appear to be a significant risk factor for breast cancer. Oral contraceptives are significantly protective against endometrial and ovarian cancer. Hormonal contraceptives can be used in women with a family history of breast cancer but should avoided in women with breast cancer.

References

1. Sondik EJ, Young JL, Horm JW. 1985 Annual Cancer Statistics Review. Bethesda, MD, National Institutes of Health, 1986.
2. Mulvihill JJ, Byrne J. Genetic counseling of the cancer survivor. Semin Oncol Nurs 1989;5:29–35.
3. Drasga RE, Einhorn LH, Williams SD, Patel DN, Stevens EE. Fertility after chemotherapy for testicular cancer. J Clin Oncol 1983;1:179–83.
4. Kedia KR, Morkland C, Fraley EE. Sexual function after high retroperitoneal lymphadenectomy. Urol Clin North Am 1877;4:523–7.
5. Nijman JM, Jager S, Boer PW, Kremer J, Oldhoff J, Koop HS. The treatment of ejaculation disorders after retroperitoneal lymph node dissection. Cancer 1982;50:2967–76.
6. Narayan P, Lange PH, Fraley EE. Ejaculation and fertility after extended retroperitoneal lymph node dissection for testicular cancer. J Urol 1982;127:685–8.
7. Lange PH, Narayan P, Vogelzang NJ, Schafer RB, Kennedy BJ, Fraley EE. Return of fertility after treatment for nonseminomatous testicular cancer: Changing concepts. J Urol 1983;129:1131–5.
8. Stillman RJ, Schinfeld JS, Schiff I. Ovarian failure in long-term survivors of childhood malignancy. Am J Obstet Gynecol 1981;139:62–6.
9. LeFloch O, Donaldson SS, Kaplan HS. Pregnancy following oophoropexy and total nodal irradiation in women with Hodgkin's disease. Cancer 1976;38:2263–8.
10. Jaffe N, Sullivan MP, Ried H, Boren H, Marshall R, Meistrich M, Maor M, da Cunha M. Male reproductive function in long-term survivors of childhood cancer. Med Pediatr Oncol 1988;16:241–7.
11. Howard GC. Fertility following cancer therapy. Clin Oncol Roy Coll Radiol 1991;3:283–7.
12. Asbjornsen G, Molne K, Klepp O, Aakvaag A. Testicular function after radiotherapy to inverted "y" field of malignant lymphomas. Scand J Haematol 1976;17:96–100.
13. Rowley MJ, Leach DR, Warner JGA, Heller CG. Effect of graded doses of ionizing radiation on the human testis. Radiat Res 1974;59:665–78.
14. Clifton DK, Bremner WJ. The effect of testicular x-irradiation on spermatogenesis in man: A comparison with the mouse. J Androl 1983;4:387–492.
15. Kinsella TJ, Trivette G, Rowland J, Sorace R, Miller R, Fraass B, Steinberg SM, Glatstein E, Sherins RJ. Long-term follow-up of testicular function following radiation therapy for early stage Hodgkin's disease. J Clin Oncol 1989;7:718–24.
16. Thomas PRM, Winstantly D, Peckham MJ, Austin DE, Murray MAF, Jacobs HS. Reproductive and endocrine function in patients with Hodgkin's disease: Effects of oophoropexy and irradiation. Br J Cancer 1976;33:226–31.
17. Sieber SM, Adamson RH. Toxicity of antineoplastic agents in man: Chromosomal aberrations, anti-fertility effects, congenital malformations, and carcinogenic potential. Adv Cancer Res 1975;40:1300–3.
18. Shalet SM. Effects of cancer chemotherapy on gonadal function of patients. Cancer Treat Rev 1980;7:141–52.
19. Sherins R, Winokur S, Devita VT. Surprisely high risk of functional castration in women receiving chemotherapy for lymphoma. Clin Res 1975;23:343A.
20. Waxman J. Chemotherapy and the adult gonad: A review. J R Soc Med 1983;76:144–8.
21. Gershenson DM. Menstrual and reproductive function after treatment with combination chemotherapy for malignant ovarian germ cell tumors. J Clin Oncol 1988; 6:270–5.

22. Pektasides D, Rustin GJS, Newlands ES, Begent RHJ, Bagshawe KD. Fertility after chemotherapy for ovarian germ cell tumours. Br J Obstet Gynaecol 1987;94:477–9.
23. Schilsky RL. Male fertility following cancer chemotherapy. J Clin Oncol 1989;7:295–7.
24. Whitehead E, Shalet SM, Blackledge G, Todd I, Crowther D, Beardwell CG. The effects of Hodgkin's disease and combination chemotherapy on gonadal function in the adult male. Cancer 1982;49:418–22.
25. Lendon M, Hann IM, Palmer MK, Shalet SM, Morris Jones PH. Testicular histology after combination chemotherapy in childhood for acute lymphoblastic leukaemia. Lancet 1978;2:439–41.
26. Wallace WH, Shalet SM, Lendon M, Morris-Jones PH. Male infertility in long term survivors of childhood acute lymphoblastic leukemia. Int J Androl 1991;14:312–9.
27. Redman JR, Bajorunas DR, Goldstein MC, Evenson DP, Gralla RJ, Lacher MJ, Koziner B, Lee BJ, Straus DJ, Clarkson BD, Feldschuh R, Feldschuh J. Semen cryopreservation and artificial insemination for Hodgkin's disease. J Clin Oncol 1987;5:233–8.
28. Fossa SD, Aass N, Molne K. Is routine pre-treatment cryopreservation of semen worthwhile in the management of patients with testicular cancer? Br J Urol 1989;64:524–9.
29. Siris ES, Leventhal BG, Vaitukaitis JL. Effects of childhood leukemia and chemotherapy on puberty and reproductive function of girls. N Engl J Med 1976;294:1143–6.
30. Rivkees SA, Crawford JD. The relationship of gonadal activity and chemotherapy-induced gonadal damage. JAMA 1988;259:2123–5.
31. Mulvihill JJ, Byrne J. Genetic counseling of the cancer survivor. Semin Oncol Nurs 1989;5:29–35.
32. Clayton PE, Shalet SM, Price DA, Morris Jones PH. Testicular damage after chemotherapy for childhood brain tumours. J Pediatr 1988;112:922–6.
33. Clayton PE, Shalet SM, Price DA, Jones PH. Ovarian function following chemotherapy for childhood brain tumors. Med Pediatr Oncol 1989;17:92–6.
34. Byrne J, Mulvihill JJ, Myers MH, Connelly RR, Naughton MD, Krauss MR, Steinhorn SC, Hassinger DD, Austin DF, Bragg K, Holmes GF, Holmes FF, Latourette HB, Weyer PJ, Meigs JW, Teta MJ, Cook JW, Strong LC. Effects of treatment on fertility in long-term survivors of childhood and adolescent cancer. N Engl J Med 1987;317:1315–21.
35. Byrne J, Fears TR, Gail MH, Pee D, Connelly RR, Austin DF, Holmes GF, Holmes FF, Latourette HB, Meigs JW, Strong LC, Myers MH, Mulvihill JJ. Early menopause in long-term survivors of cancer during adolescence. Am J Obstet Gynecol 1992;1666:788–93.
36. Hinterberger-Fischer M, Kier P, Kalhs P, Marosi C, Geissler K, Schwarzinger I, Pbinger I, Huber J, Spona J, Kolbabek H. Fertility, pregnancies and offspring complications after bone marrow transplantation. Bone Marrow Transplant 1991;7:5–9.
37. Gritz ER, Wellisch DK, Wang HJ, Siau J, Landsverk JA. Long term effects of testicular cancer on sexual functioning in married couples. Cancer 1989;64:1560–7.
38. Jacobs C, Donaldson SS, Rosenberg SA, Kaplan HS. Management of the pregnant patient with Hodgkin's disease. Ann Intern Med 1981;95:69–75.
39. Barry RM, Diamond HD, Cramer LF. Influence of pregnancy on the course of Hodgkin's disease. Am J Obstet Gynecol 1962;84:445–54.
40. Shalev O, Heyman S, Hod G, Adato P. Chronic granulocytic leukemia in pregnancy. A case report and review of the literature. Acta Obstet Gynecol Scand 1980;59:563–5.
41. Gallenberg MM, Loprinzi CL. Breast cancer and pregnancy. Semin Oncol 1989;16:369–76.
42. Sutton R, Buzdar AU, Hortobagyi GN. Pregnancy and offspring after adjuvant chemotherapy in breast cancer patients. Cancer 1990;65:847–50.
43. Rissanen PM. Carcinoma of the breast during pregnancy and lactation. Br J Cancer 1968;22:663–8.
44. Green DM, Zevon MA, Lowrie G, Seigelstein N, Hall B. Congenital anomalies in children of patients who received chemotherapy for cancer in childhood and adolescence. N Engl J Med 1991;325:141–6.
45. van der Kolk BM, Mulder NH, Mantingh A, Vandenberg E, Schraffordt Koops H, DeVries EG, Willemse PH, Sleijfer DT. Children born after their fathers had been treated with chemotherapy for testicular cancer. Eur J Obstet Gynecol Reprod Biol 1990;34:167–70.
46. Li FP, Fine W, Jaffe N, Holmes GE, Holmes FF. Offspring of patients treated for cancer in childhood. J Natl Cancer Inst 1979;62:1193–7.
47. Hawkins MM, Smith RA, Curtice LJ. Childhood cancer survivors and their offspring studied through a postal survey of general practitioners: Preliminary results. J R Coll Gen Pract 1988;38:102–5.

48. Mulvhill JJ, Byrne J, Steinhorn SA. Genetic disease in offspring of survivors of cancer in the young (abstract). Clin Genet 1986;39:72.
49. Mulvihill JJ, Myers MH, Connelly RR, Byrne J, Austin DF, Bragg K, Cook JW, Hassinger DD, Holmes FF, Holmes GF, Krauss MR, Latourette HB, Meigs JW, Naughton MD, Steinhorn SC, Strong LC, Teta MJ, Weyer PJ. Cancer in offspring of long-term survivors of childhood and adolescent cancer. Lancet 1987;2:813–7.
50. Aviles A, Diaz MJC, Torras V, Garcia EL, Guzman R. Non-Hodgkin's lymphomas and pregnancy: Presentation of 16 cases. Gynecol Oncol 1990;37:335–7.
51. Lilleyman JS, Hill AS, Anderson KJ. Consequences of acute myelogenous leukemia in early pregnancy. Cancer 1977;40:1300–3.
52. Daly H, McCann SR, Hanratty TD. Successful pregnancy during combination chemotherapy for Hodgkin's disease. Acta Haematol 1980;64:154–6.
53. Nicholson HO. Cytotoxic drugs in pregnancy. J Obstet Gynaecol Br Commonw 1968;75:2263–8.
54. Bender RA, Young RC. Effects of cancer treatment on individual and generational genetics. Semin Oncol 1978;5:47–56.
55. Kozlowski RD, Steinbrunner JV, MacKenzie AH, Clough JD, Wilek WS, Segal AM. Outcome of first trimester exposure to low dose methotrexate in eight patients with rheumatic disease. Am J Med 1990;88:589–92.
56. Greenberg LH, Palos V, Tanaka KR. Congenital anomalies probably induced by cyclophosphamide. JAMA 1964;188:423–6.
57. Toledo TM, Harper RC, Moser RH. Fetal effects during cyclophosphamide and irradiation therapy. Ann Intern Med 1971;74:87–91.
58. Coates A. Cyclophosphamide in pregnancy. Aust N Z J Obstet Gynaecol 1970;10:33–4.
59. Murray CL, Reichert JA, Anderson J, Twiggs LB. Multimodal cancer therapy for breast cancer in the first trimester of pregnancy. JAMA 1984;252:2607–8.
60. Sweet DL, Kinzie J. Consequences of radiotherapy and antineoplastic therapy for the fetus. J Reprod Med 1976;17:241–6.
61. Johnson IR, Filshie GM. Hodgkin's disease diagnosed in pregnancy. Br J Obstet Gynaecol 1977;84:791–2.
62. Parvez D, Salter LM, Armentrout SA. Successful pregnancy during chemotherapy for acute leukemia. Cancer 1981;47:845–6.
63. Hatcher RA, Stewart F, Trussell J, Kowal D, Guest F, Stewart GK, Cates W. Contraceptive Technology: 1990-1992. 15th rev ed. New York, Irvington Publishers, 1990.
64. Thomas DB, Noonan EA. Risk of breast cancer in relation to use of combined oral contraceptives near the age of menopause. WHO Collaborative Study of Neoplasia and Steroid Contraceptives. Cancer Causes Control 1991;2:389–94.
65. Thomas DB. Oral contraceptives and breast cancer: Review of the epidemiologic literature. Contraception 1991;43:597–642.
66. Romieu I, Berlin JA, Colditz G. Oral contraceptives and breast cancer. Review and meta-analysis. Cancer 1990;66:2253–63.
67. Contraceptive Technology Update. What is the risk of breast, cervical cancer with OCs? 1989;9:125.
68. Herbst AL, Berek JS. Impact of contraception on gynecologic cancers. Am J Obstet Gynecol 1993;168:1980–5.
69. Staffa JA, Newschaffer CJ, Jones JK, Miller V. Progestins and breast cancer: An epidemiologic review. Fertil Steril 1992;57:473–91.
70. Lower dose pills. Popul Rep [A] 1988;7:1.
71. Holck S. Hormonal contraceptives and the risk of cancer. World Health Stat Q 1987;40:225–32.
72. Huggins GR, Zucker PK. Oral contraceptives and neoplasia: 1987 update. Fertil Steril 1987;47:733–61.
73. Khoo SK. Cancer risks and the contraceptive pill: what is the evidence after nearly 25 years of use? Med J Aust 1986;144:185–90.
74. Monsonego J, Magdelenat H, Catalan F, Coscas Y, Zerat L, Sastre X. Estrogen and progesterone receptors in cervical human papillomavirus related lesions. Int J Cancer 1991;48:533–9.
75. Lassise DL, Savitz DA, Hamman RF, Baron AE, Brinton LA, Levines RS. Invasive cervical cancer and intrauterine device use. Int J Epidemiol 1991;20:865–70.
76. Schlesselman JJ. Cancer of the breast and reproductive tract in relation to use of oral contraceptives. Contraception 1989;40:1–38.

77. Endometrial cancer and combined oral contraceptives. The WHO Collaborative Study of Neoplasia and Steroid Contraceptives. Int J Epidemiol 1988;17:263–9.
78. Grimes DA. The safety of oral contraceptives: Epidemiologic insights from the first 30 years. Am J Obstet Gynecol 1992;166:1950–4.
79. Drife J. Benefits and risks of oral contraceptives. Adv Contracept 1990;6:15–25.
80. Cancer and Steroid Hormone Study of the Centers for Disease Control and the National Institutes of Child Health and Human Development. The reduction in risk of ovarian cancer associated with oral-contraceptive use. N Engl J Med 1987;316:650–5.
81. Grunberg SM, Weiss MH, Spitz IM, Ahmadi J, Sadun A, Russell CA, Lucci L, Stevenson LL. Treatment of unresectable meningiomas with the antiprogesterone agent mifepristone. J Neurosurg 1991;74:861–6.

14

Human Immunodeficiency Virus Infections

Perhaps the newest serious chronic illnesses affecting the reproductive age group are human immunodeficiency virus (HIV) infections and acquired immunodeficiency syndrome (AIDS). Eighty-four percent of women with HIV infection are in their reproductive years and HIV can have a tremendous impact on a pregnancy and offspring.[1] Since 1981, over 250,000 cases of AIDS have been recorded in the United States, with an estimated 1.5 million individuals infected with HIV. Worldwide more than one-third of the over 10 million persons infected with HIV are women.[2] In the United States, women accounted for an increasing proportion of total cases between 1988 (10.4%) and 1991 (12.8%)[3] and by 1991 HIV/AIDS was expected to be one of the five leading causes of death in reproductive age women.[4] Heterosexual contact also accounted for an increasing proportion of total cases each year between 1988 and 1991 (30%, 32%, 35%, and 37%).[3] The current predictions are for a doubling of heterosexual AIDS cases by 1995.[5] While the major mode of transmission for women is intravenous (IV) drug use, heterosexual transmission of HIV is increasingly rapidly. Of cases reported during 1990 to 1991, 3.1% of cases in men and 34.8% in women were classified as heterosexual transmission.[5] From 1990 to 1991 the number of reported cases of AIDS increased by 15% in women, compared with 3.6% in men.[6] For adolescents and young adults between 13 and 24, 13.4% of cases during 1989 to 1991 were due to heterosexual transmission compared to only 8.4% of cases before August 1989.

The risk of transmission of HIV appears higher for male-to-female contact than for female-to-male contact. In one study that followed long-term partners of HIV-infected individuals, the risk was 20% for female partners of infected men, versus only 1.4% (1/72 partners) in male partners of infected women.[7] Heterosexual transmission also seems to be enhanced when women have genital ulcer disease. Alarmingly high rates of HIV-infected pregnant women have been reported in some areas of the United States such as urban New York City.[8] In one study from an inner-city hospital in Brooklyn, New York, 2% (20/1000) of cord blood samples were positive for HIV.[9]

Fertility and HIV Infections

There is no current evidence that HIV infection or AIDS affects fertility unless superimposed problems exist, such as heroin addiction.[10]

Pregnancy Effects on HIV Infections

Pregnancy has the potential to worsen the immunosuppressive effects of HIV infection although the effects of pregnancy on HIV infections are not well understood. Pregnancy itself is immunosuppressing, particularly in the second and third trimesters of gestation, with a reduced T4/T8 ratio and decreased lymphoproliferative response.[11,12] However, there is only a small amount of information on the effects of HIV combined with pregnancy. In a study comparing infected and noninfected high-risk pregnant women, pregnancy appeared to accelerate HIV-induced depletion of $CD4^+$ cells.[13] In this study, 102 women who were either drug abusers or of Haitian origin were prospectively studied for immunological changes during and after pregnancy. In the 63 women who were HIV negative, $CD4^+$ cell counts fell until 8 weeks before delivery and rapidly increased just before delivery. However, among the 37 HIV-positive pregnant women, levels of $CD4^+$ cells fell during pregnancy and did not recover before or after delivery. In addition $CD8^+$ cell levels were higher in HIV-infected women. Uncontrolled studies have shown that 45 to 74% of asymptomatic HIV-infected pregnant women become symptomatic 28 to 60 months following delivery.[14–17] In one report, 12 of 16 mothers developed AIDS or AIDS-related complex (ARC) over a 30-month follow-up after they had given birth to infants with AIDS or ARC.[14] Several women who developed fulminant cases of AIDS during pregnancy have also been reported; however, cause and effect have not been proved.[18–20] Conversely, in two prospective studies examining the effects of pregnancy on HIV infection in populations primarily composed of IV drug abusers or partners of IV drug abusers, pregnancy did not seem to accelerate the course of the infection.[16,21]

HIV Effects on Pregnancy

HIV can also have a profound effect on pregnancy. In one study, 31% of pregnancies were associated with premature rupture of the membranes; 32%, with low birthweight; and 32%, with preterm births.[22] Other studies demonstrated an increased rate of premature deliveries and low-birth-weight infants in HIV-infected women.[23,24] However, these studies were often uncontrolled and this population often has higher rates of substance abuse. When high-risk asymptomatic HIV-positive women are compared to other pregnant high-risk women, spontaneous abortions, ectopic pregnancy, preterm delivery, stillbirth, birthweight, and gestational age are similar.[25–27] These case-controlled studies did not suggest that asymptomatic HIV infection is associated with an increased risk of adverse pregnancy outcomes in IV drug users. Minkoff et al. compared 126 seronegative women and 91 seropositive women who became pregnant and gave birth during the study period.[28] The two groups had identical rates of obstetric complications and there were no differences in birthweight, gestational age, head circumference, or Apgar scores among live infants.[28] Overall, while some studies found an association between HIV status and pregnancy outcome, others, after controlling for maternal drug use, did not. In the studies that did indicate differences, nutritional and socioeconomic status were not well controlled.

Transmission to the fetus occurs in about 20 to 50% of pregnancies of HIV-infected mothers.[29] Transmission may occur either in utero, at the time of birth, through exposure to maternal blood or body fluids, or through breast milk.[29] Some recent evidence suggests that spread is more likely to occur close to or at delivery rather than secondary to HIV transmission across the placenta.[30] On the other hand, the early onset of clinical and immunological features in 80 to 90% of infected children suggests possible intrauterine transmission rather than transmission at delivery.[31] Also, case reports exist of first- or second-trimester aborted fetuses from HIV-infected women who have HIV-1 infection in the fetus or placenta.[32–34] There is also some evidence to suggest that the risk of transmission is associated with certain antibodies such as GP-120, with detection of the antibody negatively correlated to the risk of infection in the fetus.

The diagnosis of HIV infection can be difficult in newborns. Most of the current tests to diagnose HIV infection use IgG antibodies which cross the placenta. Until the age of 15 months, when maternal antibodies disappear, the only form of diagnoses is either appearance of fulminant AIDS, isolation of the virus, or HIV antibodies in association with abnormal laboratory values or physical findings in the infant. Quinn et al. reported on the clinical utility of an IgA serological assay for early diagnosis in children. This test had a low sensitivity in the first months of life but a 97.6% sensitivity and 99.7% specificity after 3 months of life.[35] Landesman et al. also found the HIV IgA assay to be of significant value in the early months of life, with a positive predictive value for noninfected children of 100%.[36] This test may prove a better alternative as maternal IgA antibodies do not pass through the placenta to the fetus. Recently, viral culture and p24 antigen were examined for use in diagnosing HIV infections in neonates.[37] Burgard et al. found the viral culture to be 48% sensitive and 100% specific at birth and 75% sensitive and 100% specific at 3 months in those infants who became positive after 18 months of age.[37] The p24 antigen was only 18% sensitive at birth and 100% specific. However, the presence of p24 antigen at birth correlated with the early development of severe HIV-related disease.

Transmission of the virus to a fetus has been associated with characteristic findings including growth failure, microcephaly, prominent forehead, flattened nasal bridge, prominent eyes, blue sclerae, oblique eyes, flattened columella, triangular philtrum, and patulous lips.[38] However, some of these abnormalities may be related to concomitant drug use and viral infections.

Medications for HIV Infections and Pregnancy

Appropriate medications should be utilized to treat HIV-infected women who are pregnant unless there is strong documented evidence that would suggest fetal problems. Currently, there are few, if any therapies that should be avoided in an HIV-infected women.[10] Prophylaxis for *Pneumocystis carinii* pneumonia in HIV-infected pregnant women with low CD4 counts should be given. Aerosolized pentamidine may have the advantage of low serum levels and less fetal exposure.[10] Zidovudine (AZT) is generally used in individuals with low CD4+ counts. In those pregnant women with counts under 200/mm^3, AZT is being encouraged, while in those women with counts between 200 and 500/mm^3, the decision is more optional. If possible, therapy should be deferred until after organogenesis is complete (14 weeks of gestation). While animal studies seem somewhat reassuring in regards to teratogenicity,[10] some negative effects have been noted. One study in rats found nonmetastasizing vaginal tumors in 10% of those animals exposed to the drug for their entire lives. Other studies showed that AZT given to mice during gestation yielded fewer fetuses and greater numbers of resorptions, indicating a direct toxic effect on the developing mouse embryo.[39,40] Most other prenatal care is similar to that for non–HIV-infected individuals, with minor exceptions like the avoidance of elective placement of scalp electrodes.

Contraception and HIV Infections

Discussions regarding safe sex and contraception are crucial in HIV-infected individuals. Contraception discussion in many women who are infected with HIV is only focused on abstinence or safe sex with the intent to prevent viral spread, with little consideration for the preventing of unwanted pregnancies. Most discussions center on the utilization of barrier methods. However, when unwanted pregnancies become an issue, barrier methods are not necessarily adequate contraception. Some individuals infected with HIV will choose to abstain from intercourse, while others will continue to be sexually active. Those individuals who remain sexually active need maximal protection both from pregnancy, from sexually transmitted diseases, and from spreading the virus. The practitioner must consider the effect of the method on the course of HIV as well as the efficacy in preventing pregnancy. Since most women have been advised to use barrier methods, very few studies exist on the use of oral contraceptives in these women. Minkoff and DeHovitz reported that in pilot surveys of HIV-infected women, a large percentage would like to use both a barrier method and oral contraceptives.[10]

Barrier methods, in addition to providing contraception, can help to prevent spread of the HIV virus and provide some protection against the acquisition of other sexually transmitted diseases. Contraceptives that potentially provide some protection include the spermicides, the diaphragm, the cervical cap, and the male and female condom. It appears that nonoxynol 9 in sponge form and probably in other forms cannot be relied to protect against HIV transmission.[3,41] Diaphragms and cervical caps are also unlikely to provide adequate protection against HIV and other sexually transmitted diseases.[3] The female condom may provide more adequate protection but has only recently become available in the United States. While protection against HIV spread has not been established for the female condom, if the device is used properly and semen does not spill into the vagina, the polyurethane should theoretically prevent transmission of HIV as well as other sexually transmitted diseases in areas covered by the condom.

Hormonal contraceptives can provide more complete protection against pregnancy in HIV-infected women. The suggestion exists that oral contraceptives enhance HIV acquisition among prostitutes.[42] In addition, in another study, HIV-positive women who used oral contraceptives were found to be more likely to shed the virus.[43] The increased shedding was also reported to be correlated to cervical ectopy and pregnancy. It was not clear whether the increased shedding was related directly to the contraceptives' hormones or if the risk was related to the pill increasing cervical ectopy.

The other issue is the intrinsic safety of oral contraceptives in already infected individuals. In vitro and animal studies have suggested that reproductive hormones may alter the immune response but studies have shown both enhancement and depression.[10,44,45] Current available information does not suggest any contraindications to hormonal contraceptive use in HIV-infected women unless they have other known contraindications. No information is available that would contraindicate longer-acting contraceptives including Norplant and depomedroxyprogesterone acetate (DMPA) but more studies are needed. The physician should be aware of possible drug interactions between oral contraceptives and such medications as rifampin as discussed in Chapter 16. At present, recommended combinations include hormonal contraceptives (oral contraceptives, Norplant implant, and injectable DMPA) and latex condoms, or sterilization and latex condoms.[46] Recommendations to women whose partners will not use condoms include abstinence, spermicides, or female condoms.

The intrauterine device is probably not recommended in HIV-infected women. The device could cause increased infectivity due to increased bleeding. The string could cause abrasions of the penis during intercourse.[10]

Summary

1. HIV infections in women and heterosexual transmission of HIV infections are increasing.
2. Fertility rates are not affected by HIV infection or AIDS.
3. Pregnancy may accelerate the course of HIV infection and AIDS but this has not been well confirmed. Confounding factors such as substance abuse often exist.
4. HIV may be associated with significant effects on pregnancy including a higher prevalence of premature rupture of membranes, low birthweight, and preterm births. However, after controlling for substance abuse, some studies show no differences between HIV-infected and noninfected women.
5. Transmission to the fetus occurs in about 20 to 50% of pregnancies of HIV-infected mothers. HIV infection in the fetus has been associated with growth failure and multiple congenital abnormalities.
6. Appropriate medications should be utilized to treat HIV-infected pregnant women.
7. HIV-infected individuals who choose to remain sexually active need maximal protection from pregnancy, from sexually transmitted diseases, and from spreading the virus. Hormonal contraceptives appear safe in these individuals along with the use of barrier methods. Oral contraceptives may enhance the shedding of virus from infected women. The intrauterine device would not be recommended because of the possibility of increased bleeding or abrasions of the penis, leading to an increased risk of transmission.

References

1. Ellerbrock TV, Lieb S, Harrington PE, Bush TJ, Schoenfisch SA, Oxtoby MJ, Howell JT, Rogers MF, Witte JJ. Heterosexually transmitted human immunodeficiency virus infection among pregnant women in a rural Florida community. N Engl J Med 1992;327:1704–9.

2. Laurence J. Women and AIDS: An overview and specific disease manifestations. The AIDS Reader 1991;September/October:153–9.
3. Guinan ME. HIV, heterosexual transmission, and women. JAMA 1992;268:520–1.
4. Chu SY, Buehler JW, Berkelman RL. Impact of the human immunodeficiency virus epidemic on mortality in women of reproductive age, United States. JAMA 1990;264:225–9.
5. Allen JR, Setlow VP. Heterosexual transmission of HIV: A view of the future. JAMA 1991;266:1695–6.
6. Update: AIDS—United States, 1991. MMWR 1992;41:463–8.
7. Paidian N, Shiboski S, Jewell N. Female-to-male transmission of human immunodeficiency virus. JAMA 1991;266:1664–7.
8. Neinstein LS. Adolescent Health Care. A Practical Guide. Baltimore, Williams & Wilkins, 1991, pp 437–69.
9. Landesman S, Minkoff H, Holman S, McCalla S, Sijin O. Serosurvey of human immunodeficiency virus infection in parturients. JAMA 1987;258:2701–3.
10. Minkoff HL, DeHovitz JA. Care of women infected with the human immunodeficiency virus. JAMA 1991;266:2253–8.
11. Sridama V, Pacini F, Yang SL, Moawad A, Reilly M, DeGroot LJ. Decreased levels of helper T cells: A possible cause of immunodeficiency in pregnancy. N Engl J Med 1982;307:352–6.
12. Koonin LM, Ellerbrock TV, Atrash HK, Rogers MF, Smith JC, Hogue CJR, Harris MA, Chavkin W, Parker A, Halpin GJ. Pregnancy-associated deaths due to AIDS in the United States. JAMA 1989;261:1306–9.
13. Biggar RJ, Pahwa S, Minkoff H, Mendes H, Willoughby A, Landesman S, Goedert JJ. Immunosuppression in pregnant women infected with human immunodeficiency virus. Am J Obstet Gynecol 1989;161:1239–44.
14. Scott GB, Fischl MA, Klimas N, Fletcher MA, Dickinson GM, Levine RS, Parks WP. Mothers of infants with the acquired immunodeficiency syndrome: Evidence for both symptomatic and asymptomatic carriers. JAMA 1985;253:363–6.
15. Minkoff HL, Nanda D, Menez R, Fikrig S. Pregnancies resulting in infants with acquired immunodeficiency syndrome or AIDS-related complex: Follow-up of mothers, children and subsequently born siblings. Obstet Gynecol 1987;69:288–91.
16. Schoenbaum EE, Selwyn PA, Feingold AR. The effect of pregnancy on progression of HIV related disease (abstract THP.140). In Abstracts of the III International Conference on Acquired Immunodeficiency Syndrome. Washington, DC, US Dept of Health and Human Services and the World Health Organization, 1987.
17. Deschamps MM, Pape JW, Desvarieux M, Williams-Russo P, Madhaven S, Ho JL, Johnson WD Jr. A prospective study of HIV-seropositive asymptomatic women of childbearing age in a developing country. J Acquir Immune Defic Syndr 1993;6:446–51.
18. Jensen LP, O'Sullivan MJ, Gomezdel-Rio M, Setzer ES, Gaskin C, Penso C. Acquired immunodeficiency (AIDS) in pregnancy. Am J Obstet Gynecol 1984;148:1145–6.
19. Minkoff H, DeRegt RH, Landesman S, Schwarz R. Pneumocystis carinii pneumonia associated with acquired immunodeficiency syndrome in pregnancy: A report of three maternal deaths. Obstet Gynecol 1986;67:284–7.
20. Wetli CV, Roldan EO, Fojaco RM. Listeriosis as a cause of maternal death. An obstetric complication of the acquired immunodeficiency syndrome (AIDS). Am J Obstet Gynecol 1983;147:7–9.
21. The New York City Collaborative Study Group for Vertical Transmission of HIV: Human immunodeficiency virus (HIV) infection during pregnancy: A longitudinal study (abstract TP.55). In Abstracts of the III Conference on Acquired Immunodeficiency Syndrome. Washington, DC, US Dept of Health and Human Services and the World Health Organization, 1987.
22. Minkoff H, Nanda D, Menez R, Fikrig S. Pregnancies resulting in infants with acquired immunodeficiency syndrome or AIDS-related complex. Obstet Gynecol 1987;69:285–7.
23. Rubinstein A, Sicklick M, Gupta A, Bernstein L, Klein N, Rubinstein E, Spigland I, Fruchter L, Litman N, Lee H, Hollander M. Acquired immunodeficiency with reversed T4/T8 ratios in infants born to promiscuous and drug-addicted mothers. JAMA 1983;249:2350–6.
24. Gloeb DJ, O'Sullivan MJ, Efantis J. Human immunodeficiency virus infection in women. I. The effects of human immunodeficiency virus on pregnancy. Am J Obstet Gynecol 1988;159:756–61.

25. Minkoff H, Willoughby A, Mendez H. Human immunodeficiency virus in pregnant women and their offspring. Presented at the meeting of the Society for Perinatal Obstetricians, Las Vegas, February 1988.
26. Selwyn PA, Schoenbaum EE, Feingold AR. Perinatal transmission of HIV in intravenous drug users. Presented at the Third International Conference on AIDS, Washington, DC, June 1987.
27. Johnstone FD, MacCallum L, Brettle R, Inglis JM, Peutherer JF. Does infection with HIV affect the outcome of pregnancy? Br Med J (Clin Res) 1988;296:467.
28. Minkoff HL, Henderson C, Mendez H, Gail MH, Holman S, Willoughby A, Goedett JJ, Rubinstein A, Stratton P, Walsh JH. Pregnancy outcomes among mothers infected with human immunodeficiency virus and uninfected control subjects. Am J Obstet Gynecol 1990;163:1598–604.
29. Dinsmoor MJ. HIV infection and pregnancy. Med Clin North Am 1989;73:701–11.
30. Ehrnst A, Lindgren S, Dictor M, Johansson B, Sonnerborg A, Czajkowski J, Sundin G, Bohlin AB. HIV in pregnant women and their offspring: Evidence for late transmission. Lancet 1991;338:203–7.
31. European Collaborative Study. Children born to women with HIV-1 infection: Natural history and risk of transmission. Lancet 1991;337:253–60.
32. Peutherer JF, Rebus S, Smith I, Johnstone FD. Detection of HIV in the fetus: A study of six cases (abstract 7235). Presented at the Fourth International Conference on AIDS, Stockholm, Sweden, June 1988.
33. Sprecher S, Soumenkoff G, Puissant F, Degueldre M. Vertical transmission of HIV in a 15 week fetus (letter). Lancet 1986;2:288–9.
34. Jovaisas E, Koch MA, Schafer A, Stauber M, Loewenthal D. LAV/HTLV-III in 20 week fetus (letter). Lancet 1985;2:1129.
35. Quinn TC, Kline RL, Halsey N, Hutton N, Ruff A, Butz A, Boulos R, Modlin JF. Early diagnosis of perinatal HIV infection by detection of viral-specific IgA antibodies. JAMA 1991;266:3439–42.
36. Landesman S, Weiblen B, Mendez H, Willoughby A, Goedert JJ, Rubinstein A, Minkoff H, Moroso G, Hoff R. Clinical utility of HIV-IgA immunoblot assay in the early diagnosis of perinatal HIV infection. JAMA 1991;266:3443–6.
37. Burgard M, Mayaux MJ, Blanche S, Ferroni A, Guihard-Moscato ML, Allemon MC, Ciraru-Vigneron N, Firtion G, Floch C, Guillot F, Lachassine E, Vial M, Griscelli C, Rouzioux C. The use of viral culture and p24 antigen testing to diagnose human immunodeficiency virus infection in neonates. N Engl J Med 1992;327:1192–7.
38. Marion RW, Wiznia AA, Huthceon RG, Rubenstein A. Fetal AIDS syndrome score: Correlation between severity of dysmorphism and age at diagnosis of immunodeficiency. Arch Dis Child 1987;141:429–31.
39. Toltzis P, Marx CM, Kleinman N, Levine EM, Schmidt EV. Zidovudine-associated embryonic toxicity in mice. J Infect Dis 1991;163:1212–8.
40. Gogu SR, Beckman BS, Agrawal KC. Amelioration of zidovudine-induced fetal toxicity in pregnant mice. Antimicrobial Agents Chemother 1992;36:2370–4.
41. Kreiss J, Ngugi E, Holmes K. Efficacy of nonoxynol 9 contraceptive sponge use in preventing heterosexual acquisition of HIV in Nairobi prostitutes. JAMA 1992;268:477–82.
42. Plummer FA, Simonsen JN, Cameron DW, Ndinya-Achola JO, Kreiss JK, Gakinya MN, Waiyaki P, Cheang M, Piot P, Ronald AR. Cofactors in male-female sexual transmission of human immunodeficiency virus type 1. J Infect Dis 1991;163:233–9.
43. Clemetson DBA, Moss GB, Willerford DM, Hensel M, Emonyi W, Holmes KK, Plummer F, Ndinya-Achola S, Roberts PL, Hillier S. Detection of HIV DNA in cervical and vaginal secretions: Prevalence and correlates among women in Nairobi, Kenya. JAMA 1993;269:2860–4.
44. Sthoeger ZM, Chiorazzi N, Lahita RG. Regulation of the immune response by sex hormones. I: In vivo effects of estradiol and testosterone on poke-weed mitogen induced human B-cell differentiation. J Immunol 1988;41:91–8.
45. Kalland T, Strand O, Forsberg J. Long term effects of neonatal estrogen treatment on mitogen responsiveness of mouse spleen lymphocytes. J Clin Invest 1979;63:413–21.
46. Hatcher RA, Stewart F, Trussell J, Kowal D, Guest F, Stewart GK, Cates W. Contraceptive Technology: 1990-1992. 15th rev ed. New York, Irvington Publishers, 1990.

15

Substance Abuse

Another special problem with potential serious sequelae for a mother and infant is substance abuse. In urban areas, as many as 59% of pregnant women consume alcohol, 44% smoke cigarettes, 28% have used marijuana, 17% have used cocaine, and 4% have used opiates.[1] Both legal substances such as caffeine, nicotine, and alcohol and illegal drugs such as cocaine, heroin, benzodiazepines, barbiturates, cannabis, hallucinogens, and amphetamines can be toxic to a pregnant woman and her offspring. The toxicity of these drugs may include intrauterine growth retardation, fetal death, and teratogenesis. Gillogley et al. performed universal urine testing for cocaine, amphetamines, and opiates on 1643 women admitted to an obstetric service for a 1-year period.[2] During that time, 20.5% tested positive. In infants born to the positive group there was a significant decrease in birthweight, head circumference, length, and gestational age even after controlling for smoking, prenatal care, and prior preterm births. However, it is often difficult to assess a drug's effect on the user and an infant because of numerous cofactors. These include variations in drug purity and potency, malnutrition and poor prenatal care in the mothers, a high prevalence of other infections (e.g., sexually transmitted disease and human immunodeficiency virus [HIV] infection), and the use of multiple drugs by most substance-abusing individuals.

Important principles regarding the effect of drugs on the neonate include the following[3]:

1. The timing of the drug use may be critical, with the first 8 weeks of pregnancy being the most important for embryonic development.
2. Physiological changes occurring with pregnancy, such as alterations in plasma proteins and hormonal changes, can affect drug levels.
3. Placental function is a crucial component in determining a drug's effect on the fetus.

4. Exposure of the fetus to drugs may have serious effects on the newborn and in later life.

At the present time, little is known about the long-term effects of maternal drug use on the child, such as intellectual capacity, learning behavior, and risk of addiction during adolescence and adulthood.

Table 15–1 reviews commonly reported teratogenic effects of abused drugs. The largest identified syndrome of teratogenesis is the fetal alcohol syndrome secondary to alcohol ingestion.[4] This syndrome is the leading cause of mental retardation, with reported rates in the US population between 0.75 per 1000 live births to 2.2 per 1000 live births.[5] Table 15–2 lists the common alcohol-related birth defects, which include structural abnormalities, prenatal and/or postnatal growth retardation, behavioral changes, and the neonatal abstinence syndrome. There is also evidence of a relationship between heavy alcohol use and low birthweight.[6–10] Coles et al. examined the long-term effects of alcohol use by comparing a group of children born to either women who drank throughout pregnancy, a group that stopped drinking in the second trimester, or a group of nondrinkers.[11] The mean age at follow-up was 5 years 10 months. The children in the continued-to-drink group had more alcohol-related birth defects and had more consistent deficits in intellectual functioning including sequential processing (short-term memory and encoding) and overall mental processing.

The diagnosis of fetal alcohol syndrome includes the presence of

1. Facial dysmorphogenesis (microcephaly, short palpebral fissures, epicanthal folds, maxillary hypoplasia, cleft palate, and micrognathia)
2. Prenatal and postnatal growth retardation
3. Central nervous system abnormalities including mental retardation

In addition to these, several organ systems may be affected, leading to joint abnormalities and cardiac lesions, especially atrial septal defect and ventricular septal defect. Liver abnormalities such as hepatic fibrosis have also been reported.[12]

The prevalence of serious problems in heavy drinkers can be quite high. In one study, 33% of infants born to heavily alcoholic mothers had the fetal alcohol syndrome and an additional 33% had features consistent with alcohol-related problems.[6] With moderate alcohol consumption, an estimated 11% of infants of women drinking between 1 and 2 oz of alcohol per day during the first trimester have problems consistent with alcohol effects.[7]

The use of cigarettes by pregnant women with and without other substance abuse problems is common, with between 22 and 38% of pregnant women smoking throughout their pregnancy. Nicotine is associated with significant problems, including a 34% higher perinatal death rate[13] and an increased risk of preeclampsia, abruptio placentae, and placenta previa.[14] Numerous retrospective and prospective studies have proved an association between smoking in pregnant women and low birthweight.[15–20] These

Table 15–1 Commonly Reported Teratogenic Effects of Abused Drugs

Specific Fetal Effects	Opiates	Alcohol	Other Sedative-Hypnotic Drugs	Cocaine	Other Stimulants	Hallucinogens	Marijuana	Nicotine
Structural nonspecific growth retardation	X	X	—	X	—	—	X	X
Specific dysmorphic effects	—	X	—	X	—	—	—	—
Behavioral	X	X	X	X	X	X	X	X
Neurobiochemical (abstinence syndrome)	X	X	X	—	—	—	—	—
Increased fetal and perinatal mortality	X	X	—	X	—	—	—	X
Women reporting use in pregnancy (varies with population).%	5	>50	<5	≤20	<5	<5	5–34	>50

Reprinted by permission of the *Western Journal of Medicine* (Hoegerman G, Wilson CA, Thurmond E, Schnoll SH. Drug-exposed neonates. 1990;152:559–64).

Table 15–2 Alcohol-Related Birth Defects

Structural changes
  Prenatal growth retardation
  Microcephaly
  Short palpebral fissure
  Indistinct philtrum
  Hypoplastic maxilla and flattened midface
  Thin vermillion border
  Cardiac defects

Behavioral changes
  Mild to moderate mental retardation
  Delayed motor and language
  Increased irritability
  Decreased ability to habituate

Neurobiochemical changes
  Neonatal abstinence syndrome

Reprinted by permission of the *Western Journal of Medicine* (Hoegerman G, Wilson CA, Thurmond E, Schnoll SH. Drug-exposed neonates. 1990;152:559-64).

infants also have an increased risk of growth retardation, prematurity and respiratory tract infections, and sudden infant death syndrome.[3,12]

Marijuana use has also been suggested to be associated with an increase in fetal problems including congenital malformations and lower infant birthweight.[21,22] However, most of the studies involving marijuana use have used small study populations and a retrospective design.

Cocaine use in the United States is a significant problem. It is estimated that as many as 10 million individuals in the United States have used cocaine and 5 million use it regularly.[23] Women aged 18 to 34 make up 15% of all regular users of recreational cocaine.[24,25] In addition, surveys have indicated that between 3.4 and 10% of pregnant women use cocaine.[1]

Significant obstetric and neonatal complications have been associated with cocaine use in pregnancy. These include spontaneous abortion, low birthweight, intrauterine growth retardation, stillbirth, microcephaly, childhood neurobehavioral deficits, sudden infant death syndrome, cerebral infarct, abruptio placentae, and birth defects.[1,15,26] Volpe reviewed the effects of cocaine use on the fetus and reported on several teratogenic effects of cocaine on the development of the brain.[27] These included microcephaly in 16% of exposed infants and disturbances of midline proencephalic development and neuronal migration (agenesis of corpus callosum, absence of septum pellucidum, septo-optic dysplasia, and neuronal heterotopias). Little and Snell studied the pattern of fetal growth retardation in fetuses exposed to cocaine as opposed to fetuses exposed to alcohol or no drugs.[28] In cocaine-exposed infants, head circumference was reduced more than birthweight, which was similar to that in alcohol-exposed infants. The decrease in head circumference was similar in alcohol- and cocaine-exposed infants. The vasoconstrictive properties of cocaine may be responsible for some of the problems such as abruptio placentae and cerebral infarctions.

Evidence also exists that there are behavior differences in cocaine-exposed infants. The most common reported behaviors include lethargy, poor social responsivity, irritability, hypertonicity, tremulousness, and disorganized patterns of feeding and sleeping.[15] Chasnoff et al. evaluated the relationship between the timing of cocaine use in pregnant women and complications.[29] This study compared women who only used cocaine in the first trimester with those who used cocaine throughout pregnancy and a normal matched group of obstetric patients with no history of drug use. Only the group who used cocaine throughout pregnancy had evidence of an increased rate of preterm delivery, low-birthweight infants, and a decrease in head circumference. Both groups of women who used cocaine had significant impairment of orientation, motor, and state regulation behaviors on the Neonatal Behavioral Assessment Scale. However, much more needs to be learned about the long-term effects of cocaine exposure on infants and children, which is still under investigation. As yet it is difficult to directly link the toxic effect of cocaine to specific long-term behavioral outcomes because most studies have had either small sample sizes, confounding factors, or lack of long-term follow-up.

Other teratogenic problems associated with cocaine use in pregnant mothers are of some controversy. Birth defects reported in some studies include genitourinary malformations, prune-belly syndrome, limb reduction defects, cardiovascular defects, and cerebral infarcts.[1,25] A recent case-control study demonstrated a statistically significant association of cocaine use with urinary tract defects (4.39 odds ratio).[29] Results from animal studies are mixed. While congenital defects are found and are similar to defects found in humans, the malformations do not show a relationship to doses, and the defects appear to come in random fashion during development and not at characteristic time periods. It appears that cocaine is probably a weak teratogen but potentially affects a large population. The mechanism for the toxicity is probably through vasoconstriction and local hemorrhage.[30]

Amphetamines, while not as popular as cocaine, are an important drug of abuse. The most commonly form of abuse is the pure form of methamphetamine hydrochloride called "ice." Fewer reports are available on the effects of methamphetamine during pregnancy than with cocaine. However, there have been reports on newborns of decreased body weight, length, and head circumference. In addition, in animal studies methamphetamine has produced exencephaly, cleft palate, and eye anomalies.[31]

Complications in pregnant women and their offspring from narcotic addiction result less from the physiological changes of the drug and more from associated life-style problems. These include intravenous drug use, malnutrition, high exposure to sexually transmitted diseases including HIV infection, and the lack of prenatal care. All of this puts them at increased risk for local abscesses, hepatitis, thrombophlebitis, endocarditis, and other infections.

Commonly used depressants include the barbiturates and diazepam. Barbiturates have not been associated with teratogenicity although a neonatal withdrawal syndrome can occur several days to 2 weeks after delivery. Research on the teratogenicity of diazepam has been conflicting, with some reports finding an increased incidence and others finding no association.[32–34]

PCP (phencyclidine), a common hallucinogen of abuse, has been associated with abnormal neonatal behavior including lethargy, floppiness, nystagmus, and tremors.[35] However, PCP has not been associated with teratogenicity in humans.

The inhalation of toluene-based solvent continues to be another popular form of substance abuse. These substances are readily available in spray paint and glue preparations. The effects of toluene use during pregnancy have not been frequently reported. However, use during pregnancy can be significantly toxic. In one study of 21 newborns exposed to toluene in utero, there was a significant increase in preterm labor or delivery (86%), perinatal death (14%), and growth retardation.[36] Metabolic acidosis secondary to renal tubular acidosis was a common complication in these women. There was also an increase in growth retardation and developmental delay in these infants in their childhood.

Over 50% of infants born to mothers with street drug or alcohol addiction will demonstrate evidence of neonatal abstinence syndrome. This includes signs of irritability; autonomic system dysfunction such as yawning, sneezing, and low-grade fever; gastrointestinal abnormalities such as diarrhea and vomiting; and failure to thrive and increased apnea. The most common treatment has been to use phenobarbital, 2 to 4 mg/kg orally or intramuscularly every 8 hours.[3] For opiate withdrawal, methadone and diazepam have been used. Whichever drug is used, it should be tapered by 10 to 20% per day.

Breast-feeding is another potential problem for mothers with a substance abuse problem. Amphetamines, cocaine, heroin, marijuana, nicotine, and PCP can all cause problems to newborns who breast-feed.[3,37]

The choice of a contraception in women who are abusing drugs is complicated by several factors. For women who are abusing drugs and are living on the streets, contraception may be a low priority compared to other nonmedical and medical needs.[38] These women may also fail to seek medical attention and fail to insist that their partners use condoms.[38] In addition, many of these women are at increased risk of contacting a sexually transmitted disease and are thus in need of contraception to prevent both conception and sexually transmitted diseases. For noncompliant women who are abusing drugs, a progestin implant or depomedroxyprogesterone acetate (DMPA) used in conjunction with condoms may be the best solution.

Concern has arisen that methadone may reduce oral contraceptive effectiveness by increasing the clearance of hormones through hepatic enzyme induction.[38] However, there are no clinical data available that support a decreased effectiveness rate of oral contraceptives in these women. While the intrauterine device is a consideration, it is associated with other problems in this population because of the higher risks of contracting a sexually transmitted disease.

References

1. Frank DA, Zuckerman BS, Amaro H, Aboagye K, Bauchner H, Cabral H, Fried L, Hingson R, Kayne H, Levenson SM, Parker S, Reece H, Vinci R. Cocaine use during pregnancy: Prevalence and correlates. Pediatrics 1988;82:888–95.
2. Gillogley KM, Evans AT, Hansen RL, Samuels SJ, Batra KK. The perinatal impact of cocaine, amphetamine, and opiate use detected by universal intrapartum screening. Am J Obstet Gynecol 1990;163:1535–42.
3. Hoegerman G, Wilson CA, Thurmond E, Schnoll SH. Drug-exposed neonates. West J Med 1990;152:559–64.
4. Zimmerman EF. Substance abuse in pregnancy: Teratogenesis. Pediatr Ann 1991;20:541–7.
5. Abel EL, Sokol RJ. Incidence of fetal alcohol syndrome and economic impact of FAS-related anomalies. Drug Alcohol Depend 1987;19:51–70.
6. Olegard R, Sabekg M, Aronsson M, Sandin B, Johansson AR, Carlsson C, Kyllerman M, Iversen K, Hrbek A. Effects on the child of alcohol abuse during pregnancy. Retrospective and prospective studies. Acta Paediatr Scand Suppl 1979;275:112–21.
7. Hanson, JW, Streissguth AP, Smith DW. The effects of moderate alcohol consumption during pregnancy on fetal growth and morphogenesis. J Pediatr 1978;92:457–60.
8. Little RE, Streissguth AP. Effects of alcohol on the fetus: Impact and prevention. Can Med Assoc J 1981;125:159–64.
9. Jones KL, Smith DW, Streissguth AP, Myrianthopoulos NC. Outcome in offspring of chronic alcoholic women. Lancet 1974;1:1076–8.
10. Little RE, Asker RL, Sampson PD, Renwick JH. Fetal growth and moderate drinking in early pregnancy. Am J Epidemiol 1986;123:270–8.
11. Coles CD, Brown RT, Smith IE, Platzman KA, Erickson S, Falek A. Effects of prenatal alcohol exposure at school age. I. Physical and cognitive development. Neurotoxicol Teratol 1991;13:357–67.
12. Hill LM. Effects of drugs and chemicals on the fetus and newborn (part 2). Mayo Clin Proc 1984;59:755–65.
13. Weisberg E. Smoking and reproductive health. Clin Reprod Fertil 1985;3:175–86.
14. Henderson CE, Mullin PP. Alcohol and substance abuse in pregnancy. In Cherry SH, Merkatz IR, eds. Complications of Pregnancy: Medical, Surgical, Gynecologic, Psychosocial, and Perinatal. 4th ed. Baltimore, Williams & Wilkins, 1991, pp 160–71.
15. Singer LT, Garber R, Kliegman R. Neurobehavioral sequelae of fetal cocaine exposure. J Pediatr 1991;119:667–71.
16. Kleinman JC, Madans C. The effects of maternal smoking, physical stature, and education attainment on the incidence of low birth weight. Am J Epidemiol 1985;121:843–55.
17. Picone TA, Allen LH, Olsen PN, Ferris ME. Pregnancy outcome in North American women. II. Effects of diet, cigarette smoking, stress, and weight gain on placentas, and neonatal physical and behavioral characteristics. Am J Clin Nutr 1982;36:1214–24.
18. Shinon PH, Klebanoff MA, Rhoads GG. Smoking and drinking during pregnancy: Their effects on preterm birth. JAMA 1986;255:82–4.
19. Wainwright RL. Change in observed birth weight associated with change in maternal cigarette smoking. Am J Epidemiol 1983;117:668–75.
20. Naeye RL. Influence of maternal cigarette smoking during pregnancy on fetal and childhood growth. Am J Obstet Gynecol 1981;57:18–21.

21. Greenland S, Staish D, Brown N, Gross SJ. The effects of marijuana use during pregnancy. Am J Obstet Gynecol 1972;143:408–13.
22. Hingson R, Alpert J, Day N, Dooling E, Kayne H, Morelock S, Oppenheimer E, Zuckerman B. Effects of maternal drinking and marijuana use on fetal growth and development. Pediatrics 1982;70:539–46.
23. Fishburne PM. National Survey on Drug Abuse: Main Findings. Washington, DC, National Institute of Drug Abuse, 1980. US Dept of Health and Human Services publication no. ADM 80-976.
24. Chasnoff IJ, Landress HJ, Barrett ME. The prevalence of illicit-drug or alcohol use during pregnancy and discrepancies in mandatory reporting in Pinellas County, Florida. N Engl J Med 1990;322:1202–6.
25. Little BB, Snell LM, Klein VR, Gilstrap LC. Cocaine abuse during pregnancy: Maternal and fetal implications. Obstet Gynecol 1989;73:157–60.
26. Donovan J. Randomized controlled trial of antismoking advice in pregnancy. Br J Prev Soc Med 1977;31:6–12.
27. Volpe JJ. Effect of cocaine use on the fetus. N Engl J Med 1992;327:399–407.
28. Little BB, Snell LM. Brain growth among fetuses exposed to cocaine in utero: Asymmetrical growth retardation. Obstet Gynecol 1991;77:361–4.
29. Chasnoff IJ, Griffith DR, MacGregor S, Dirkes K, Burns KA. Temporal patterns of cocaine use in pregnancy: Perinatal outcome. JAMA 1989;261:1741–4.
30. Webster WS, Brown-Woodman PDC. Cocaine as a cause of congenital malformations of vascular origin: Experimental evidence in the rat. Teratology 1990;41:689–97.
31. Vorhees CV, Acuff-Smith KD. Prenatal methamphetamine-induced anophthalmia in rats. Neurotoxicol Teratol 1990;12:409.
32. Safra JM, Oakley GP. Association between cleft lip with or without cleft palate and prenatal exposure to diazepam. Lancet 1975;2:478–80.
33. Rosenberg L, Mitchell A, Parsell J. Lack of relation of oral cleft to diazepam use during pregnancy. N Engl J Med 12983;309:1281–5.
34. Shinon P, Mills J. Oral cleft and diazepam use during pregnancy. N Engl J Med 1984;311:919–20.
35. Golden NL, Sokol RJ, Rubin JL. Angel dust: Possible effects on the fetus. Pediatrics 1980;65:18–20.
36. Wilkins-Haug L, Gabow PA. Toluene abuse during pregnancy: Obstetric complications and perinatal outcomes. Obstet Gynecol 1991;77:504–9.
37. Committee on Drugs, American Academy of Pediatrics. Transfer of drugs and other chemicals into human milk. Pediatrics 1989;84:924–36.
38. Hankoff LD, Darney PD. Contraceptive choices for behaviorally disordered individuals. Am J Obstet Gynecol 1993;168:1986–9.

16

Medications

Women with special medical problems may be on multiple medications. These medications may have effects on fertility and pregnancy. In addition, some of these medications may interact with contraceptive devices or vice versa.

Medications during Pregnancy

Many medications, such as anticonvulsants and steroids, have already been dealt with in the chapters on specific illnesses. This section summarizes this information and includes information about other medications not previously discussed. Several articles have reviewed the effects of various medications during pregnancy.[1-8]

Medication exposure during pregnancy and the postpartum period can potentially cause problems during preconception, the first-trimester period of organogenesis, the second and third trimesters during fetal development, the labor and delivery period, and the breast-feeding period. Potentially, a drug given to men or women before conception can cause embryonic maldevelopment.[3] Usually a drug given during the first 7 days after conception will cause either a miscarriage or no problems. The period of organogenesis beginning at about 14 days after conception is most commonly related to drug-associated congenital abnormalities. Thus, avoidance of drugs, when possible, during this time period is recommended. The risk for birth defects in the second and third trimesters is much smaller. However, certain medications, such as tetracycline, can still cause problems during this time period.

While many drugs have been suggested to be associated with fetal malformations, only about 30 medications currently used in the United States have been proved to be associated with teratogenic effects. To help to clarify the risk of medications to pregnant women, the Food and Drug Administration (FDA) has revised the literature on medications to place drugs in one of five categories (Table 16–1).

Antibiotics

Many women with a chronic illness are placed on antibiotics at some time during the course of their illness and often for extended periods of time. Most antibiotics cross the placental barrier and thus carry the potential for toxicity. The teratogenicity of most antibiotics is not known as most studies were conducted in animals and may not reflect the effects of these medications in humans. Because of physiological changes during pregnancy, there is a net drop in maternal antibiotic levels of about 10 to 50% in late pregnancy and the immediate postpartum period. Table 16–2 reviews the safety and risks of antimicrobial agents in pregnancy.

PENICILLINS

In general, these are considered safe although data on newer drugs such as mezlocillin and penicillins with clavulanic acid are limited. Penicillins are usually the drug of choice in pregnant women when they provide adequate coverage.

CEPHALOSPORINS

These are also considered safe during pregnancy and have not been associated with teratogenic effects, although less is known about third-generation cephalosporins.

Table 16–1   FDA Pregnancy Categories

CATEGORY	DESCRIPTION
A	Medications for which controlled studies in women fail to demonstrate a risk to the fetus.
B	Either (a) animal studies have not demonstrated a fetal risk, but no adequate human studies have been done, or (b) animal studies have uncovered some risk that has not been confirmed in controlled studies in humans.
C	Either (a) animal studies have revealed adverse fetal effects, but not adequate controlled studies have been done in humans, or (b) studies in humans and animals are not available.
D	Medications that are associated with birth defects in humans, but with potential benefits that outweigh their known risks.
X	Medications contraindicated in pregnant patients because of known occurrence of fetal abnormalities demonstrated in human or animal studies. Potential risks for these medications clearly outweigh their potential benefits.

Table 16-2 Safety and Potential Risks of Major Categories of Antimicrobial Agents in Pregnancy

ANTIMICROBIAL AGENTS	USE IN PREGNANCY[a]	Maternal	Fetal/Neonatal
		POTENTIAL TOXICITY	
Antibacterial			
Aminoglycosides	Use with caution	Oto- and nephrotoxicity	Eighth-nerve toxicity
Cephalosporins	Considered safe	Allergic reactions	None known
Chloramphenicol	Relatively contraindicated	Bone marrow depression; aplastic anemia	Gray syndrome
Ciprofloxacin	Relatively contraindicated		May be associated with cartilage erosion
Clindamycin	Use with caution	Allergic reactions; pseudomembranous colitis	None known
Erythromycin base	Considered safe	Allergic reactions	None known
Erythromycin estolate	Relatively contraindicated	Cholestatic hepatitis	None known
Methenamine mandelate	Considered safe	None known	None known
Metronidazole	Use with caution	Blood dyscrasia; neuropathy; intolerance to alcohol	No known teratogenicity in humans
Nalidixic acid	Relatively contraindicated	Toxic psychosis, seizures	Increased intracranial pressure; papilledema; bulging fontanelles
Nitrofurantoin	Use with caution	Neuropathy; hemolysis (G6PD deficiency)	Hemolysis (G6PD deficiency)
Penicillins	Considered safe	Allergic reactions	None known
Sulfonamides	Use with caution	Allergic reactions	Kernicterus; hemolysis (G6PD deficiency)
Tetracyclines	Relatively contraindicated	Hepatotoxicity; pancreatitis; renal failure	Tooth discoloration and dysplasia; inhibition of bone growth
Trimethodprim	Relatively contraindicated	Allergic reactions	Folate antagonism; potentially teratogenic
Antimycobacterial			
Ethambutol hydrochloride	Use with caution	Optic neuritis	None known
Isoniazid	Use with caution	Hepatotoxicity in rapid acetylators	Possible neuropathy and seizures
Rifampin	Use with caution	Hepatotoxicity; hypoprothrombinemia; bleeding	No known teratogenicity in humans
Antifungal			
Amphotericin B	Use with caution	Nephrotoxicity; anemia; hypokalemia; idiosyncratic reactions	No known teratogenicity; reversible azotemia and hypokalemia
Flucytosine	Relatively contraindicated	Hepatotoxicity; marrow aplasia	Potential teratogenicity

Griseofulvin	Relatively contraindicated	Allergic reactions; hepatotoxicity	Potential teratogenicity
Ketoconazole	Relatively contraindicated	Hepatitis; adrenal suppression	Safety not established
Miconazole nitrate	Relatively contraindicated	Hyperlipidemia; hyponatremia and thrombocytosis	Safety not established
Antiviral			
Acyclovir sodium	Use with caution (life-threatening infections only)	Nephrotoxicity with dehydration	None known
Amantadine hydrochloride	Relatively contraindicated	Anxiety, hallucinations and psychosis	Potential teratogenicity
Vidarabine	Relatively contraindicated	Neurotoxicity with tremor and hallucinations; thrombocytopenia and leukopenia	Potential teratogenicity
Zidovudine	Relatively contraindicated		May be fetotoxic
Antiparasitic			
Chloroquine phosphate	Considered safe	Ototoxicity	None at recommended doses
Iodoquinol (diiodohydroxyquin)	Use with caution	Iodine hypersensitivity	None known
Diloxanide furoate	Relatively contraindicated	None	Safety not established
Emetine hydrochloride	Relatively contraindicated	Cardiotoxicity	Fetal damage
Furazolidone	Use with caution	Allergic reactions; monoamine oxidase inhibition agranulocytosis; hemolysis (G6PD deficiency)	Hemolysis (G6PD deficiency)
Mebendazole	Relatively contraindicated	Leukopenia; abdominal pain	Potential teratogenicity
Niclosamide	Use with caution	None	Safety not established
Paromomycin sulfate	Considered safe	Gastrointestinal disturbance	None known
Pentamidine isethionate	Use with caution	Hypotension, hypoglycemia, blood dyscrasia	No known teratogenicity
Piperazine citrate	Use with caution	Allergic reactions; seizures; visual disturbance	None known
Praziquantel	Considered safe	Sedation, dizziness	Safety not established
Primaquine phosphate	Relatively contraindicated	Hemolysis (G6PD deficiency)	Hemolysis (G6PD deficiency)
Pyrimethamine and dapsone	Relatively contraindicated	Hemolysis; agranulocytosis	Hemolysis; methemoglobinemia
Pyrimethamine and sulfadoxine	Relatively contraindicated	Allergic reactions; blood dyscrasia	Potential teratogenicity
Quinacrine hydrochloride	Relatively contraindicated	Hemolysis; toxic psychosis; hepatotoxicity	Safety not established
Quinine sulfate	Use with caution (life-threatening infections only)	Cinchonism; hemolysis; renal failure	Optic nerve hypoplasia; congenital deafness
Spiramycin	Use with caution	Allergic reactions	None known
Thiabendazole	Use with caution	Allergic reactions; blood dyscrasia	Safety not established

a"Considered safe" implies a lack of evidence to suggest any significant toxicity exists; "use with caution" implies that reports of maternal or fetal toxic reactions exist and use should be closely monitored; "relatively contraindicated" implies that the risk of toxicity is high and there are alternative agents that may provide a more favorable risk-benefit ratio. G6PD = glucose-6-phosphate dehydrogenase.
Adapted from Chow AW et al.[3]

AMINOGLYCOSIDES

These should be used with extreme caution in pregnancy and only for serious gram-negative infections. Streptomycin and kanamycin in particular have been associated with ototoxicity in the fetus.

ERYTHROMYCIN

While erythromycin base is considered safe, erythromycin estolate is contraindicated because of the risk of cholestatic hepatitis.

METRONIDAZOLE

Because of reported teratogenic effects in animals, this antibiotic should be used only with caution in pregnancy. However, no teratogenic effects in humans have been reported.

SULFONAMIDES

Sulfa drugs should be avoided in the third trimester as they can raise bilirubin levels by competing for bilirubin-binding sites. There are no known teratogenic effects in humans. Pregnancy is considered a relative contraindication to the use of trimethoprim-sulfamethoxazole because of the drug's folate antagonism and potential teratogenic effects. It could be used in cases of life-threatening infections such as *Pneumocystis carinii.*

TETRACYCLINES

These drugs should be avoided during pregnancy as they are potentially hepatotoxic and renal toxic to the mother and can cause tooth discoloration and dysplasia in the neonate. The risk of tooth discoloration occurs after about the fourth month of gestation.

CHLORAMPHENICOL

Chloramphenicol should be avoided in pregnancy as it can cause gray syndrome in newborns associated with a high mortality.

CLINDAMYCIN

While no teratogenic effects have been reported, the drug should be reserved for serious infections with no other safer alternatives because of potential gastrointestinal side effects (pseudomembranous colitis).

NITROFURANTOIN

Nitrofurantoin should only be used with caution in pregnant women. It can potentially cause neuropathies in mothers and hemolysis in mothers or infants with glucose-6-phosphate dehydrogenase (G6PD) deficiency.

CIPROFLOXACIN (CIPRO)

This drug has not been associated with teratogenic effects. However, it may be associated with cartilage erosion of weight-bearing joints in immature animals and so its use should be avoided during pregnancy.[9]

Analgesics and Antiinflammatory Medications

Women with chronic illness may require analgesics or antiinflammatory medications during the course of their illness. Acetaminophen appears safe as an analgesic. While aspirin is relatively safe, it can be toxic in the final weeks of pregnancy when it could lead to problems with hemorrhage during delivery. There are also some reports of aspirin causing a decrease in fetal birthweight and an increase in the incidence of stillbirths.[10,11]

NONSTEROIDAL ANTIINFLAMMATORY DRUGS

At present there are no known teratogenic effects of these medications. However, their use should be limited in pregnant women, especially in the third trimester. Since these medications inhibit prostaglandin synthesis, the drugs could interfere with labor. They may also increase the risk of hemorrhagic complications at delivery.

Antiacne Medications

Some women with chronic illness are at greater risk for severe acne because of steroid use or other drugs. Oral isotretinoin (Accutane) is highly effective in treating severe cystic acne. However, the drug is a potent teratogen in humans and should not be used in pregnancy. The drug is associated with a 40% spontaneous abortion rate and 25% rate of significant fetal abnormalities with first-trimester exposure.[12] Isotretinoin is eliminated from the body rapidly and so women could discontinue therapy 1 month before becoming pregnant without a risk of birth defects.[13] Erythromycin appears safe for use during pregnancy.

Antiarrhythmics

Drugs that have been considered relatively safe to use in pregnancy, when indicated, include digoxin, quinidine, procainamide, and lidocaine. Beta-blockers appear relatively safe but there has been some concern about intrauterine growth retardation, neonatal hypoglycemia, and hyperbilirubinemia.[14,15] Verapamil appears not to be associated with teratogenic effects, although experience is more limited.

Anticoagulants

Various chronic illnesses may be associated with an increased risk of thromboembolic disease and require the use of anticoagulants. Oral anticoagulants cross the placental barrier and can cause damaging fetal effects. During the first trimester, numerous problems include facial defects, optic atrophy, microcephaly, and central nervous system defects.[16] Reported problems in the second and third trimesters include mental retardation, microcephaly, optic atrophy, and fetal death. In one review of 418 pregnancies in which warfarin derivatives were used, one-sixth ended in abortion or stillbirth, one-sixth resulted in an abnormal live-born infant, and two-thirds resulted in infants who appeared normal at birth.[16]

The alternative to using oral anticoagulants is heparin. Heparin, being a large molecule, does not cross the placenta. It has not been associated with teratogenicity or fetal hemorrhage. Heparin is the choice of many experts in anticoagulating pregnant women despite the need for subcutaneous or intravenous administration. While heparin remains the preferred anticoagulant during pregnancy, it is not clearly proved that heparin is significantly better. In the study by Hall et al., there was no overall difference in neonatal outcome whether heparin or warfarin derivatives were used.[16] Warfarin was associated with a higher incidence of early fetal loss and persistent sequelae, whereas heparin was associated with a higher incidence of perinatal, neonatal, and maternal mortality. With both drugs the normal pregnancy outcome rate was about 67%.

Anticonvulsants

See the extensive discussion in Chapter 3.

Chemotherapeutic Agents

While these drugs should be avoided if possible, there may be cases where their use must be considered for an active oncogenic problem in the mother. Several agents are known to be teratogenic in the first trimester, and include aminopterin, busulfan, chlorambucil, fluorouracil, cyclophosphamide, methotrexate, and thioguanine. See discussion in Chapter 15.

Psychotropic Medications

No psychotropic drug has been proved to be entirely safe when used during pregnancy. Antipsychotic medications, such as the phenothiazines and thioxanthenes, should only be used during pregnancy for psychotic patients with a requirement for such medication. Most reports, however, do not indicate an increased risk of major malformations secondary to these medications.[17] Tricyclic antidepressants should also be reserved for pregnant women who require this medication for treatment of acute endogenous depression. There is some controversy over whether imipramine and amitriptyline can cause fetal limb reduction defects.[17] Although controversial, first-trimester use of benzodiazepines has been associated with teratogenic effects including cleft lip and palate. Both benzodiazepines and tricyclic antidepressants have been associated with neonatal withdrawal symptoms. Lithium is known to cause teratogenic effects, with a 7% risk of cardiovascular malformation if used in the first trimester. It is also associated with neonatal effects including lethargy, hypotonia, hypothyroidism, and diabetes insipidus. It is recommended that lithium be slowly withdrawn before the time when a woman wishes to conceive.

Medication Interactions with Hormonal Contraceptives

Women with chronic illnesses are often on a multitude of different medications. It is essential that whatever contraception the woman chooses, it have little effect on the efficacy and pharmacokinetics of the drugs she is taking. Conversely, it is important that the medications used to treat the disease process do not interfere with the efficacy of the contraceptive method. While not an issue with barrier methods, drug interactions become a serious consideration predominantly with hormonal contraceptions. As discussed in other chapters, the intrauterine device (IUD) may lose some effectiveness in women taking systemic corticosteroids or other immunosuppressive medications.

Oral contraceptives have been used extensively by millions of women, with over 60 million users worldwide and 12 million users in the United States. However, the pharmacology of hormonal contraceptives and the interactions between the estrogen and progesterone components and other medications are complex areas. Clinically important drug interactions with hormonal contraceptives include those agents that can potentially reduce the efficacy of hormonal contraceptives and those agents whose effects are altered by hormonal contraceptives.[18,19] It should be remembered that oral contraceptives comprise a mixed group of medications in regard to the doses of estrogens and the types and dosages of progestins. In addition, the effects of hormonal contraceptives vary from individual to individual depending on body mass, physical activity, and other factors.[20]

Tables 16–3 and 16–4 review the most commonly reported drugs that potentially reduce or enhance oral contraceptive efficacy.[21,22] Szoka and Edgren reviewed medical papers that reported possible decreased contraceptive efficacy from drug interactions.[18] They found 22 case reports, 8 clinical studies, and 18 reports from Syntex's Adverse Drug Experience Series, for a total of 443 adverse incidents. Of the women with these problems, 149 women became pregnant and 294 experienced menstrual disturbances. Substantial numbers of cases were associated with only four categories of medications—antibiotics, anticonvulsants, antidepressants, and analgesics. Of these, 76% involved antibiotics and the largest of these were

Table 16–3   Drugs Reported To Be Possibly Associated with Reduced Oral Contraceptive Efficacy

| DRUG | DOCUMENTATION | MANAGEMENT | |
		Taking Medication 1 Week or Less	*Taking Medication Over 1 Week*
Antibiotics Rifampin	Established	Use backup method while taking drug and for 2 weeks thereafter	Switch to a nonhormonal method
Tetracycline, doxycycline	Minimal	None	None, or may increase OC dose with spotting
Penicillins, Chloramphenicol, Cephalosporins, Sulfonamides, Nitrofurantoin	Contradictory	Available evidence suggests no change, could use backup method until 1 week off antibiotics	Conservative approach is to use backup method for 1 month
Griseofulvin	Strongly suspected	Usually used for over 1 week	Either switch to nonhormonal method or use OC with 50 µg of estrogen
Anticonvulsants Phenytoin, phenobarbital Primidone, Carbamazepine, Ethosuximide	Strongly suspected	Use backup method until 2 weeks off medication	Either switch to nonhormonal method or use OC with 50 µg of estrogen; DMPA can also be used

Adapted from Goldzieher,[21] Grimes,[22] Contraceptive Technology Update.[24] OC = oral contraceptive.

antituberculous medications. The other six categories of medications all involved fewer than 10 reported incidents each. Contraceptive failures leading to pregnancy were reported for all 10 categories of drugs. However, it is impossible to extrapolate from these reports that the pregnancy rate is any higher than would be expected in a control group of women taking oral contraceptives without one of these medications. While most of the reports in this study involved pills with 50 µg of estrogen or more, there has been no increase in the reporting rate of incidents with the introduction of lower-dose oral contraceptives.

Several potential mechanisms have been reported where medications could alter the efficacy of oral contraceptives by reducing estrogen/progestin levels. These include liver enzyme induction, elevating sex hormone–binding globulin (SHBG), altering absorption, or side effects of the primary medication.[23,24]

Table 16–4   Drugs Reported To Be Possibly Associated with Enhanced Oral Contraceptive Efficacy or Increased Side Effects

DRUG	EFFECT
Vitamin C	1 g daily increases ethinyl estradiol blood levels by 50%
Co-trimoxazole	Increased ethinyl estradiol levels, norgestrel not affected

Adapted from Goldzieher,[21] Grimes,[22] and Contraception Report.[24]

Absorption

Medications may alter the absorption of contraceptive steroids by either causing vomiting or diarrhea, reducing levels of intestinal bacteria, or reducing absorption capacity of the intestinal lumen. Ethinyl estradiol is normally rapidly absorbed in humans, reaching peak levels in 120 minutes.[25] In the jejunal mucosa, about 65% of ethinyl estradiol is sulfate conjugated on first pass and eliminated. Estradiol is also excreted from the liver into bile as glucuronide or sulfate conjugates into the intestinal lumen. Here the compounds are hydrolyzed by intestinal bacteria, with the original ethinyl estradiol being reabsorbed. Antibiotics could potentially alter this enterohepatic circulation by cutting down on intestinal flora. Antibiotics can also induce diarrhea or vomiting leading to lowered absorption of oral contraceptives. Drugs such as acetaminophen that also undergo sulfation may compete with ethinyl estradiol for sulfation. This would cause less ethinyl estradiol to be conjugated, excreted, and available for reabsorption.[23] The process of absorption may also be impaired by medications that alter the absorptive process itself. Laxatives, for example, increase the rate at which medications pass over the absorptive surface. Use of antacids could potentially reduce bioavailability by interacting with the therapeutic agent. In vitro adsorption of synthetic sex steroids by the antacid magnesium trisilicate has also been reported,[26] but in vivo bioavailability appears unaffected.[27]

Elevated Sex Hormone–Binding Globulin

Some medications may increase the activity of SHBG. Contraceptive steroids are highly bound to SHBG in the blood (> 95%) so that medications that affect this binding can affect contraceptive levels. However, clinically important interactions of this type have not been well documented.

Hepatic Enzyme Induction

The most likely way in which medications alter hormonal contraceptive efficacy is the effect of certain medications on the hepatic enzyme oxidation system. Medications that speed up this enzyme system can increase the metabolism of contraceptive steroids and theoretically decrease contraceptive hormone levels and efficacy. The major drug groups that have led to concerns in this area have been antibiotics and anticonvulsants, but other potential medications that could cause enzyme induction and interfere with biotransformation of steroids include analgesics (amidopyrine, phenacetin), cytotoxic agents (cyclophosphamide), antimigraine agents (dihydroergotamine), and tranquilizers (meprobamate, chlordiazepoxide).[28]

There are several different P_{450} cytochrome oxidases which may be under separate genetic control.[29] This may explain the reason for such individual metabolic variability of contraceptive steroids. For example, with long-term treatment using 30 to 50 μg of ethinyl estradiol daily, plasma concentrations range from 6 to 190 pg/mL in different individuals.

Several studies have examined the interaction of antibiotics and hormonal contraceptives. In one study, 13 women using a combination oral contraceptive with ethinyl estradiol and levonorgestrel were studied while receiving ampicillin.[30] There were no significant changes in plasma concentrations of ethinyl estradiol, levonorgestrel, follicle-stimulating hormone (FSH), or progesterone as compared with prior cycles off ampicillin. Another study examined steroid hormone levels in 16 women taking ethinyl estradiol, 30 μg, and norethindrone, 1 mg, and either ampicillin (6 women), 500 mg twice daily for 5 to 7 days, or metronidazole (10 women), 400 mg for 6 to 8 days.[31] Neither antibiotic changed the peak or 24-hour plasma level or areas under the curve for norethindrone or ethinyl estradiol. Swenson et al., in a study of five women on oral contraceptives, examined hormone levels after 10 days of oral tetracycline, 250 mg four times a day (four women), or ampicillin, 250 mg four times a day (one woman), during the third month of oral contraceptives.[32] They found that urine excretion dropped from 51 to 35% while fecal excretion increased from 48 to 64%. More rapid elimination of ethinyl estradiol was found in three of the five women. Friedman et al. examined 11 women on two cycles of Demulen (ethinyl estradiol and ethynodiol diacetate) while taking either ampicillin or a placebo.[33] All cycles appeared anovulatory and endogenous steroid levels appeared suppressed in 10 of the 11 women. Unfortunately, these studies involved small numbers and did not examine the rate of pregnancy, the ultimate outcome. In fact, the number of reported pregnancies appears small. As of the end of 1988, Syntex reported a total of 13 pregnancies in women using its oral contraceptives combined with the recent use of antibiotics including doxycycline, nitrofurantoin, ampicillin, amoxicillin, tetracycline, erythromycin, and penicillin.[34] In another study, Back et al. reported on the pregnancies occurring in England between 1968 and 1984 in women on oral contraceptives and antibiotics.[35] There were 63 alleged interactions between antibiotics and oral contraceptives, of which 32 involved the use of penicillin; 12 involved tetracycline; 2 each involved cephalosporin, trimethoprim, and erythromycin; and 1 involved sulfonamides. While all cases are not reported, considering the enormous numbers of women who are probably on both oral contraceptives and antibiotics, the number of pregnancies appears small. Thus, it would seem that antibiotics could be prescribed without significantly altering the efficacy of oral contraceptives. However, detection of a small increase in the pregnancy rate, when pregnancy rates are so low in women using oral contraceptives, would involve a prospective study of thousands of women. The small, possible risk should be pointed out to those women on prolonged courses of antibiotics or anticonvulsants.

Rifampin, through enzyme-inducing properties and lowering estrogen and progestin levels, seems to be the major antibiotic to reduce the efficacy of hormonal contraceptives.[23] Contraceptive Technology advises switching to an effective nonhormonal method in women taking rifampin for over 1 week.[24] In those taking the rifampin for 1 week or less, Contraceptive Technology advises using a backup method while taking rifampin, and for 2 weeks afterward. For antibiotics excluding rifampin, Contraceptive Technology advises using a backup method for the first month in those women using antibiotics for over 1 week. While some practitioners advise a backup method in addition to oral contraceptives if antibiotics are taken for 1 week or less, available evidence does not support this.

User Factors

One other factor that could reduce oral contraceptive efficacy are the side effects of some medications. This could include drowsiness, nausea, or abdominal pain. These side effects could cause a woman to miss taking her oral contraceptives for several days.

In evaluating all of the currently available information, the anticonvulsants along with rifampin and griseofulvin are the major drugs of concern that lower the efficacy of hormonal contraceptives. The effect of anticonvulsants on hormonal contraceptive efficacy is discussed further in Chapter 3. Alternatives for increasing the efficacy of oral contraceptives include switching to a higher-dose oral contraceptive with 50 μg of estrogen, if there are no contraindications, or adding 1 g of vitamin C daily. Vitamin C can increase the therapeutic effect of oral contraceptive steroids by inhibiting the enzymes involved in oral contraceptive metabolism. One gram of vitamin C can increase the bioavailability of contraceptive steroids by 50% or more.[2,21]

Another potential interaction between medications and oral contraceptives is the effect of oral contraceptives on the pharmacokinetics of other medications. Tables 16–5 and 16–6 review possible reported problems and management. In these studies, oral contraceptives were reported to potentially augment bioavailability in some cases and to decrease bioavailability in others.[20] In most cases, the reports involved oral contraceptives inhibiting microsomal enzymes and thus inhibiting the metabolism of other drugs, potentially leading to enhanced bioavailability and drug toxicity.

Table 16–5   Altered Pharmacokinetics of Drugs by Oral Contraceptives

	BIOAVAILABILITY		
TYPE OF DRUG	*Augmented*	*Decreased*	AUTHORS
Analgesics			
Acetaminophen		Induced conjugation	Abernethy and Greenblatt[53]
Aspirin		Induced conjugation	Miners et al., 1981, 1986[54]
Morphine		Induced conjugation	Mitchell et al., 1983[55]
Antihypertensives			
Metoprolol			
Oxprenolol	Inhibited oxidation		Kendall et al., 1982[56]
Propranolol			Kendall et al., 1984[57]
Anticoagulants			
Warfarin	Inhibited oxidation		De Teresa et al., 1979[58]
			MacLeod and Sellers, 1976[59]
Antidepressants			
Imipramine	Decreased clearance		Abernethy et al., 1984[37]
Antiasthmatic			
Theophylline	Inhibited oxidation		Gardner and Jusko, 1986[50]
Aminophylline	Inhibited oxidation		Roberts et al., 1983[51]
Antiepileptics			
Phenytoin	Inhibited oxidation		Kutt and McDowell, 1968[60]
Barbiturates	Inhibited oxidation		Tephly and Mannering, 1969[61]
Glucocorticoids			
Cortisol	Decreased clearance		Marks et al., 1961[62]
			Legler and Benet, 1986[63]
			Shaw et al., 1983[64]
			Boekenoogen et al., 1983[65]
			Kozower et al., 1974[66]
			Frey et al., 1984, 1985[67,68]
Lipid-lowering drugs			
Clofibrate		Increased conjugation	Miners, 1984[69]
Tranquilizers			
Alprazolam			Stoehr et al., 1984[70]
Triazolam			Ochs et al., 1987[71]
Chlordiazepoxide	Decreased clearance		Roberts et al., 1979[72]
Nitrazepam	Inhibited oxidation		Jochemsen et al., 1982[73]
Diazepam	Decreased clearance		Giles et al., 1981[74]
			Abernethy et al., 1982, 1984[37,52]
			Routledge et al., 1981[75]
Lorazepam		Increased clearance	Patwardhan et al., 1983[76]
Oxazepam		Increased conjugation	Stoehr et al., 1984[70]
			Patwardhan et al., 1983[76]

Adapted from Teichmann.[20]

There have been concerns of changes in antibiotic levels in women on oral contraceptives. However, studies to date with ampicillin have not found altered antibiotic levels in women on both medications.[31,36] There is an increased risk of liver toxicity with the combination of hormonal contraceptives and troleandomycin, so that this combination should be avoided.

Benzodiazepines have been found to have either increased or decreased clearance. Benzodiazepines (such as imipramine) that undergo oxidation have a decreased clearance and the potential for augmented activity.[20] Conversely those benzodiazepines that are predominantly conjugated may have a higher clearance rate with the potential for decreased activity.[37–40] It is far from substantiated that these metabolic alterations have any significant clinical effect but they should be watched for in those women on the combination of oral contraceptives and benzodiazepines. If evidence of toxicity is present, then the dose of antidepressants should be reduced. In women on oral contraceptives and imipramine, the dose of imipramine should be reduced by about one-third.

A decreased oxidation rate is also found with the combination of phenytoins/barbiturates and oral contraceptive pills, which could alter the bioavailability of anticonvulsants.[20] In addition, estrogens and progesterones themselves can have pro- and anticonvulsant effects on the brain. Thus, the effects of oral contraceptives on seizure activity can be quite complex, including the effects of altered pharmacokinetics and the direct effects of estrogen and progesterone on the brain. However, as discussed in detail in Chapter 3, clinical effects are usually minimal. However, if symptoms of anticonvulsant toxicity occur, the dose should be altered.

Some women with chronic illnesses are on long-term anticoagulation because of thromboembolic problems or artificial heart valves. Warfarin can have its metabolic oxidation pathway inhibited by oral contraceptives and thus its bioavailability could potentially be enhanced. However, since combination oral contraceptives also stimulate various coagulation agents such as factors VII and X, the net effect of the combination or combined oral contraceptives and warfarin (Coumadin) could be either an enhancement or a weakening of the anticoagulation effect.

While it would be unusual for women with significant hypertension to be placed hormonal contraceptives, women with mild hypertension may be on both medications. As listed in Table 16–5, some potential interactions could occur. Beta-blockers can have inhibited oxidation leading to higher bioavailability. This is not true for acebutolol, as it undergoes unmetabolized renal excretion.

Another common medication used in women with chronic illnesses is glucocorticoids. Spangler et al. reported a twofold to 20-fold increase in the antiinflammatory effects of topical hydrocortisone in oral contraceptive users.[41] It has been suggested that estrogens can influence the ratio of free and protein-bound glucocorticoids.[20] The mechanism may involve not only an alteration in protein binding between cortisol-binding globulin

**Table 16–6   Management of Drugs Whose Activity May
Be Modified by Oral Contraceptive Use**

DRUG	MANAGEMENT
Analgesics	
Acetaminophen	Because of potentially decreased bioavailability, larger doses of analgesic may be required.
Aspirin	Because of potentially decreased bioavailability, larger doses of analgesic may be required.
Meperidine	Because of potentially increased bioavailability, smaller doses of analgesic may be required.
Antibiotics	
Troleandomycin/TAO	Risk of liver toxicity, so avoid use of combination oral contraceptives simultaneous with TAO.
Anticoagulants	
Warfarin (Coumadin)	Watch for increased or decreased anticoagulation effect. If problems with adequate anticoagulation, avoid estrogen-containing methods.
Antidepressants	
Imipramine	Because of increased bioavailability, decrease dosage by about one-third.
Antihypertensives	
Beta-blockers including atenolol, metoprolol, propranolol	Increased effect, so monitor pulse for excessive bradycardia, may need lower dose.
Guanethidine	Decreased effect, so use low dose
Methyldopa	of oral contraceptives or progestin-only methods.
Bronchodilators	
Aminophylline	Potential for increased theophylline bioavailability. Carefully monitor for drug side effects and begin with two-thirds normal starting dose, reduce dose if toxicity develops. There may be no change in those women who smoke.
Corticosteroids	Potential for increased bioavailability, so watch for potentiation of effects and decrease dose, if necessary.
Tranquilizers	
Group A; Alprazolam Chlordiazepoxide (Librium) Diazepam (Valium) Benzodiazepine Triazolam	Because of potential increased effect, watch closely for effects, may need to reduce dose.
Group B Lorazepam (Ativan) Oxaline, temazepam (Levanxol, Normison) Oxazepam	Dosage change not usually required.

Adapted from Goldzieher,[21] Grimes,[22] and Teichmann.[20]

and cortisol but also a decrease in inhibition of oxidation of the corticos-teroid. The clinical relevance of these findings has not been well studied.

Women with chronic illnesses may be relatively deficient in certain vitamins because of inadequate nutritional intake. Oral contraceptives have been reported to decrease the concentrations of zinc, folic acid, and vitamins B_1, B_6, B_{12}, and C.[42–49] This is not a problem in women on a normal diet but in women who may be already nutritionally depleted, it could become clinically relevant.

Theophylline metabolism can be reduced by oral contraceptives by the reduction of both oxidation and clearance rates.[50] It is recommended to reduce the dose of aminophylline by one-third for those women on oral contraceptives. However, as smoking increases enzyme induction, these effects on theophylline may not be seen in those women who smoke and are on oral contraceptives.[51,52]

Summary

1. The potential exists for certain medications to reduce the efficacy of oral contraceptives through primarily inducing the oxidase system of the liver or through altering the enterohepatic circulation. The most frequently described interactions have been between oral contraceptives and anticonvulsants, rifampin, and griseofulvin. The limited number of clinical studies seems to indicate a minimal clinical impact in most individuals. However, the potential interactions should be discussed with these women, particularly those taking anticonvulsants, rifampin, or griseofulvin.

2. The pharmacokinetics of certain medications can be altered through effects on absorption or altering hepatic enzyme induction. However, there are often many counteracting effects associated with using a medication in combination with oral contraceptives, so that the net clinical effect is usually negligible. Despite this, women with chronic diseases on these combinations of medications should be monitored closely for changes in the therapeutic effects of the medication while on oral contraceptives.

References

1. Karboski JA. Medication selection for pregnant women. Drug Ther 1992;1:53–61.
2. Hill LM. Effects of drugs and chemicals on the fetus and newborn (part 2). Mayo Clin Proc 1984;59:755–65.
3. Chow AW, Jewesson PJ. Use and safety of antimicrobial agents during pregnancy. West J Med 1987;146:761–4.
4. Cefalo RC. Drugs in pregnancy: Which to use and which to avoid. Drug Ther 1983;13:167–75.
5. Aselton P, Jick H, Milunsky A, Hunter JR, Stergachis A. First trimester drug use and congenital disorders. Obstet Gynecol 1985;65:451–5.

6. Katz Z, Lancet M, Skornik J, Chemke J, Mogilner BM, Klinberg M. Teratogenicity of progestogens given during the first trimester of pregnancy. Obstet Gynecol 1985;65:775–80.
7. Chernoff GF, Jones KL. Fetal preventive medicine: Teratogens and the unborn baby. Pediatr Ann 1981;10:210–7.
8. Niebyl JR. Therapeutic drugs in pregnancy. Postgrad Med 1984;75:165–72.
9. Schluter G. Toxicology of ciprofloxacin. In New HC, Weuta H, eds. Proceedings of 1st International Ciprofloxacin Workshop. Amsterdam, Excerpta Medica, 1986, p 61.
10. Rudolph AM. Effects of aspirin and acetaminophen in pregnancy and in the newborn. Arch Intern Med 1981;141:358–63.
11. Lewis RN, Schulman JD. Influence of acetylsalicylic acid, an inhibitor of prostaglandin synthesis, on the duration of human gestation and labour. Lancet 1973;2:1159–61.
12. Lammer EJ, Chen DT, Hoar RM, Agnish ND, Benke PJ, Braun JT, Curry CJ, Fernhoff PM, Grix AJ Jr, Lott IT. Retinoic acid embryopathy. N Engl J Med 1985;313:837–41.
13. Shalita AR, Armstrong RB, Leyden JJ, Pochi PE, Strauss JS. Isotretinoin revisited. Cutis 1988;42:1–19.
14. Cottrill CM, McAllister RG, Gettes L, Noonan JA. Propranolol therapy during pregnancy. J Pediatr 1977;91:812–4.
15. Pruyn SC, Phelan JP, Buchanen GC. Long-term propranolol therapy in pregnancy. Maternal and fetal outcome. Am J Obstet Gyencol 1979;135:485–9.
16. Hall JG, Pauli RM, Wilson KM. Maternal and fetal sequelae of anticoagulation during pregnancy. Am J Med 1980;68:122–40.
17. Leiter G. Teratogenesis and drugs in pregnancy. In Cherry SH, Merkatz IR,eds. Complications of Pregnancy: Medical, Surgical, Gynecologic, Psychosocial, and Perinatal. 4th ed. Baltimore, Williams & Wilkins, 1991, pp 148–55.
18. Szoka PR, Edgren RA. Drug interactions with oral contraceptives: Compilation and analysis of an adverse experience report database. Fertil Steril 1988;49:31S–8S.
19. Derman R. Oral contraceptives: A reassessment. Obstet Gynecol Surv 1989;44:662–8.
20. Teichmann AT. Influence of oral contraceptives on drug therapy. Am J Obstet Gynecol 1990;163:2208–13.
21. Goldzieher JW. Hormonal Contraception: Pills, Injections and Implants. 2nd ed. London, Ontario, EMIS-Canada, 1989, pp 44–9.
22. Grimes DA, ed. Drug Interactions with Oral Contraceptives: A Review of Known and Suspected Interacting Agents. The Contraception Report. Liberty Corner, NJ, Emron Inc. Vol III, No. 5, 1992, pp 9–13.
23. Fotherby K. Interactions with oral contraceptives. Am J Obstet Gynecol 1990;163:2153–9.`
24. Contraceptive Technology Update: How Some Drugs Reduce Contraceptive Efficacy. American Health Consultants, Atlanta, GA, 1993;15:62–4, S2–S4.
25. Hanker JP. Gastrointestinal disease and oral contraception. Am J Obstet Gynecol 1990;163:2204–7.
26. Khalil SAH, Iwunagwu M. The in vitro uptake of some oral contraceptive steroids by magnesium trisilicate. J Pharm Pharmacol 1976;28(suppl):47.
27. Joshi JV, Sankolli GM, Shah RS, Joshi UM. Antacid does not reduce the bioavailability of oral contraceptive steroids in women. Int J Clin Pharmacol Ther Toxicol 1986;24:192–5.
28. Khoo Sk, Correy JF. Contraception and the high risk women. Med J Aust 1981;1:60–8.
29. Lu AYH, West SB. Multiplicity of mammalian microsomal-cytochromes P450. Pharmacol Rev 1980;31:277–92.
30. Back DJ, Breckenridge AM, MacIver M, Orme M, Rowe PH, Staiger CH, Thomas E, Tija J. The effects of ampicillin on oral contraceptive steroids in women. Br J Clin Pharmacol 1982;14:43–8.
31. Joshi JV, Joshi UM, Sankholi GM, Krishna V, Manklekar A, Chowdhury V, Hazari K, Gupta K, Sheth UK, Saxena BN. A study of interaction of low-dose combination oral contraceptive with ampicillin and metronidazole. Contraception 1980;22:643–52.
32. Swenson L, Goldin B, Gorback SL. Effect of antibiotics on fecal/urinary excretion of ethinyl estradiol, an oral contraceptive (abstract). Gastroenterology 1980;78:1332.
33. Friedman CI, Huneke AL, Kim MH, Powell J. The effect of ampicillin on oral contraceptive effectiveness. Obstet Gynecol 1980;55:33–7.
34. Fleischer AB Jr, Resnick SD. The effect of antibiotics on the efficacy of oral contraceptives: A controversy revisited. Arch Dermatol 1989;125:1562–4.
35. Back DJ, Grimmer SFM, Orme MLE, Proudlove C, Mann RD, Breckenridge AM. Evaluation of Committee on Safety of Medicines Yellow Card Reports on oral contracep-

tive-drug interactions with anticonvulsants and antibiotics. Br J Clin Pharmacol 1988;25:527–32.

36. Philipson A. Plasma and urine levels produced by an oral dose of ampicillin administered to women taking oral contraceptives. Acta Obstet Gynecol Scand 1979;58:69–71.

37. Abernethy DR, Greenblatt DJ, Shader RI. Imipramine disposition in users of oral contraceptive steroids. Clin Pharmacol Ther 1984;35:792–7.

38. Gringas M, Beaumont G, Grieve A. Clomipramine and oral conntraceptives: An interaction study—Clinical findings. J Int Med Res 1980;8:76–80.

39. Luscombe DK, John V. Influence of age, cigarette smoking and the oral contraceptive on plasma concentrations of clomipramine. Postgrad Med J 1980;56:99–102.

40. Prange AJ. Estrogen may well affect the response to antidepressants. JAMA 1972;219:143–4.

41. Spangler AS, Antoniadas HN, Sotman SL, Inderbitzin TM. Enhancement of the anti-inflammatory action of hydrocortisone by estrogen. J Clin Endocrinol 1969;29:650–5.

42. Webb JL. Nutritional effects of oral contraceptive use. A review. J Reprod Med 1980;25:150–6.

43. Schenker JG, Jungreis E, Polishuk WZ. Oral contraceptives and correlation between copper and ceruloplasmin levels. Int J Fertil 1972;17:28–32.

44. Rhode BM, Cooper BA, Farmer FA. Effect of orange juice, folic acid and oral contraceptives on serum folate in women taking a folate-restricted diet. J Am Coll Nutr 1983;2:221–30.

45. Rivers JM, Devine MM. Plasma ascorbic acid concentrations and oral contraceptives. Am J Clin Nutr 1972;25:684–9.

46. Luhby AL, Brin M, Gordon M, Davis P, Murphy M, Spiegel H. Vitamin B6 metabolism in users of oral contraceptive agents I. Abnormal urinary xanthurenic acid excretion and its correction by pyridoxine. Am J Clin Nutr 1971;24:684–93.

47. Aly HE, Donald EA, Simpson MH. Oral contraceptives and vitamin B6 metabolism. Am J Clin Nutr 1971;24:297–303.

48. Heilmann E. Oral Kontrzeptiva und Vitamine. Dtsch Med Wochenschr 1979;104:144–6.

49. Basu TK. Drug and vitamin interactions in adult. Int J Vitam Nutr Res 1984;54:157–68.

50. Gardner MJ, Jusko WJ. Effects of oral contraceptives and tobacco use on the metabolic pathways of theophylline. Int J Pharmacol 1986;33:55–64.

51. Roberts RK, Grice J, McGuffie C, Heilbronn L. Oral contraceptive steroids impair the elimination of theophylline. J Lab Clin Med 1983;33:55–64.

52. Abernethy DR, Greenblatt DJ, Divoll M, Arendt R, Ochs HR, Shader RI. Impairment of diazepam metabolism by low-dose estrogen-containing oral contraceptive steroids. N Engl J Med 1982;306:791–2.

53. Abernethy DR, Greenblatt DJ. Impairment of antipyrin metabolism by low-dose oral contraceptive steroids. Clin Pharmacol Ther 1981;29:106–10.

54. Miners JO, Grgurinovich N, Whitehead AG, Robson RA, Birket DJ. Influence of gender and oral contraceptive steroids on the metabolism of salicylic acid and acetylsalicylic acid. Br J Clin Pharmacol 1986;22:135–42.

55. Mitchell MC, Hanew T, Meredith CG, Schenker S. Effects of oral contraceptives steroids on acetaminophen metabolism and elimination. Clin Pharmacol Ther 1983;34:48–53.

56. Kendall MJ, Quarterman CP, Jack DB, Beeley L. Metoprolol pharmacokinetics and the oral contraceptive pill. Br J Clin Pharmacol 1982;14:120–2.

57. Kendall MJ, Jack DB, Quarterman CP, Smith SR, Zaman R. Beta-adrenoceptor blocker pharmacokinetics and the oral contraceptive pill. Br J Clin Pharmacol 1984;17:87S–9S.

58. de Teresa E, Vera A, Ortigosa J, Pulpon LA, Arus AP, de Artaza M. Interaction between anticoagulants and contraceptives: An unsuspected finding. Br Med J 1979;2:1260–1.

59. MacLeod SM, Sellers EM. Pharmacodynamic and pharmacokinetic drug interactions with coumarin anticoagulants. Drugs 1976;11:461–70.

60. Kutt H, McDowell F. Management of epilepsy with diphenylhydantoin sodium JAMA 1968;203:969–972.

61. Tephly TR, Mannering GJ. Inhibition of drug metabolism by steroids. Med Pharmacol 1969;4:10–14.

62. Marks LJ, Benjamin G, Duncan FJ, O'Sullivan VI. Comparative effects of ethinyl estradiol, 17 alpha ethinyl-19-nortestosterone and methyl-testosterone on the plasma clearance of infused cortisol. J Clin Endocrinol Metab 1961;21:826–32.

63. Legler UF, Benet L. Marked alterations in dose-dependent prednisolone kinetics in women taking oral contraceptives. Clin Pharmacol Ther 1986;39:425–9.

64. Shaw MA, Back DJ, Aird SA, Grimmer SF, Orme MC. Urinary concentrations of steroid glucuronides in women taking oral contraceptives. Contraception 1983;28:69–75.
65. Boekenoogen SJ, Szefler SJ, Jusko WJ. Prednisolone disposition and protein binding in oral contraceptive users. J Clin Endocrinol Metab 1983;56:702–9.
66. Kozower M, Veatch L, Kaplan MM. Decrease clearance of prednisolone, a factor in the development of corticosteroid side effects. J Clin Endocrinol Metab 1974;38:407–12.
67. Frey BM, Schaad HJ, Frey FJ. Pharmacokinetic interaction of contraceptive steroids with prednisone and prednisolone. Eur J Clin Pharmacol 1984;26:505–11.
68. Frey BM, Frey FJ. The effect of altered prednisolone kinetics in patients with the nephrotic syndrome and women taking oral contraceptive steroids on human mixed lymphocyte cultures. J Clin Endocrinol Metab 1985;60:361–9.
69. Miners JO. Gender and oral contraceptive steroids as determinants of drug glucuronidation: Effects on cloribric acid elimination. Br J Clin Pharmacol 1984;18:240–3.
70. Stoehr GP, Kroboth PD, Juhl RP, Wender DB, Phillips JP, Smith RB. Effect of oral contraceptives on triazolam, temazepam, alprazolam, and lorazepam kinetics. Clin Pharmacol Ther 1984;36:683–90.
71. Ochs HR, Greenblatt DJ, Friedman H, Burstein ES, Locniskar A, Harmatz JS, Shader RI. Bromazepam pharmacokinetics: Influence of age, gender, oral contraceptives, cimetidine, and propranolol. Clin Pharmacol Ther 1987;41:562–70.
72. Roberts RK, Desmond PV, Wildinson GR, Schenker S. Disposition of chlordiazepoxide: Sex differences and effects of oral contraceptives. Clin Pharmacol Ther 1979;25:826–31.
73. Jochemsen R, van der Graaff M, Boeijinga JK, Breimer DD. Influence of sex, menstrual cycle and oral contraception on the disposition of nitrazepam. Br J Clin Pharmacol 1982;13:319–24.
74. Giles HG, Sellers EM, Naranjo CA, Frecker RC, Greenblatt DJ. Disposition of intravenous diazepam in young men and women. Eur J Clin Pharmacol 1981;20:207–13.
75. Routledge PA, Stargel WW, Kitchell BB, Barchowsky A, Shand DG. Sex-related differences in the plasma protein binding of lidocaine and diazepam. Br J Clin Pharmacol 1981;11:245–50.
76. Patwardhan RV, Mitshell MC, Johnson RF, Schenker S. Differential effects of oral contraceptive steroids on the metabolism of benzodiazepines. Hepatology 1983;3:248–53.

17

Adolescents, Women over 35, and Postpartum Women

Three other special conditions that can affect decision making around pregnancy and contraception include those women who recently delivered a baby and those women at both ends of the reproductive age spectrum, i.e., adolescents and women over 35 years old. The largest increases in births in the United States and the highest percentages of unintended pregnancies have been among women in these two age groups. The high rates of unintended pregnancies have also led to high rates of abortions in these two age groups, with almost one abortion for every live birth among younger adolescents and one abortion for every two live births in women over 40.

Adolescents

Sexual Activity

Teens have high rates of sexual activity. By the time adolescents are 16 years, 29% of boys and 17% of girls have had sexual intercourse.[1] By the time they are 18 years, 65% of boys and 54% of girls are sexually active.[1] Reported rates are even higher in the study of never-married urban females reported from the National Survey of Family Growth in 1988[2] and Sonenstein's data in males.[3] In these studies, 50% of males had sexual intercourse by age 16 and 72% by age 18. For females, the rates were 34% and 70%, respectively. Rates of sexual intercourse by age and race for white and black teens are reported in Table 17–1. The trends in sexual activity among US teens is reported in Table 17–2.

Table 17–1   Percentage of Never-Married Metropolitan-Area
Females Ever Having Had Sexual Intercourse, by Age, 1988

AGE (YR)	TOTAL	WHITE	BLACK
Total	53	52	60
15	27	27	27
16	34	30	49
17	52	49	67
18	70	71	71
19	78	78	80

Data from National Survey of Family Growth.[2]

Pregnancy

Adolescents are at high risk for getting pregnant. Each year about 11% of adolescent women become pregnant,[1] with close to 1 million pregnancies and ½ million births among adolescents. Of these pregnancies about 47% end in a live birth, 40% end in a therapeutic abortion, and 13% in a miscarriage.[4] Of adolescent pregnancies, 80 to 90% are among unmarried teens and more than 75% of pregnancies among unmarried women aged 15 to 19 are unintended.[5] Between 1950 and 1985, the nonmarital birthrate among adolescents younger than 20 years rose by 300% for whites and 16% for blacks. Among married adolescents, about 87% of pregnancies were carried to term.

The pregnancy rate among African American adolescents is about double that of white women aged 15 to 19. In addition, white adolescents more frequently abort, resulting in much higher birthrates among African American teens. Pregnancy rates are much higher in the United States than in Canada and European countries.[6] US pregnancy rates in teens are double those in Britain, France, and Canada, three times that in Sweden, and seven times higher than that in Holland.[7]

Teenagers have the highest rates of abortions relative to pregnancies. Over 50% of pregnancies in unmarried adolescents result in a therapeutic abortion. They also tend to delay seeking an abortion so that abortions are often done at a later gestational age. Twenty-seven percent of abortions in adolescents less than 15 years old were done after 13 weeks of gestation and 14.7% occurred at later than 16 weeks' gestation.[8]

There are potential associated negative sequelae for some adolescents who become pregnant. The majority of health risks associated with teenage childbearing are secondary to either socioeconomic factors, other associated health behaviors such as substance abuse, or lack of prenatal care.

Adolescents who become pregnant during early puberty, who receive late or no prenatal care, or who drink, smoke, or use drugs are at risk for adverse medical outcomes.[1] Maternal mortality is 2.5 times higher among females under 15 as compared to mothers aged 20 to 24. Adolescents who

Table 17–2 Trends in Percentage of US Never-Married Metropolitan-Area 15- to 19-Year-Old Females Ever Sexually Active

	1971	1976	1979	1982	1988
Total	30	43	50	45	53
White	26	38	47	43	52
Black	54	66	66	54	60

Note: Data calculated from 1971, 1976, and 1979 National Surveys of Young Women and 1982 and 1988 National Surveys of Family Growth.

Adapted from Hofferth SL, et al. Premarital sexual activity among U.S. teenage women over the past three decades. Fam Plann Perspect 1987;19:46, and National Survey of Family Growth.[2]

become pregnant while in high school are also at higher risk of dropping out of school and becoming dependent on welfare or becoming single parents.[1] Teenage parents are more likely to have a lower socioeconomic status, have low-paying jobs, or be unemployed than those who delay childbearing. Teens who marry because of pregnancy are three times more likely to divorce. In addition, teen mothers have more children.

Consequences to infants include an increased risk of low-birthweight babies in mothers less than 15 years old and 1.5 times the risk in mothers aged 15 to 17.[9] The infant mortality rate is 2.4 times higher for babies born to women under 15 than babies born to women in their early 20s. Because of the risk of sexually transmitted diseases (STDs), human immunodeficiency virus (HIV) infection, and substance abuse in teen mothers, these areas should be discussed and evaluated in pregnant teens.

Contraception

About 50% of American adolescents do not use contraception the first time they have intercourse.[10] Of those who use contraception, about 47% use the condom, 27% rely on withdrawal, and only 17% use the pill.[11] In addition, about 25% use no contraceptive at their last intercourse and 50% do not use condoms during their last intercourse.[8] Early counseling interventions become important, as 20% of premarital teen pregnancies occur within the first month after commencing sexual intercourse and 50% within the first 6 months.[12] Only about one in seven adolescents visits a family planning clinic before sexual activity begins; most wait 9 months or more.

There are many reasons given by adolescents for the lack of contraceptive use.[9] These include

- Perception of low risk including teens believing that they are too young to get pregnant or that the risk is very low
- Inability to access contraception because of lack of information, concerns about confidentiality, and concerns about cost or transportation
- Lack of knowledge regarding correctly using contraceptive techniques

- Fear of side effects
- Ambivalence about being sexually active
- Refusal by partner to use contraception
- Desire to have a baby to become independent, prove fertility, or rebel against family

Because of the high rate of sexual activity and resultant problems including sexually transmitted disease and pregnancy, sexuality and contraception are important areas to cover in evaluating adolescent patients. This can be sensitive information to obtain from an adolescent. At Childrens Hospital of Los Angeles, the HEADSS interview has been used to help obtain this information from the teen.[13] Before this interview, the teen is explained the reasons for asking some of these sensitive questions and is reassured about confidentiality. This interview includes:

- *Home:* Where is the teen living? How is the teen getting along with parents and siblings?
- *Education:* Is the teen in school? Where does the teen go to school and what are recent grades? In what subjects is the teen doing well (or poorly) in school? What are the teen's plans after school?
- *Activities:* What does the teen do after school hours? What does the teen do for fun? What sports or hobbies is the teen involved with.
- *Drugs:* What types of drugs are used by the teen's peers or family members? What types of drugs does the teen use?
- *Sexuality:* Is the teen dating? What are the degree and types of sexual experiences? Is the teen involved in a sexual relationship? Does the teen prefer sex with the same, opposite, or both sexes? Has the teen had sexual intercourse and how many partners has the teen had? Has the teen had any sexually transmitted diseases? Does the teen use contraception and with what frequency? The area of sexual or physical abuse should also be addressed, particularly if there are any significant problems in any part of this psychosocial interview. Clues to possible prior abuse include: runaway behavior, changes in school grades, lack of friends, substance abuse, early onset of sexual intercourse, or history of suicide attempts.
- *Suicide:* Has the teen had prior suicide attempts? Is there any current suicidal ideation?

Important considerations for health care providers who are providing contraception to adolescents include:

- Reassuring confidentiality to adolescents in the area of contraception if needed
- Becoming familiar with local community resources serving the special needs of teens
- Having services that are teen-friendly, i.e. after school hours

Abstinence is a legitimate form of contraception for teens. Adolescents need to be aware that this is a reasonable alternative to sexual intercourse. Because of media and peer pressure, many teens feel that all other adolescents are sexually active. Adolescents need to be reminded that even by the age of 19, about 25% of teens have not had intercourse. In addition, teens need to be reassured that despite being sexually active with one partner, they do not need to be sexually active with every partner.

Barrier methods in adolescents have several positive effects. Condoms in particular are associated with decreased rates of STDs, pelvic inflammatory disease (PID), and prevention of HIV transmission. In addition, condoms have the advantage of being relatively cheap and accessible. The use of condoms for STD prevention in particular needs to be stressed with adolescents despite the use of other contraceptive devices such as oral contraceptives.

Vaginal spermicides also have the advantage of not requiring a prescription and are easy to use. However, because of their lower effectiveness and lower protective value in preventing HIV and STDs, they should be used in conjunction with a condom. Teens need careful instruction on the correct use of spermicides, including timing, insertion, and use of the applicator. The contraceptive sponge has the advantage of not requiring an application just before intercourse. However, it also has a lower effectiveness rate and protective value against STDs and HIV than do condoms. Diaphragms are not an ideal method for most adolescents because the technique requires high motivation and comfort with one's body.

Oral contraceptives have several advantages with teens. Oral contraceptives are highly effective when taken regularly. In addition, several problems that occur after the onset of puberty can be helped by the use of oral contraceptive pills. These include abnormal uterine bleeding, dysmenorrhea, and acne. Dysmenorrhea is common in adolescents, occuring in 45 to 60% of postpubescent women, with 10% of these individuals having severe enough symptoms to keep them out of school or other activities 1 to 3 days per month.[14] Approximately 50% of adolescents are anovulatory in the first 2 years following menarche, leading to problems with cycles that are either too frequent or too heavy. Oral contraceptives can decrease dysmenorrhea by suppressing ovulation and with cycling can decrease abnormal uterine bleeding. Oral contraceptives can also decrease the rates of PID. The potential drawbacks include poor compliance because of the need for daily pill taking.

Many adolescents are reluctant to go on oral contraceptives because of concerns about side effects including cancer, weight gain, and acne. Misconceptions and reassurance about oral contraceptive use become important in the counseling of teens, as well as a discussion of the positive effects of oral contraceptives.

Other alternative hormonal contraceptives in this age group include the Norplant implant and intramuscular depomedroxyprogesterone acetate

(DMPA). Contraceptive effectiveness and side effects in adolescents on DMPA were reviewed by Cromer et al. in a retrospective chart review of 86 teens.[15] No pregnancies were found in this study, which included over 1,000 woman-months. The continuation rate was 72% at 1 year, 56% at 2 years, and 18% at 3 years. The side effects recorded on the teen's charts included: 43% with amenorrhea, 42% with fatigue, 38% with headache, 35% with depression, 20% with nausea, 18% with nonmenstrual bleeding and 15% with spotting. Fifty-six percent of the teens were "very happy" with DMPA. Another side effect that needs to be evaluated in this population is the prevalence and degree of weight gain. DMPA appears to be a very effective contraceptive in the adolescent population and may have a high rate of acceptance. Further studies of DMPA in this population are needed.

Some data is available on the use of the Norplant implant in adolescents. O'Connell et al. reported on short-term follow up of adolescent Norplant users.[16,17] They found that the contraceptive was well-tolerated with side effects being minimal. Weight gain was noted to be a mean of 1.46 kg at 3 months. Among 307 adolescent Norplant users, eight pregnancies were noted. However, in retrospect it was discovered that these teens were pregnant at the time of insertion. This suggests the importance of a sensitive pregnancy test before placement since the histories from some adolescents may be inaccurate. Adequate counseling of teens before the procedure is important to allay concerns about the surgical procedure and other side effects. It is also important to discuss the probable menstrual changes that will occur.

With any of the hormonal contraceptives, it is important to consider that none of these methods prevent the transmission of HIV and other STDs. Thus, counseling regarding condom use becomes very important.

Lastly, the intrauterine device (IUD) is a poor choice of contraceptive in adolescents because of the higher risk of STDs and the possible complications of PID, including infertility.

Older Reproductive Age

There are increasing numbers of reproductive women in the over 35 age group as the postwar baby boom children are reaching their 30s and 40s.[18] In 1980, the largest group of reproductive women were 20 to 24 years of age; in 1990 the largest group were 30 to 34; and in the year 2000, the largest group is predicted to be 40 to 44.[18] In 1991 there were more women (29.8 million) aged 30 to 44 than women aged 15 to 29. In addition to these higher numbers of older reproductive age women, many women of reproductive age are delaying childbirth until their 30s. By delaying childbirth, these women need increasing periods of contraceptive use. Women over 35 who have delayed childbearing are at increased risk for ovarian, endometrial, and breast cancer. Infertility rates are increased in women over 35.[19]

Pregnancy

With the shift of the population toward an older reproductive age, and with the delay in childbearing in recent decades, a dramatic increase has occurred in birth rates in the past decade among United States women over 35 years of age. U.S. birth rates in women between 35 and 39 fell from a peak of 50 to 60 live births per 1,000 women to a low of about 20 per 1,000 women in 1980. By 1990, however, this rate had climbed dramatically to about 30 per 1,000.[20] In women in their late 30s, 56% of pregnancies are unintended, with 77% of pregnancies in women in their early 40s unintended. This population also has a high abortion rate, with 55% of unintended pregnancies in women in their late 30s ending in an abortion and 59% among women in their early 40s. Except for teenagers, women aged 40 and above have the highest abortion ratio.[14]

Women of older reproductive age have higher rates of spontaneous abortion, ectopic pregnancy, trisomic anomalies, low birth weight, macrosomia, abruptio placentae and labor dysfunction.[19,21,22] While women of advancing reproductive age are at increased risk for maternal and fetal morbidity and mortality, much of this risk can be explained by coexisting medical complications.[19]

Contraception

Contraceptive services rank high on the list of services requested by women in the later reproductive years. Women 35 to 40 and over have often completed their families but still require years of contraception.

Women over 40 have one of the highest rates of noncontraception use, yet at the same time they have a maternal mortality rate that is 10 times the rate of women in their 20s.[23] In women 45 to 49 the maternal mortality rate is even higher, 50 times the risk of women in their twenties.[24] Women over 40 also have abortion rates similar to those in adolescents. Much of our knowledge regarding safety and side effects of contraceptives in women over 35 is limited because reproductive research is usually carried out in women under this age.[25]

The National Survey of Family Growth reported that two-thirds of women between 40 and 44 either have had a surgical sterilization, are infertile, or have a partner who has undergone sterilization.[26] In women in this age group, 25% use reversible methods and 8% use no method. In women between the ages of 35 and 39, 60.5% have chosen sterilization.[8] The most common reversible contraceptive used by women over the ages of 35 to 40 is the condom.[27] The next most popular choices are the diaphragm and other barrier methods.

Hormonal contraception methods including injectables, implants, and oral contraceptives have a low prevalence of use in women over 35. Oral contraceptive use in women 35 to 39 has been about 5%, dropping to 3% in women aged 40 to 44.[27] In past years, health care practitioners have been somewhat reluctant to utilize oral contraceptives in women over 35 years of age. Much of this concern arose from older studies demonstrating elevated cardiovascular risk. These studies utilized higher doses of estrogen and progestins and also included women who would no longer have been advised to use oral contraceptives. Even in these studies, most of the risk was in women who had other independent risk factors, such as smoking. More recent studies do not indicate an increased cardiovascular risk in properly screened women. In January 1990, the Food and Drug Administration (FDA) recommended eliminating the age limit on oral contraceptive use and requested manufacturers to modify labeling to read that the benefits of pill use after age 40 may exceed the possible risks.

Women over 35 who smoke should not be placed on oral contraceptives because of the higher risk of thromboembolism.[28] In women over 35 to 40, cardiovascular risk factors should be examined very closely before contemplating oral contraceptives. However, oral contraceptives in appropriately chosen women, even if they are over the age of 35 or 40, provide effective and safe contraception with risks smaller that those posed by pregnancy.

Oral contraceptive use may have significant benefits in women over 35. It provides safe and easily reversible contraception. It decreases the risk of ovarian and endometrial cancer. Oral contraceptives may also lower the rates of dysmenorrhea, irregular bleeding, and abnormal uterine bleeding. In addition, after menopause, women are at increased risk of osteoporosis. Women who have taken oral contraceptives long-term prior to menopause seem to have higher bone densities than women who do not use oral contraceptives.[29–31]

One question that arises in women on oral contraceptives is the appropriate time to make the transition from oral contraceptives to hormonal replacement therapy (HRT). There does not appear to be an exact age that is most appropriate for the switch. It is probably reasonable to choose a year between about 48 and 50 years of age to stop oral contraception. If a woman's menstrual cycles resume within several months, then a decision could be made to either go back on oral contraceptives for a couple more years or to use a nonhormonal contraceptive until she is postmenopausal. If the woman wants to go back on oral contraceptives, then she could return for 1 to 2 years and stop again. If a woman's periods do not resume, then starting HRT with estrogen and progesterone would be appropriate to lower the risk of osteoporosis and possibly lower the risk of cardiovascular disease.

The Norplant implant and injectable DMPA can also provide safe, effective and reversible contraception for women over age 35. Both of these methods can be associated with irregular menses or heavy bleeding, which could be a negative in perimenopausal women who may already be experiencing irregular bleeding.

The IUD can be a safe and effective form of contraception in women over age 35. IUDs, however, are used by less than 5% of women aged 35 to 44.[27] IUDs are best utilized in women who have completed their families and are in a stable monogamous relationship. This situation and the fact that the IUD does not interfere with any metabolic system often makes the IUD an ideal contraceptive in women over 35.

Contraception in Postpartum and Breast-Feeding Women

A last group of women who have special concerns about contraception are those women who are postpartum and/or breast-feeding. Most couples resume sexual intercourse after the first or second postpartum month, and many begin sooner.[32,33] Breast-feeding has had a comeback in the United States with an increase from a low of 22% in 1972 to over 60% in 1982, with a small drop since to about 52% in 1989.

Breast-feeding stimulates prolactin which appears to suppress ovulation through several postulated mechanisms: direct suppression of ovarian steroid production, suppression of ovarian responsiveness to luteinizing hormone (LH), suppression of the positive feedback of estrogen on the midcycle rise of LH and follicle-stimulating hormone (FSH), and reduction of the pulsatile release of gonadotropin-releasing hormone.[6,34] In non-breast-feeding women, gonadotropin levels appear to approach normal levels by 3 to 5 weeks after delivery. In one study, the mean time to first ovulation in non-breast-feeding women was 45 days postpartum and as early as 28 days in some cases.[35] The return of ovulation in breast-feeding women can vary from as early as 9 weeks to as late as 18 months.[36] The duration of anovulation and/or amenorrhea is dependent on whether the women is fully breast-feeding or only partially breast-feeding.[37] With frequent, continuous breast stimulation there is a greater contraceptive effect. The pregnancy data in breast-feeding women who use no contraception show that 1.7% become pregnant in the first 6 months of breast-feeding, with 7% becoming pregnant by 12 months and 13% by 24 months.[38] In another study, the risk in amenorrheic, breast-feeding women was 0.9% at 6 months and 17% at 12 months.[39] This compared to menstruating, breast-feeding women who had pregnancy rates of 36% at 6 months and 55% at 12 months. Thus, the major risk appears to be among breast-feeding women who are having menstrual cycles or to those amenorrheic women who are over 6 months postpartum. The maximum protective effect of breast-feeding is achieved when a woman is fully breast-feeding, meaning no supplemental feedings or pacifier, and the woman remains amenorrheic. With these two conditions, breast-feeding appears more than 98% effective for 6 months.[40] The longer a woman breast-feeds, the greater the risk that menses will occur while still breast-feeding and that ovulation will occur before the first menstrual cycle.

Women may regain fertility before they have detected their menstrual cycle returning. Speroff and Darney recommend a contraceptive method by the end of the *third postpartum month* in a woman who is fully breast-feeding and by the end of the *third postpartum week* in the woman who is partially breast-feeding or not breast-feeding.[41] This rule applies to full-term or near full-term pregnancies. Women who have an early miscarriage or therapeutic abortion can begin any hormonal contraceptive immediately. Speroff and Darney recommended moving up the first postpartum visit to the third week since this time is more appropriate for contraceptive counseling and treatment than the sixth week, which might be too late to prevent pregnancy.[41]

Non-breast-feeding Women

Non-breast-feeding women should begin contraception immediately postpartum or by the third postpartum week. In non-breast-feeding women, combination oral contraceptives can be begun during the third to fourth postpartum week. It is recommended to avoid combination oral contraceptives before this time because of the higher risk of thromboembolic problems immediately after delivery.[42]

Diaphragms and cervical caps must be refitted postpartum and this should wait until the sixth week postpartum. Episiotomy sites may still be tender, making fitting of these devices difficult. These devices, along with the sponge, should not be used until 6 weeks after delivery. Lubricated condoms are the contraceptive of choice until other methods can be started. If sterilization is contemplated, discussion should begin before delivery.

Breast-feeding Women

Amenorrheic, fully breast-feeding women should begin contraception by the third month. Partially breast-feeding women, i.e., those using supplements or those breast-feeding infrequently (more than 6 hours between feedings) should begin contraception by the first postpartum examination or sooner.

Controversy exists over the use of hormonal contraceptives in breast-feeding women. The progestin-only pill has been recommended for years for lactating women and does not appear to have any adverse effects. These pills can be started immediately postpartum or at the first postpartum visit between 3 and 6 weeks. The combination of the progestin-only pill and breast-feeding have almost 100% contraceptive efficacy. Because the progestin-only pill may actually increase milk production, it can be started soon after delivery.[43] The progestin pill should be continued throughout the period of breast-feeding and then can be switched to a combination oral contraceptive pill.

Combination oral contraceptives have been discouraged from use in lactating women because of concerns that the estrogen component can decrease the milk supply.[24] Breast-feeding women on oral contraceptives have a lower incidence of breast-feeding after the sixth postpartum month and have a shorter lactating period compared to controls (3.7 months versus 4.6 months).[44-46] There is some indication that lower dose combination pills may have less or no effect on breast-feeding.[47] There is no evidence that combination oral contraceptives harm a nursing infant.[48] The total dose consumed by a nursing infant is equal to one pill for every 4 years of full lactation.[48] Controversy still exists over when the combination pill can be started. Recommendations have ranged from waiting until an infant has been weaned, to 6 months postpartum, to as soon as 6 weeks postpartum when lactation is established.[6]

The Norplant implant and DMPA have also been advocated for use in lactating women. Controversy exists over how soon to begin these hormones. Wyeth-Ayerst, the Norplant manufacturer, and Upjohn Company, which manufactures DMPA, have recommended waiting 6 weeks after delivery before starting these hormones. The Population Council, in a summary of scientific data on Norplant, state that levonorgestrel is transferred to newborns via breast milk but that no evidence exists of any significant effects on the health of infants when the hormones are used beginning 6 weeks after childbirth.[49] The Population Council still recommends the 6-week waiting period. The World Health Organization also recommends waiting 6 weeks postpartum with DMPA because of the irregular bleeding associated with DMPA and the more frequent bleeding associated with the postpartum period.[50]

Other experts feel that there is no reason to withhold these hormones for 6 weeks. Speroff and Darney, in their recent guide to contraception, recommend the early use, either immediately postpartum or no later than 3 weeks postpartum, of Norplant and DMPA for breast-feeding mothers.[41] *Contraceptive Technology Update* also agrees with the early use of Norplant for lactating women.[49]

The IUD can be an excellent method of contraceptive in postpartum women who are breast-feeding. Both the copper IUD (T380A) and the progestin IUD appear safe in breast-feeding women.[51,52] The amount of progestin in the progestin-releasing IUD appears small enough to not affect milk production or the infant. The copper IUDs are safe between 4 and 8 weeks postpartum with normal rates of pregnancy and expulsions.[53] Studies are currently underway to investigate the safety and efficacy of inserting the IUD immediately postpartum.

Barrier methods are safe in the postpartum period and do not alter breast-feeding. However, they require a highly motivated couple. Vaginal dryness is common postpartum so that lubricated condoms may be very helpful. Condoms have the additional benefit of providing significant protection against the introduction of bacteria into the vagina helping to avoid postpartum endometritis. The cap, sponge, and diaphragm may be used after about 6 weeks when postpartum bleeding has stopped. Spermicides including foams, creams, and suppositories would appear safe starting immediately postpartum. While there are no known effects of spermicides on breast-feeding, studies in animals have reported that nonoxynol-9 can be absorbed through skin and secreted in breast milk.[54]

For women who do not want any further children, tubal ligation is an option, or, alternatively, vasectomy in the male partner.

Summary

1. Adolescents are at high risk for unintended pregnancy with a low prevalance of effective contraception use in all sexual encounters.
2. There are potential negative sequelae for adolescents who become pregnant although many of these are associated with inadequate prenatal care and other health risk behaviors.
3. Barrier methods are important to discuss with teens, particularly the condom, which can reduce rates of STDs and HIV transmission.
4. Oral contraceptives are safe and effective for use in most adolescents. The Norplant implant and DMPA are other good alternatives in this age group. The IUD is discouraged in the teen population because of the high risk of STDs.
5. Women over the age of 35 are at high risk of an unintended pregnancy. Pregnancies in these women are asssociated with higher rates of obstetrical complications.
6. Acceptable contraceptive devices in women over 35 include combined oral contraceptives, the Norplant device, DMPA, the IUD, and barrier methods. The combination oral contraceptive pill is no longer discouraged in appropriately selected women over age 35.
7. In postpartum women, ovulation can occur before the first menstrual cycle. Women who fully breast-feed should begin contraception by the third postpartum month, while other breast-feeding women should begin by 3 to 6 weeks postpartum.
8. In non-breast-feeding women, combination pills can be started between the third and fourth postpartum week. Diaphragms and cervical caps should be refitted at about 6 weeks postpartum. Lubricated condoms should be used before other methods can be started and may alleviate problems associated with postpartum vaginal dryness.

9. In breast-feeding women, combination oral contraceptives should be avoided until either the infant is weaned or until about 6 months postpartum. The progestin-only contraceptive can be started soon after pregnancy. The Norplant implant and DMPA can be utilized 6 weeks postpartum although some authorities advocate its use immediately postpartum. The IUD can be inserted 4 to 8 weeks postpartum.

References

1. Gans JE, Blyth DA, Elster AB, Gaveras LL. America's Adolescents: How Healthy Are They? Chicago, American Medical Association, 1990.
2. Sonenstein FL, Pleck JH, Ku LC. Sexual activity, condom use and AIDS awareness among adolescent males, Fam Plann Perspect 1989;21:152.
3. National Survey of Family Growth, National Center for Health Statistics, Hyattsville, MD, 1988.
4. Henshaw SK, Van Vort J. Teenage abortion, birth and pregnancy statistics: An update. Fam Plann Perspect 1989;21:85.
5. Hayes CD (ed). Risking the future: Adolescent sexuality, pregnancy, and childbearing, vol 1. Washington DC, National Academy Press, 1987.
6. Hatcher RA, Stewart F, Trussell J, Kowal D, Guest F, Stewart GK, Cates W. Contraceptive Technology 1990–1992, 15th ed. New York, Irvington Publishers, 1990.
7. Jones EF, Forrest DJ, Goldman N, Henshaw KS, Lincoln R, Rosoff JI, Westoff CF, Wulf D. Teenage pregnancy in developed countries: Determinants and policy implications. Fam Plann Perspect 1985:17:53.
8. Sulak PJ, Haney AF. Contraceptive challenges at the beginning and end of the reproductive years: Adolescence and advanced reproductive age. Am J Ob Gyn 1993;168:2042–8.
9. Neinstein LS. Teenage Pregnancy in Adolescent Health Care: A Practical Guide. Baltimore, Urban and Schwarzenberg, 1991, pp 561–76.
10. Hofferth SL, Hayes CD (eds). Risking the Future: Adolescent Sexuality, Pregnancy and Childbearing, vol. 2. Washington, DC, National Academy Press, 1987.
11. Pratt W, Mosher W, Bachrach C, Horn M. Understanding U.S. Fertility: Findings from the National Survey of Family Growth, Cycle III. Popul bull 1984;39:1–42.
12. Zelnik M, Kantner JE. Sexual activity, contraceptive use, and pregnancy among metropolitan area teenagers: 1971–1979 Fam Plann Perspect 1980:12:230.
13. Neinstein LS. The Office Visit and Interview Techniques in Adolescent Health Care: A Practical Guide. Baltimore, Urban and Schwarzenberg, 1991, pp 45–56.
14. Neinstein LS. Dysmenorrhea and Premenstrual Syndrome in Adolescent Health Care: A Practical Guide. Baltimore, Urban and Schwarzenberg, 1991, pp 653–60.
15. Cromer BA, Smith D, Blair JM, et al. Depo-Provera: Effectiveness, side effects, and satisfaction in adolescents. Presented at NASPAG Seventh Annual Meeting, April 16–18, 1993, Colorado Springs, CO.
16. O'Connell BJ, Hillard P, Bacon J. Norplant contraceptive use in the adolescent population. Presented at NASPAG Seventh Annual Meeting, April 16–18, 1993, Colorado Springs, CO.
17. O'Connell BJ, Craighill M, Emans SJ. Pregnancy detection in adolescent Norplant users. Presented at NASPAG Seventh Annual Meeting, April 16–18, 1993, Colorado Springs, CO.
18. Grimes DA (ed). The contraception report: Reproductive health in the perimenopause. Liberty Corner, NJ, Emron Inc. March 1993, pp 5–10.
19. Newcomb WW, Rodriguez M, Johnson JW. Reproduction in the older gravida. A literature review. J Reprod Med 1991;36:839–45.
20. National Center for Health Statistics, Vital Statistics of the United States, DHEW, Washington D.C. 1992.
21. Mishell DR Jr. Oral contraceptives for women over the age of 35. Int J Fertil 1991; 36(Suppl 2):55–64.

22. Grimes DA. OCs and your older patient. Dialogues in Contraception 1988;2:1–3,6.
23. Wharton C, Blackburn R. Lower-dose pills. Popul Rep 1988;26(3), Series A(7).
24. Luukkainen T. Contraception after thirty-five. Acta Obstet et Gynecol Scand 1992;71:169–74.
25. Dialogues in contraception: FDA panel recommends removing age ceiling for OC use: 1990:2:1–4.
26. Forrest JD, Singh S. The sexual and reproductive behavior of American women, 1982–1988. Fam Plann Perspect 1990;22:206–214.
27. Mosher WD. Contraceptive practice in the United States, 1982–1988. Fam Plann Perspect 1990;22:198–205.
28. Williams RS. Benefits and risks of oral contraceptives. Postgrad Med 1992;92:155171.
29. Kleerekoper M, Brienze RS, Schultz LR, Schultz CC. Oral contraceptive use may protect against low bone mass. Arch Intern Med 1991;151:1971–1976.
30. Recker RR, Davies KM, Hinders SM, Heaney RP, Stegman MR, Kimmel DB. Bone gain in young adult women. JAMA 1992;268:2403–2408.
31. Kritz-Silverstine D, Barrett-Connor E. Bone mineral density in postmenopausal women as determined by prior oral contraceptive use. Am J Public Health 1993;83:100–102.
32. Ford K, Labbok M: Contraceptive usage during lactation in the United States: An update. Am J Publ Health 1987;77:79–81.
33. Richardson AC, Lyon JB, Graham EE. Decreasing postpartum sexual abstinence time. Am J Obstet Gynecol 1976;126:416.
34. Sauder SE, Frager M, Case GD, Kelch RP, Marshall JC. Abnormal patterns of pulsatile luteinizing hormone secretion in women with hyperprolactinemia and amenorrhea: Responses to bromocriptine. J Clin Endocrinol Metabl 1984;59:941–948.
35. Gray RH, Campbell OM, Zacur HA, Labbok MH, MacRae SL. Postpartum return of ovarian activity in non-breast-feeding women monitored by urinary assays. J Clin Endocrinol Metal 1987;64:645–650.
36. McGregor JA. Lactation and contraception. In: Neveille MC, Neifert MR, eds., Lactation, Physiology, Nutrition, and Breast-feeding. New York, Plenum Press, 1983:405–421.
37. Kennedy KI, Rivera R, McNeilly AS. Consensus statement on the use of breast-feeding as a family planning method. Contraception 1989;39:477–496.
38. Short RV, Lewis PR, Renfree MB, Shaw G. Contraceptive effects of extended lactational amenorrhoea: Beyond the Bellagio consensus. Lancet 1991;337:715–717.
39. Diaz S, Aravena R, Cardenas H, Casado ME, Miranda P. Contraceptive efficacy of lactational amenorrhea in urban Hilian women. Contraception 1991;43:335–352.
40. Kennedy KI, Rivera R, McNeilly AS. Consensus statement on the use of breast-feeding as a family planning method. Contraception 1989;39:477–496.
41. Speroff L, Darney P. A Clinical Guide for Contraception. Baltimore, Williams and Wilkins, 1992.
42. Howie PW, Evans K, Forbes CD, Prentice CRM. The effects of stilboestrol and quinestrol upon coagulation fibrinolysis during the puerperium. Br J Obstet Gynaecol 1975;82:968.
43. McCann MF, Moggia AV, Hibbins JF, Potts M, Becker C. The effects of a progestin-only oral contraceptive (levonorgestrel 0.03 mg) on breast-feeding. Contraception 1989;40:635–648.
44. Nilsson S, Mellbin T, Hofvander T, Sundelin C, Valentin J, Nygren KG. Long term follow-up of children breast-fed by mothers using oral contraceptives. Contraception 1986;34:443–457.
45. Diaz S, Peralta O, Juez G, Herreros C, Casado ME: Fertility regulation in nursing women: III. Short-term influence of a low-dose combined oral contraceptive upon lactation and infant growth. Contraception 1982:27:1–11.
46. Peralta O, Diaz S, Juez G, Herreros C, Casado ME, Salvatierra AM, Miranda P, Duran E, Croxatto HB. Fertility regulation in nursing women: V. Long term influence of a low-dose combined oral contraceptive initiated at day 90 postpartum upon lactation and infant growth. Contraception 1983;27:27–38
47. Lonnerdal B, Forsum E, Hambraeus L. Effect of oral contraceptives on composition and volume of breast milk. Am J Clin Nutri 1980;33:816–824.
48. Labbok MH. Consequences of breast-feeding for mother and child. J Biosoc Sci (Suppl) 1985;9:43–54.
49. Contraceptive Technology Update: Are Norplant, Depo-Provera good options for nursing mothers? Atlanta, GA, American Health Consultants, March 1993:46–48.

50. World Health Organization. Injectable contraceptives. Geneva, WHO, 1990.
51. Wenof M, Aubert JM, Reyniak JV. Serum prolactin levels in short-term and long-term use of inert plastic and copper intrauterine devices. Contraception. 1979;19:21.
52. Chi IC, Potts M, Wilkens LR, Champion CB. Performance of the copper T-380A intrauterine device in breast-feeding women. Contraception 1989;39:603–618.
53. Mishell DR Jr, Roy S. Copper intrauterine contraceptive device event rates following insertion 4 to 8 weeks postpartum. Am J Obstet Gynecol 1982;143:29–35.
54. Chrapil M, Eskelson CD, Stiffel U, Owen JA, Droegemueller W. Studies on nonoxynol-9, intravaginal absorption, distribution, metabolism and excretion in rats and rabbits. Contraception 1980;22:325–336.

Index